Praise for *CAVEWORLD*:

"Here is a work of emotional havoc, horse sense, and deep deferential insight. Gnade's litanies on American life are a sand-shower blasting you clean with their dirt ... moving through *Caveworld* you will see your own ghosts and have them exorcised."
—Andrew Mears, of band Pet Moon, formerly of Youthmovies and Foals, author of *Kettle Drum*

"Adam Gnade's body of work is haunting, inspirational, fierce, and tender. Few American writers have been able to give us all the pain and bullshit and euphoria of growing up, without either romanticizing it or trivializing it. *Caveworld* captures the search for life that all of us have felt, and are still feeling, and wrestles it to the ground with brutal beauty. I saw myself here, at times in ways that I'd rather have not, and you will too."
—Will Potter, journalist and author of *Green is the New Red*

"Reminiscent of Saul Bellow, *Caveworld* is a story told with energy and love for the characters and places. Easily his best work yet."
—Bart Schaneman, journalist and author of *Trans-Siberian*

"*Caveworld* digs like an archaeologist (into the ghosted past, into the hot earth, into the culture, into the psyche), uncovering a fossil fragment that leads not only to an ancient skeleton but connects to an entire modern kingdom: dark and unacknowledged in broad San Diego sunlight, yet now verified, human and undeniable. For this kingdom of his characters, Adam Gnade never claims to hold the key, but he holds the pen: He writes everything, archiving, dusting, scraping away in an accessible language that both proves and dignifies the gnarled record of life revealed to us in this novel that has everything and nothing to do with the exploration of caves."
—Rich Baiocco, author of *Death in a Rifle Garden*

Other titles by Adam Gnade:

Seasons Loving Nothing

Hymn California

The Darkness to the West

Hey Hey Lonesome

The Heat and the Hot Earth

Hymn California

They Will Stand On You and Spit (w/ Bart Schaneman)

The Growling Mouth

The Do-It-Yourself Guide to Fighting the Big Motherfuckin' Sad

Ringside!: A Companion Piece to The Do-It-Yourself Guide to Fighting the Big Motherfuckin' Sad

CAVEWORLD

a novel

Adam Gnade

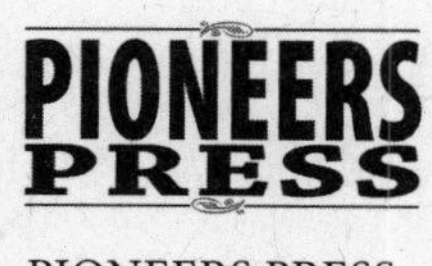

PIONEERS PRESS

PUNCH DRUNK PRESS

PIONEERS PRESS
816 North Main Street #200
Lansing, KS 66043
www.pioneerspress.com

Cover artwork: Joshua Krause
Cover & book design: Rio Safari

ISBN: 978-1-939899-18-7

Printed in the United States of America

December 2013

BOOK ONE

THE LIGHT IN THE WINDOW

"They blew us to pieces and the pieces came back together, and when the pieces came back together, they blew us back apart."
—Ed Distler, *A Book of Lists*

NEW YORK CITY

1978

JANUARY 5TH

It was just after midnight when I left the restaurant and walked to the train alone. It had been raining all day, but the rain had stopped and the streets were wet and the gutters full and the lights of cars and storefronts were shining red and neon blue in the puddles.

I walked past the arcade and the laundry. Rey Bar Diner and Aunt Marla's Pizza were full but there was no one on the street. From outside Marla's, you could see the red glow of candles on tables and the shapes of people moving, and further back the blinking square of light where the jukebox and cigarette machines sat between the restrooms. A block past Marla's I crossed the street and there was the market with its yellow canvas awning and the light in the window and the rows of fruit on display outside in wooden stands.

You could smell the pineapples. It was faint at first then ripe and heavy as you passed. A good smell. I picked one up and cradled it in my arm and went inside for Alka-Seltzer, humming "Alka-Seltzer to the *res*cue."

There was a girl my age talking to the boy behind the counter. She bought a can of Coke and I couldn't hear them talk but I could tell they knew each other. When I got up close she said, "Jean's back at home now and she needs Grandma's new number before I go to Kelly's." She had braces on her teeth. "You should bring some steaks for Sunday." (*Schteaks*, she said.)

"Steaks? Okay. Potatoes?"

"Sure. Yeah. Potatoes."

"Bread? White bread?"

"I think she's got some. Get some anyway."

"Cool." The boy bent over the counter and wrote something on a scrap of paper and slid it to her and said, "Bye, sis."

She smiled at him, and as she walked past me, she stopped and turned. "Five steaks, right? Don't forget. Jean's back home."

"Right. Five steaks."

"Five." She held up five fingers and he laughed.

She was pretty. Little rectangular wire glasses and freckles and a lot of blonde hair parted down the middle and tucked behind her ears, heart-shaped face, eyes so green they were unnatural, alien, like bottle glass. She was as tall as I am and she wore a tan coat with a belt. A raincoat. No, something else. Something English. I loved her. For a second. Maybe I didn't. I felt like I did. For a second.

The girl walked out the door, and as the bell rang, the man walked in.

He had the shotgun on the boy before I had time to think and he was talking fast. "The register. Open the register."

The boy said it was empty. "Less than a dollar," he said. "My sister had me break a twenty. I'm cleaned out."

The man said something in Italian and then he said, "Open it."

And the boy said, "There's nothing, nickels, quarters."

And the man said, "*Show me*," and the boy went for something under the counter.

This happened fast. The boy holding a pistol in both hands, his arms outstretched. The man with his shotgun braced at his shoulder.

The man swore and shook his head but the boy smiled and you could tell he was confident now.

The man said, "Put the gun down and there won't be no problems."

And the boy said, "No. *You* put the gun down and you can leave." The man looked at me and swore again and when he swore there was spit on his bottom lip and he licked it off.

The boy said, "Let him go," (jerking his head in my direction). "Let him go."

The man looked at me again and said, "What, him?" And when the boy turned to look at me, the man took a big step forward and shot the boy.

That was three days ago and I'm as far from New York City as I've been in years, but that man's face won't leave me. Hair short like mine, black like mine, but receding at the temples. The big chin and jaw—hinge-jawed like a snake—the sweat at his brow, sweat like baby oil, a heavy brow, pockmarks on the cheeks. His mouth a girl's mouth, thick, pursed. The flatness of his stare. Nothing behind it. A wall behind muddy iris. I see the buckshot hit the boy and I see the boy's head break open and spray across me like the streak of a garden hose. And the man. The gun on me. The smell of gunpowder and blood and oniony sweat. "*Kneel*."

I knelt on the floor, the pineapple in my arms like a football.

He pressed the gun barrel against my forehead and I dropped the pineapple. He pumped another shell into the chamber and looked me in the eyes, nodded, and backed out. He left. He left me on my knees.

The bell dinged.

That was it.

Missouri's a world away from Queens. My uncle's farmhouse back by the river and trees. The snow falling outside. The smell of the fireplace and coffee brewing. My uncle and his cousin talking in the kitchen about someone called Tate Jayfers who'd got drunk the night before and shot a horse.

"The horse was called J.R."

"What'd it stand for?"

"What?"

"What'd J.R. stand for?"

"Why would I know *that*?"

Tomorrow I leave for the coast. My brother knows I'm coming but he doesn't know why. I asked and he said there was a room and that was that.

I left New York after the shooting. I went straight to my dorm and I packed up my books and some of my clothes and wrapped it all in a blanket and slung the blanket over my shoulder.

On the way out I passed a boy from my physics class in the hallway and he fell back against the wall and his eyes were big and he was shaking, and then I remembered the shirt. I'd washed the blood off my face and took off my jacket but I'd forgotten to change the shirt. The boy turned and ran down the hall and then I was running and then I was outside and a half-hour later I was driving away from my life and away from Tami and New York City and having this one set of dreams and believing in a certain order of truths that now seem baseless.

The drive across was hard. The heater cut out in Louisville and I was lost for hours in West Virginia. The whole country was out on the road and everything was sleet and ice and big rigs passing and bad accidents and eerie blue-white snow in the darkness and headlamps blooming in my rear-view and brakelights flashing red.

When the heater died, I pulled over at a pancake diner and put on two pairs of jeans and two sweaters and buttoned my coat to my neck and drove clear to Weston, Missouri, stopping only for coffee and gas. When I got to my uncle's farm, I pulled into the drive and it was dark and a light came on in the house and then another, and my uncle stepped out onto the porch in his pajamas and ski jacket with a rifle in his hands.

When he saw who it was, he set the gun against the railing and jogged out through the snow to meet me.

Inside, they put me at the table and made a plate of corned beef hash with a fried egg on top and a side of canned peaches, and then my aunt brought us coffee and my uncle sat down and told me all about my cousins in ag school and Clara's work with the farm bureau and how they were fighting the county.

I told him about my classes at Columbia and then I told him about the man and the boy and he said, "Well. I *swear*," and went to the icebox and came back with a couple of beers. "You can stay with me and Clara as long as you need. You know you and Jakey were always good as my own kids. You got a place and a job out here on the farm if you want it."

I told him I was bound for California to live with Jake and his wife Sorel and start school in the fall and he said, "*Well*, that sounds like a good plan, too."

We drank the beers he brought and then he asked if I wanted a cigarette and I said I didn't smoke and he said he was going to have one anyway and I said that was fine.

He went to bed and I heard him and Clara talking until late.

I tried to sleep but I saw the man's face whenever I'd start to drift off.

4

He came back to me and he knew all about me, every piece of my history and all of my future. It drained right out of me and into the flatness of his eyes. Behind his eyes, a whole store and wealth of information about me. He had me and he could find me when he wanted. Which is bullshit. I know. But I see him and that's enough to get me thinking. So here I am, 4 a.m., writing this in the easy chair by the fire, watching the snow fall from the window. California? California.

SAN DIEGO

TWENTY YEARS LATER

10 P.M.

The moon is white and round on the hood of the Mazda as Joey Carr and Tyler Monahan drive down Market Street and it warbles on the black waters of the bay as they round the shipyard and make their way past the harbor warehouses and dry-docked sailboats and construction cranes.

Behind 7-Eleven in Golden Hill they smoke crystal in the car, then Tyler lights a cigarette and rolls down the window and looks pale and sad and tired.

The woman on the radio is singing "Aaand ayii-eeee-iiiiii will always love you-oooh-oooh," and Joey laughs and Tyler laughs and Joey turns the dial to talk radio and mutters something about the hurricane and shuts it off. Silence. The ticking of the engine as it cools and the wet static crackle of electric lines and the sunscreen smell of coconut air freshener and it's October but Joey's back to a thousand beach days with his aunt and uncle and afternoons falling asleep on towels in the sand (warm below him, almost hot) and breeze and sun on his face, the sea stretching out below, dark blue and wind-tossed and sparkling in the sun. He can smell the salt and drying kelp and Tyler's cigarette is now Joey's uncle's.

"You know how it is." Tyler stabs his cigarette into the ashtray below the radio until it's a wad of filter. He takes the filter and flicks it out the window. "It just happened before I knew it was happening."

Joey checks his hair in the rearview mirror. "How old were you?" His hands are shaking. "We should do a couple lines."

"She was thirteen and I was fifteen." Tyler looks straight ahead, holding the wheel like he's still driving, staring down the yellow-lit alley, the dark-painted garage doors framed by white stucco, a silver trash can with a black plastic bag bulging out and its lid on top, tilted like a beret. "Maggie and I were in Pismo Beach on vacation with my parents."

"Pismo's nice."

"It was. We go every year."

"I heard somewhere that you can drive on the beach." Joey shuts his eyes and clicks his car seat back until he's lying down. "I've always wanted to drive on the beach. Sorry. Go on."

"It's okay. We were . . . we were eating and then she and I were holding hands under the dinner table. Just like that."

"Was it a restaurant?"

"At the place my parents rented, a house on the beach."

"Fancy pants."

"It was bad because she was my sister's best friend, which is weird because they're nothing alike. I guess it was school. They were at Kroc together before Mission Bay. The only thing they had in common was *Beavis and*

Butthead and church and potato burritos and then Maggie stopped going to church."

Tyler chops up a line on his ATM card and bends over and does it and then cuts one for Joey.

"Here. Yours."

Joey sits up and leans down over the gear shift and snorts it and then they sit back and Joey's thoughts race and Tyler talks and Joey sees Tyler asking Maggie out and he sees their first kiss. And it's Maggie sitting up in the bleachers at night under the lights next to Tyler's sister wrapped in a Navajo blanket sharing a plaid thermos of hot apple cider and Tyler kicking a soccer ball into the net and falling on his back and everyone standing up to cheer and Tyler getting up and running across the field back to his side and smiling up at Maggie and Maggie smiling back. The grass bright green and black all around, the lights hot-white.

"Then, four years," he says softly, "four *years*." Tyler holds the wheel, his arms locked out straight. "You haven't met her so you don't know." His jaw goes tense, gritting. "I wish it would've . . . y'know, would've played out differently . . . or something. I don't know, I still love her and it's weird because we're not together anymore but we still . . . we're still hanging *out* all the time and we still . . . sometimes we . . . *do* stuff. But she's doing stuff with *other* guys now. I just . . . I don't know what to *do*."

Joey sees the light through the curtains in Maggie's bedroom and he hears a dog barking at dinnertime. A gray and white cat moves through the weeds outside her window stalking a fat, green Japanese beetle and a lawnmower kick-starts, and then the distant snap of firecrackers as they burst off in a string. It's a summer evening where she is and Joey can smell hotdogs grilling until they're covered in dry, black bubbles. *Fucking hotdogs,* he thinks. *Give me hotdogs now.* He thinks of chili dogs, chili dogs with cheese, with onions, the hotdogs with cheese injected into the middle (*gross*), baseball games, big foam #1 fingers that say Padres!, black iron grills with tripod legs like alien invaders, Hebrew National commercials, and the job Nicole had where she dressed up like a meatball and handed out sausage samples up and down University Avenue. He says, "You going to the party?"

"No. Maybe. I guess I will. I don't think Chente likes me."

"No, don't worry, he does."

"He's . . . I don't know. I'll be there. Maggie wants to go. She likes his band."

"What's she doing these days?"

"These days?"

"Y'know, what's she up to?"

Joey's eyes are closed and Tyler's talking now and Joey sees what Tyler describes. It's a sunlit glare of images, the rows of houses and the green of lawns blinding, and Maggie squinting up at the sky, the black makeup smear around her eyes to make them glow darkly, a wrist lined in rubber bracelets. Maggie off in her head—seventeen, dark green eyes, a band of black around the iris, a mop of brown hair in tumbling curls, quiet and obsessed in gray stovepipe jeans, beat-up sneakers, and a white camisole shirt.

Joey sits back in his seat and his jaw is twitching and it's Maggie cutting through the front yards and palm-tree-lined streets of her neighborhood. Past Tyler's house, his bright blue Mazda in the driveway, shiny, pod-like, uncool. Past cars parked with sun on their windows. Past the mailbox on the corner, past garden hoses in green, sun-warmed coils (the smell of fresh-cut grass and dry dust and sprinkler water). Past sleeping dogs chained in yards, past the mailman, who stops to watch her as she walks away, her shadow on the sidewalk stretching behind her in the shape of a knife.

Maggie walking through the Circle K parking lot on a muggy evening holding a soda cup with a tall red straw, and now pulling the straw up, slurping at it as she moves past the flower stand and the Blockbuster, shuffling along, shoes scuffed, small and anonymous in a world of strip malls and taco shops and a sky with no clouds, a vast blue dome stretching high above her.

1978

JANUARY 7TH

The drive from Missouri was fine. It was snowy the rest of the way, but as I crossed into California it looked like spring. I took a mountain pass and it was raining, and then I was driving down into a big green valley and the road was empty and wet and clean and the sun was coming through the clouds in great slanted rays. There was nothing out there—no homes or stores or gas stations or billboards. It was hills and scrub-brush and rocky land and the highway and me. I turned the radio to the '50s station and drove until I hit the city.

Pacific Beach was smaller than I imagined. Low buildings. Beach apartments. Ratty houses and shops. People out walking. Kids and dogs in yards. Sprinklers.

I knew my brother lived on a street called Cass and that it ran north-south, but I didn't have a map so I drove west down Garnet Avenue hoping to run into it.

Garnet looked like the sleepy main street in any small town: a pizza parlor with a line of Chianti bottles in the window, a barber shop with the spinning pole, a sandwich place full of people and a couple of guys my age smoking cigarettes out front, laughing about something.

After a few blocks I passed Jake's street, but I could tell I was near the ocean and I wanted to see it, so I kept driving until I found the shore.

At the foot of Garnet, I parked in front of a seedy-looking bar and walked out onto the pier. My heart beat fast. I was excited. Excited to see it.

After growing up near the big, gray, stormy Atlantic, the Pacific looked like a lake. It was calm and blue and the surf was small, and I stood against the white-painted railing and watched the waves roll in and the surfers paddle to catch them.

The air was fresh and salty and clean and the coastline was low-lying and gray-brown. To the north, the land came out into a small rocky point. South was beach-sand as far as you could see, shoreline with a boardwalk and houses, and then it was like staring into fog or pure light—the coast filtered away into haze and glare and mist and you saw nothing.

Below me the old, gray footboards of the pier creaked and groaned and you could see light in the cracks between them and then green water below. Above was pure empty blue, not a cloud in sight, and there were noisy seagulls drifting and crying out and coming down to rest on the pier railing.

California.

My new life.

I walked to the end of the pier. There was an old Mexican man fishing and he was pulling something up, reeling it in. As I walked closer, he braced himself against the railing and he leaned into it and talked under his breath. "C'mon on, sweetheart," he said, turning the reel, "C'mon now, c'mon, sweetheart, c'mon," and just as I thought he had it, his rod bent forward like a horseshoe and his line went tense, tight, and then snapped in two.

1998

CHENTE'S PARTY, 1 A.M.

Joey gets to the party late and walks through the house looking for Tyler. The front room is dark and faces move around him: unfamiliar kids who narrow their eyes and stare at him, frowning. *Cholos* with hairnets and Dickies and flannels. Loud voices ("No way, you *love* to lie!"), laughing girls who look mean. The hallway is packed with bodies and Joey pushes through them into the kitchen and someone says, "Chill out, whiteboy."

The kitchen is lit brightly and people stand around the keg holding red plastic cups, counting down to something, and it's "One!" and "Two! Three! FOUR! FIVE! *SIX!*" and Joey squeezing into the living room and the living room full of people jammed together in front of the band, drinking and loud. Someone claps him on the back and he turns around. "Joey Carr, in the flesh!"

It's Javier, the new busboy from work. Joey smiles and they try a complex handshake but they mess it up and Javier shrugs and laughs, "Iss all good, Carr. We good. You know what? I'm *drunk*!"

Chente is just visible above the crowd and Joey stands on his toes and cranes his neck above the shoulders in front of him. Chente Ramirez, black hair slicked back and shining, guitar strapped on, red-brown face pouring sweat. Joey moves closer so he can see. Chente tuning his guitar, frowning. The bassist messing with the dials on his bass amp and the drummer with his sticks crossed in his lap, looking down at his hands, out of breath, shoulders and chest heaving, sweating, keyed-up, waiting for the next song.

"*Pues, pues . . . un más!*" Chente shouts back at his band. He looks down at his guitar neck as he twists one of the tuning pegs and hits the top string with his thumb.

Chente's drummer leans forward and says something to the bassist and the bassist shakes his head, handing him a bottle of Cuervo tequila.

"*Órale, cabrones,*" Chente says into the microphone. "One more. One more." The mic feeds back and Chente steps away from it and frowns. "Okay, hold on. *Órale, ahora mismo vamos a tocar una nueva canción. Esta canción se llama—*"

"*Chingate,* Chente Ramirez!" shouts a deep, hoarse voice from the back of the crowd. "Fuck you *and* your new songs! Jus' shut up and *play, cabrón*."

Chente starts to say something into the mic but then he laughs and shakes his head. "Okay, okay, this song goes out to . . . to José Morales in the back for all his love and support and kind words over the years."

"Thas riiight, *carnalito*," shouts the voice. "*Es la neta, guey!* Play some fucking rock 'n' *roll!*"

Chente looks back at his drummer and nods his head.

The drummer sets his sticks on the snare and sits up straight and cracks his neck and rolls his shoulders and now he's ready. He picks up his drumsticks again and nods at Chente.

Chente turns to face the mic, addressing the crowd: "You tired of working jobs that make you feel dead?!" The mic feeds back again.

The crowd shouts "Yeah!" bottles in hand, swaying, happy. The whole middle row staggers to the side and Joey's caught up in it, and he laughs as they begin to fall and then they're pulled back up again. Someone shoves a beer up to his mouth and it conks his front teeth, but another hand grabs it away and throws it at the wall and it shatters and the crowd spills forward as one mass. He tastes blood.

"You sick of teachers and bosses who act like *cops*?!" Chente shouts and the crowd yeah's back at him again. "Well, this one's for you! One, two, *tres, quatro*!" And they kick into the song and it's loud and fast and rhythmic and the people begin to dance and shove and knock against each other and a pit forms in front of the band.

Joey breaks away and pulls himself through the wall of bodies.

He sees Tyler at the back of the room and Tyler smiles and waves, standing on his tiptoes.

"Hey! Tyler! You made it! It's *crazy* up there!"

"What?!"

"I just—" Joey puts his hand on Tyler's shoulder and talks in his ear. "I just got here. It's crazy up there. What's goin' on?"

"Nothing. We're just about to leave."

"No, *stay*."

"Maybe."

"C'mon, Tyler. You should. Please? I just got here."

"Oh, wait. Joey, this is Maggie."

And Maggie steps out from behind Tyler, and Joey tries to talk but he's thought so much about her all night after hearing Tyler's story. His voice stops in his throat. Maggie—her green eyes sparkling, dark hair in twin braids, her face glowing fresh white like she's just come in from the rain, her lips glossed with a shiny coat of pink. She's wearing a brown corduroy rancher's coat lined with wool on the collar and cuffs, and her jeans are tight and gray and they lead down to flat-soled buckle shoes. Over her shoulder is the strap of a green army satchel covered in activist pins and she's holding the strap in one hand at her chest and a big clear bottle in a brown bag in the other. Her eyes trained straight on Joey. She smiles and shakes her head.

"So *you're* the bad Joey Carr getting Tyler into all this trouble."

"I'm the Joey—I mean—I'm Joey."

She laughs. "I'm Maggie."

"I'm Joey."

"Yeah, I know, silly." She smiles and puts her hand out to shake but instead of shaking Joey goes in for a hug and she steps back and he fumbles forward and gets confused and offers the bottle of tequila. "Here." His voice cracks and it comes out high. He tries to lower it. "*Tequila*."

"Fuck *yeah*. Awesome. Trade me." She hands Joey her bottle and then unscrews the plastic cap off the tequila. "To Chente's band." She takes a small sip and makes a face and then takes another sip, this one better. Her next sip is a gulp and Joey's heart swells and like a thunderclap he's in love.

4 A.M.

Later on, the crowd thins out and Chente and his bandmates pack up their equipment and move it to the back bedroom.

Joey and Maggie—talking in the middle of the living room about

Chente. Tyler off smoking in the backyard. Joey saying, "No, seriously. We drove around the Gaslamp with a megaphone pretending to be preachers."

"With a *megaphone*?"

"Yep. I was 'Pastor Brother' and Chente was 'Pastor *Carnal*,' which means 'brother' or 'buddy' in Spanish. Y'know, just yelling from the truck window at people coming out of the fratty bars. Giving sermons from the truck as we drove along the strip. Silly stuff. 'Jesus died for a six-pack of Diet *Pepsi!*' and 'Jesus loves you so much he took off his beard and did a head-spin on a tortilla.' Chente just comes up with that stuff off the top of his head. It was fine until someone threw a D battery at us."

"D batteries are big, right?"

"They're huge."

"Ouch."

"Everyone else went wild and was, like . . . like, cheering us on and following the truck and waving at us. It was crazy."

A tall, older guy in a maroon tracksuit and a white fisherman's hat comes out of the kitchen, turns, and heads straight for Maggie.

"Now hey, *Miss Little*," he says, towering over them, looking Maggie up and down. "Now hey." He smiles and his left front tooth is gold with a tiny diamond pot leaf in the middle, and Joey thinks, *You're great*.

"Hay is for horses," Maggie says and smiles.

The man moves closer and leans down to her. "It is indeed. Allow . . . allow me to *introduce* myself," he says, a hand on his chest, bowing his head, "My name Kevrone Berry Smith. Son of Lando Calrissian. Owner of a Lonely Heart. Lord of the Dance. King of *all* this shit. Listen: K-e-v. R-o-n-e. *Kevrone*. And hello to you, you sexy little . . . you little . . . majestical . . . little baby *deer* . . . little walkin', talkin' little . . . hey girl . . . you little *thing*. You a emerald. You a diamond. Ughn! Agh! Hoo!"

Joey nervous, looking around.

"Hi," she says blushing red. "I like your name."

"Now, now, Miss Little, I live up the block. In the *big* house next to the daycare. Big ol' Jabba's Palace house, I like *Star Wars,* I do. Now, now, I'm kind of the . . . I'm the *boss* around this place. Somebody gots to tell these lazy Mexicans what to do. Naw, naw, I'm playing now, we all friends, Mexicans and me, we cool, you know me, haha. I'm a honorary Mexican anyway. I'm a *icon* around here."

"I should—"

"Miss Little, hush up, hush. Now that we . . . now that we *friendly,* as it were, how 'bouts me and you go back in Dr. *Señor* Chente Ramirez San's state-sanctioned love-nest sex-den bedroom and—"

Maggie frowned. "I don't think so. I'm sorry. I just . . . I just want to hang out with my friend here. Y'know, we're just hanging out . . . here right now." Maggie looks at Joey, who stands stalk-still, powerless, fighting inside himself.

"—and smoke us some of this greasy, *naaaahsty,* dirty, fuh, fuh, fuh-*filthy, sticky-ass*—"

"I mean, I'm just talking to my friend and I want to stay here and—"

"—buckwild-Michael-Jordan-Bugs-Bunny-*Space-Jam*-Gorbachev-Chernobyl-nuclear weedy weedsy *weed* and talk abouts some *fine* things for while." He shows Maggie a Ziplock bag of grass, then sniffs it, and shouts a joyful "Hooo!" before stuffing it back in his pocket.

"I don't really smoke weed or anyth—" she starts to say, but then Tyler's pushing through the crowd and he's standing next to her, saying:

"She's with me." Tyler stands up as straight as he can. "She's with me." His voice is high and unsteady. "She's still my . . . she's . . . my *girlfriend.* We're dating." Tyler nods and rakes a nervous hand through his white-blonde hair and it falls back along the sides of his face. His eyes go wide and then he pulls back together and tries again. "She's my girlfriend."

"So hey now, Scarecrow Wizard of Oz." Whispering "*muhfucka,*" Kevrone grins, waving him away. "Miss Little, let's say I take you back there right now and we gets to know each other, as it were. *I'm loyal.* Any fool here can vouch for me and *my* ways. I ain't here to trick *nobody*. N-o-b-o-d-*y*," he spells the word out and adds emphasis to the last letter. "My aim is nothin' but *true . . . blue,* Miss Little."

Joey's mind spins as he fights for a solution. "Tequila," he says. He holds the bottle in the man's direction.

"Aw *hell* yeah, son." Kevrone opens the bottle with a dainty twist of the cap and turns it upside down and swallows like he's drinking water.

"Bottom's up, Kevy," grunts Chente under the weight of the bass amp he's carrying. He walks sideways along the wall, holding the amp and moves past Joey and Maggie and grins at Joey and shakes his head. "Joey, *carnal*, stick around, alright? I wanna talk to you about something."

"Okay." Joey shrugs at Chente.

"Hooo! Shit, *son*!" sputters Kevrone. He hands the bottle back to Joey, wiping his mouth with his hand. "S-h-i-t. Shit with wings on its back and little headlights. Shit that climb outta the toilet and whup your ass for shittin' it out to *begin* with, sayin' 'You muh*fucka*.' Shit that'd drive a truck into your house and bust down the wall and steal your *TV*. Hooo! Hooo!" His eyes are glassy and red and he coughs and smiles and then coughs again. "Hooo! S-h-i-double-t excla*mation* ation ation *ation* point. Two more ation. Ation, ation," singing in falsetto, "don't forgehhhhh-eh-ehhht."

"No, no," says Joey, "have some more. It's a party."

Tyler pulls a cigarette from his pack, sticks it in his mouth, and walks away, shaking his head.

Maggie moves closer to Joey and he feels her hand on the back of his arm.

"Sure *is*," says Kervone. "A *birthday party*. Happy birthday to Kevrone Berry Smithy Smithy Smay-ithy *Smith* and his *whole* life." He takes another drink and then another and now he's distracted and wanders away, handing the bottle back to Joey without looking at him. Kevrone staggers into the kitchen. "Who got cigarettes?" he shouts. "I *know* some muhfucka got *cigarettes*." He walks out the kitchen door and into the backyard and shouts, "Hooo!" and now his voice is muffled, and then he's gone.

"Thank you, Joey Carr," says Maggie. "You saved the day."

"I can't believe that worked. Is that what 'bait and switch' means?"

"Whatever it was, that was fucking awesome. Hey Joey Carr, let's drink some more of . . . of that tequila."

"You want some more?"

"Totally. A gallon. A barrel."

"Here."

"Thanks."

"Where's Tyler?"

"He was just here." Maggie hands the bottle back.

"Did he leave?"

"I hope not. He's my ride."

Joey looks around the room. "I think he went for a cigarette. We should probably just . . . *leave* and go somewhere uh . . . I don't know. I have no idea." He turns back to Maggie and shrugs and she smiles and laughs and starts to blush, her eyes green and full of light. She reaches for the tequila again.

Okay, Joey thinks. *Okay. Here we go.*

CLAIREMONT

Tyler Monahan lives with his parents and younger sister in Clairemont, a working-class suburb on the hill overlooking the bay, and further west, the dim gray line of the Pacific. (His father, an employee of the city; his mother, a stay-at-home mom.) On Tyler's street, the houses are small and quiet and modest, the lawns tidy, geometric. Across the street and a block to the south is the house where Maggie lives with her mother and her sister and two younger cousins. When Joey finds this out, he makes a point of stopping by Tyler's as often as he can. The conversation starts with an excuse. "Hey Tyler, let's see if Maggie's mom can feed us," or "I bet Maggie's cousins have some movies we haven't seen." When Maggie's mom is at work at the mall, they sit at the patio table in the ruined, dusty backyard and drink 40s and smoke cigarettes. Sometimes they watch TV and talk and Joey tries to entertain Maggie and her cousins and her sister and make them laugh. Her sister, Jolie—fourteen, a tomboy, red hair, braces, country music fan, trailerpark voice, rabid liar, Dairy Queen employee. Molly—the baby cousin at twelve, four feet tall, big owl glasses, waist-length hair. Molly—hiding in the back of the house, refusing to bathe. Cecilie, the older cousin, sixteen, tall and dark-haired and sad. Cecilie—sleeping all day, taking endless baths, showing up like a ghost for meals, walking without sound, writing letters to her mom up in the women's prison, dreaming all day of moving back to Ohio. The four of them—too close, stuck inside, ditching school, meeting boys in the front yard, sitting in the uncut grass under the tree with bare feet, toes digging into the earth, tempestuous, sauntering, fighting over the phone ("Give it to me! Magg*ie*!"), reading for days without end, locked in the bathroom for hours, brokenhearted, crying, hungry, restless, laughing at everything, bickering over food, chasing each other around the house. Maggie—the boss, sending them off to bed, making their lunches when her mom worked early. Marla, the girls' mom—divorced and dating a man who owns a fish market in Point Loma and three rock cod boats. Marla—long red hair, smart, pretty, kind and sad-eyed, raised in Europe as an army brat, always working at the department store at UTC, in debt, cries over the phone in her room.

The house is crumbling but with a sweet, humid decay—new life in the ruins. Cecilie's wet towels drying on the tops of doors, a steamy bathroom mirror, initials and hearts drawn on it with a finger, and bath tiles warm and mildewing and towel racks tangled with curler and blow-dryer cords. Molly and Cecilie's room—piled to the walls with old suitcases, cardboard boxes marked "bedroom" and "baby stuff" and "kids," empty bottles of nail polish, books on witches and knights and pagan rituals. Molly's mattress (the bottom bunk) covered in plastic horse statues, shoes with no laces, jump ropes, P.B. Rec Center Halloween carnival prizes (bat rings, sticky spiders that cling to the walls, grinning plastic skeletons). Stuffed behind the dresser: leather belts with plastic rhinestones, woven bracelets, plastic Easter eggs (puce, lime green, yellow), stray press-on nails, crumpled-up drawings made by boys in her class where she looks like an elven princess.

Cecilie's bed (the top bunk) was pissed on by Jolie's cat and because of this she sleeps on the floor of the solarium in a My Little Pony sleeping bag. (At night she stays up late in her sleeping bag reading sci-fi and fantasy novels.) Jolie's room—a sea of trash, looks like a closet, smells like gym clothes. Empty Ritz boxes on the floor, soccer trophies, cereal bowls, miniature novelty baseball bats that are also pens. On her walls are posters of bands she doesn't like, fist-size holes she's punched, boys' names and phone numbers penciled-in next to the bed (all the i's and j's dotted by hearts and stars). Maggie's room—a big four-poster bed and a mirror and nothing else. In one corner a boombox and a stack of books. The only window opens into the side-yard and through the curtains you can see the sun. An unused door that leads to the garage is covered in a collage of Johnny Depp and Courtney Love photos cut from magazines, the occasional tooth blocked out in Sharpie, here and there a mustache or a heart. The smell in Maggie's room is incense and the smoky wax from strawberry and vanilla candles blown out. The only poster on her wall (stolen from a doctor's office) reads: "Never, *EVER* shake a baby."

Directly to the west of Clairemont is Pacific Beach where Joey lives with his aunt and uncle in a three-bedroom house two blocks from the ocean. Joey's part of Pacific Beach was once grain fields and dirt roads and farmland. From the beaches to the west to the flat lands north of Mission Bay, cattle stood in fields and ate grass within view of the sea. The soil was warm and sandy and there was marsh, and around the marsh there were farmhouses. The neighborhood grew fast when the railroad came. Before the Spanish arrived, a Kumeyaay tribe lived in a seaside village where Joey's aunt and uncle's home would be built following the second World War. But now it's Mexican restaurants and streets with swimsuit boutiques and surf shops and beach bars with neon signs. A small town grown into a tourist trap. (As a boy, Joey dug in the backyard looking for arrowheads and found shards of pottery and mysterious bones that turned out to be chicken. Once, a wheat penny, which he promptly lost.)

Joey's bedroom faces north and from his window you can see a block of pink stucco apartments with the words "Pacific Isle Manor" in cast-iron letters across the front (the 'M' and first 'C' missing for three months now, stolen by "Tall" Tim Sanders on a drunken spree as a present for his unrequited love, Melissa Carville, a bartender at Club Tremors). Joey's room has been a mess since the second day of middle school when he awoke with the realization that it was "all downhill from here," the Beach Boys' "Kokomo" playing on his clock radio. The room: twin bed with a black comforter and no sheets, dresser filled with junk, gray carpet floor piled with school books from his failed stint at City College, sneakers, a baseball glove (an unused present from his sister Macey), a black comb he's had since fourth-grade picture day. The walls plastered floor-to-ceiling in posters, pages cut from magazines, newspaper articles, fliers, self-portrait photos of himself holding the camera at arm's length and brooding melodramatically. The windowsill is lined with Dr. Pepper cans, crusts from ancient tomato sandwiches, and coffee cups growing mold. The stereo is covered in dust and on it (in a place of honor, sitting on his childhood copy of *Harriet the Spy*) is the silver and black switchblade that Chente bought him in Tijuana for his birthday.

Standing on the corner outside Joey's house, you can look out over the rooftops of P.B. and see the hills of Clairemont to the east. Through the haze it's a low, green-brown clump of land that runs in a long wavering mesa top.

Somewhere in that smudge of treetops and gray dots of buildings is Maggie's house, and when Joey stares at it just right, he can make himself see it.

1978

JANUARY 12TH

Yesterday was my birthday, and my brother and I celebrated early with fresh lobster and abalone his buddy Pat got off the coast of La Jolla. Jake says things like, "Birthdays are when you take stock of your life and figure yourself out," and, "It's time, Merc, ol' buddy. You're nineteen, you need a *job*." Jake also does things like sit on the couch and smoke dope and drink gin from the bottle until he falls asleep and I'm left sitting across from him, bored, staring down at my shoes. Jake's a drinker and the fact that I'm not makes him distrust me. I like beer okay and I'm good for one (maybe two) but beyond that I get bored and Jake says things like, "Merc, ol' buddy, you know who doesn't drink? Faggots don't drink." Our uncle Jasper, whom we both loved, was a "faggot." (I don't think Jake knows that.) Jake's life is awful and it hurts to see what he's become since I last saw him. Growing up, our family had money. And then we didn't. It happened fast. Jake and I called it "The Fall." The last time Jake and I lived together our family had a lake house and good cars and we dressed well. Now this. The *real* Fall.

The day before I got here, Jake's wife Sorel left him and moved in with a friend in Fallbrook. Jake is unemployed and he's overweight and he looks old. My brother is thirty-three. Our parents had him after the war when Dad got back from the Pacific and was in the process of starting over as a civilian.

Dad got work delivering ice in a truck and that was fine, and then there was Korea and he went back into the service, switching branches from the Marines to the Army. After that was Vietnam. As much as he tried to find a new life after the second World War, the only thing Dad knew was the service. Once Korea began, his career was the military from then on out, just like our grandfather Tate, who fought in the first World War.

We all thought Vietnam would be over fast, but we were wrong. Growing up, Vietnam was a constant presence in my life. It's only been *over*-over for a few years and not having it around feels weird. Like, it's old Uncle Vietnam War: What's he gonna do next? What's our old buddy The Endless Fucking War up to now? I was born in 1959 and my father was over there before I can remember. Then, eight years ago, my Dad was killed by a sniper as he stepped off a helicopter somewhere in the A Shau Valley. When I try to think of this, I see long grass blowing flat as the chopper lands and I see sky that's dark gray (almost volcanic, Paleozoic). I hear the whupping of the blades and the tap tap tap sound of small arms fire, but I can't see my father. I can only imagine life as he saw it. I can't picture him at all. Most days I can't see his face. I don't have much to work with.

The few memories I have of my father are distant and spread out across large blocks of time. I remember him from blurry photos and from brief weekend trips to meet up on leave, but there's nothing more than that. My brother knew him better and I've always been jealous. Jake was born in '46 so he knew Dad in the time between World War II and Korea and between Korea and Vietnam, and it made a big impression on him.

In younger pictures, Jake looks like Superman. He's tall, square-jawed, and has jet-black hair cut short and big, dark, matinee-idol eyes. In high school, he was the football team's quarterback and he helped take them all the way to Nationals in his senior year. Jake's plan after college was politics. He was going to be a senator for the state of New York. "After that, who knows?" he used to say. "President? Can you see your big brother as President of the United States?" Thing was, I could. It was no stretch of the imagination to see Jake running the country, tall and ambitious and proud and strong. He wanted the world. That was his dream but his dream didn't come true.

When Jake went into the service the year Dad died, it was too much for our mother. Mom, who was so strong when Dad was away, fell into herself, and that was it. She's out here in a home but she's not Mom anymore. She doesn't talk and they feed her and they take her to the bathroom and she sits and stares out the window until it's dark. Jake visits on Mondays, Wednesdays, and Fridays. Sometimes he drops by on Sundays to read the Bible and pray over her. I'm supposed to go tomorrow but I don't know if I will. It's been nearly eight years since I've seen her.

When Dad was killed and Jake enlisted and Mom got sick, I went to stay with Mom's sister, Joyce May, in Binghamton. My mother was born in Buffalo. I grew up in Queens but we had a summerhouse in Upstate while Dad was alive. After Dad died, it was one thing after the next. Mom put away in a home. Jake off in Vietnam. Uncle Carl selling our house in Queens for us and then the summer place in Old Forge and taking off with the money. That was it. The Fall. A fallen family. Three years later, Joyce May fractured the left side of her pelvis in a car accident and I moved back to the city and lived with some friends of my brother until high school was over.

Jake came back from Vietnam a year and a half after he went in, but no one in the family talks about why. From what I gather, he fell apart just like Mom. None of us have what my father had, the thing that made him stay in, war after war. In pictures, sitting on a tank or standing in the jungle holding his gun, our father is happy. That's what I know of him. Happy, laughing, big square glasses with thick frames and tape in the middle, his helmet askew, a cigarette dangling out the side of his mouth. It always got to me. How could my father be so happy without us? Was he happy because he loved the service or because he was away from us? Whatever it was, I felt worthless. What good am I if my own father doesn't want to be with me? I don't think that way anymore, but at the time it overwhelmed me. My father was my hero but I'm not even sure why.

Jake's asleep now. The TV on an old Technicolor Western movie—Apache braves on horses standing in a line on the ridge in black silhouette, the sky red-purple. Jake looks nothing like the Superman in those photos from before the war. His hair is long and he has a mustache and the start of a beard. Before the war, he dressed like me, in blue jeans and a t-shirt, clean-cut. Now it's slouchy brown pants, an old striped sweater with stains on the front, and a *vest* of all things.

In my bedroom, I do push-ups until I'm out of breath. Then I hit the books. Tonight I'm studying the European theater of the second World War. The British pushing for Caen. The allies holding 80 miles of Normandy coastline. Sixteen divisions now in France and a million Allied troops headed for the streets of Paris. Hitler holding Rudstedt and Rommel to blame.

It's weird, I guess. I've still got my course books and I'm still following along. The problem is I've always been in school. I graduated high school two years early at the top of my class and I went to Columbia on a full-ride scholarship to be a war historian (specializing in the Pacific Theater). Columbia, my dream. *In lumine Tuo videbimus lumen*. The golden old-world sound of the words "Kings College." Hollerith, both Roosevelts, Stephen Jay Gould, Millikan, Irwin Edman, the economist Friedman, Oscar Hammerstein, Asimov, Howard Koch, Alexander Hamilton. I wanted to be up there with them, and I got my wish.

The whole thing is a trick. I was born with a photographic memory. No one knows this besides Jake. My mind is a book of lists. I remember numbers, facts, dates, anything mathematical, jingles of car commercials, TV ads, map directions, phone numbers, license plates, conversations, all of it down to the last letter or number. I don't always understand what I hear (sometimes to my detriment) but I retain it, and because of that school was a breeze. With history, I had a leg up on everyone else. I could afford to spend my time figuring out the impetus and the repercussions of the events instead of memorizing dates, and because of that, my teachers thought I was some kind of prodigy. Now, without the structure of school, I'm lost and bored. So I read. I keep up.

Jake drinks all day and he shouts at the TV and his friends come over and listen to screeching, terrible hippie music and I shut myself in my bedroom and I read about the Panzer divisions, Manifest Destiny, the Dual Resonance Model, Quantrill's Raid, the Battle of Wuhan, the Battle of Pea Ridge, westward expansion, the Magna Carta, oil rig technology, Civil War medicine, Ernest J. King, Osami Nagano, the Japanese surrender aboard the *Missouri*, Stephen A.

Douglas' Kansas Nebraska Bill of 1854, pangenesis. I read my course books but I also read books I checked out (and I guess stole) from the Columbia library: Samuel Eliot Morison's *History of United States Naval Operations in World War II* (volumes 3 and 4), Dee Brown, Joseph Heller, Gabriele Veneziano, Elizabeth Bacon Custer's *Tenting on the Plains*, Willa Cather, James Jones, the golden boy Juliano, Wouk's great *Winds of War* and *War and Remembrance*, Ed Distler's *Ghosts and The Amazon*, Leonard Susskind, Dreiser, Iris Murdoch. I give myself tests and I write term papers that no professor will ever see.

This notebook came from a class exercise. My first semester at Columbia, I had a psych professor who had us keep journals. He told us that to truly know our subconscious motives aren't sabotaging our conscious plans, we need to deconstruct (and then *analyze*) our lives as if we were a third party. The assignment was to keep the journal for three months and at the end go back and write an analytical essay detailing our various agendas in relation to where we wanted to go with our lives (and do so from the perspective of a critical outside observer). On the first day, our professor said, "The idea is you carry your notebook wherever you go, so's not to . . . y'know, let it fall into enemy hands." (That made everyone laugh and broke the ice.) "The only way to be fully candid and, by extension, *honest*, is to keep your journal with you. It should be small enough to fit in your front pocket, or, for you ladies, in your purse or handbag or clutch or tote or whatever the fuck you're calling them these days." (More laughter. He was that kind of professor. He wore colored socks and an old McGovern Shriver pin on his tan-brown blazer.) "Write small and use all the space on the page. No filler, but don't be afraid of details." At first I kept the names out just to be safe. Now I'm not so cautious. The notebook (this is my fifth) stays with me. I write alone and I tell no one about it. (It's safer that way.) The first notebooks I burned when I was done. I'll do the same with this one. It's less about the end result than the action.

JANUARY 15TH

Made an interesting discovery today. Jake was off buying weed with his friend Herman so I had the place to myself, and I ended up going through the bookcase in the front room. The top shelf was all *National Geographic*s, (three) books about Cleopatra, and (four) big coffee-table photobooks on ancient Egypt. The second was random supermarket paperbacks, biographies, romance novels, nothing interesting. The bottom shelf was nearly empty, but I found one of Jake's photo albums and in the album was a letter to me dated August 1st, 1970, the month my mom was taken away.

When Jake was in Vietnam, I got two letters from him. This one was unsent. I present it (copied here) as a piece of family history.

One thing I should say: As infrequently as Jake wrote, at least he made the effort. Dad never wrote—to any of us.

Dear baby brother,

How's it going, little man? I hope you're well and that Mom is keeping the house together and not worrying herself sick. I've been here at the new firebase for a week now and things are fine. The food is good and the people I'm with are all great guys. You shouldn't worry about your brother out here. I'm in good hands and if there *is* fighting going on, I haven't seen it.

We do a lot of work around the base but we also get to play football and listen to the radio and have card games. It's just like back home. Only in the middle of the jungle in South East Asia. Haha.

Tell Mom and J.M. thanks for the packages they sent. I shared them. Of course.

Between you and me, I want you to watch out for Mom and make sure she's taking it easy. Oh, and remind Carl about fixing the washer when he's there. I don't want Mom getting overwhelmed again. You know how it is. I'm sure she's in good hands too. You're the boss now, little man. You're brave and smart. I know you'll do a great job.

Vietnam is a pretty country. Our firebase is surrounded by jungle. Deep green jungle. Right now it's the rainy season but before this it was dry and dusty and any chance we got to go into the jungle was a nice relief. You know how I hate hot, dusty places. Well, it gets DUSTY, haha. The dust here is red and fine and it gets in your eyes and sometimes the choppers whip it up so much you have to wrap a shirt around your mouth and nose and keep your head down. The sky is so blue. So empty and blue and the dust is so red. You sit around praying for rain and then when the rain comes you're praying for it to be dry again, haha.

Flying over the country is [unintelligible handwriting, "great" maybe?]. You'd like helicopters I bet. Soaring over the jungle in [another part I can't read] you see it all below you and it's thick and green and you fly over rivers with people on tiny boats who look up at you and rice patties with big black water buffalo and people carrying baskets on their backs.

We haven't been to any of the villages around here but you see them from the helicopter. Thatch huts, pigs, chickens, alot of little kids your age running around. You can't tell one Vietnamese from the next but they seem like good, hard-working people.

Merc, you're going to hear a lot of talk about what the army is doing here and you might hear people say we're doing bad things. This is not true. Don't believe what you hear. You know your brother, I wouldn't do anything like that and I wouldn't be involved with anyone who would. We're here keeping the peace and helping out. Hero-work. That's all. We're doing the right thing, little man. I hope you don't let anyone tell you otherwise. Your big brother's one of the good guys. Don't you forget that.

Well, it's about time for chow so I'm going to mosey on out and get [unreadable]. Tell mom not to worry and you don't worry either and I'll be home when this is all over and I'll bring you something nice.

Your big brother,
Jake

[Underneath his name, a drawing of a cowboy smoking a cigarette.]

1998

KENSINGTON, 2:12 A.M.

In the alley behind the bar, Chente hits the guy and he doesn't stop. The guy's on his back now and Chente's standing over him, holding him by his necktie, hitting him—hitting and then "You," (hit) "son of a," (hit). Joey tries to pull Chente off the guy because he's sure Chente's killed him, but he slips and falls on his side and the world swings around him and he throws up in his mouth and spits it out on the asphalt. Chente stops and lets go of the guy's tie and the guy's head smacks the concrete and the hollow sound it makes is terrible. Joey crawls up to the body, kneeling, placing a finger on the guy's neck to feel his pulse and the guy moans and a tear rolls down Joey's face and drops into the guy's mouth. Joey doesn't see this. He also doesn't see: 1) The black silhouette of the woman standing in the mouth of the alley with a baby in a stroller. Watching, not afraid, but sad. 2) The "Thank You For Pot Smoking" sticker on the dumpster. 3) The tabby cat ("Mr. Pretty Phil") watching from the upstairs balcony. Chente sees all three of these things. He looks down at Joey and wipes his own blood from under his nose and his eyes are fierce and white and storming.

"Joey, *move*."

"Chente, no, just—"

"Joey, *carnal*. Move."

Joey gets up and staggers to the side and tries to walk but he falls again. He grabs at the handle of the dumpster but he doesn't catch it and he's down.

The woman in the mouth of the alley walks on, pushing the stroller, singing in a soft coo, "Jimmy is a baby / Jimmy is a baby / Jimmy is a baby / Jimmy is a pup / Jimmy is a nice man / Jimmy is a sweet man / Jimmy is a kind man / Jimmy is a pup." Jimmy the baby/pup—asleep in his stroller blankets, dreaming of his father's bearded face.

The guy tries to roll to the side but Chente kicks him in the face and the guy's head jerks hard to the left, and he stops moving.

The guy's mouth is open, his white button-up shirt spotted with blood. Chente spits on him and kicks him in the side but the guy's body doesn't move. He kicks him again and it's like kicking a sack of earth.

Mr. Pretty Phil, the tabby cat, goes back inside to piss on a light blue sweater his owner left on the couch. The sticker on the dumpster still thanks you for pot-smoking.

Joey gets up and tries to run to the car but the lights dim around him and then go bright again and he falls forward onto his knees and throws up in a great yellow splash. It is the fourth (and final) time he will throw up tonight. The first three hurt coming out; this one was easy and fast.

Chente walks past him, swaying to the side, car keys in hand, jingling.

WORK, THE NEXT DAY

In the downstairs broom closet at work, the lights off, the door locked behind them, Joey tries to think about Petra while Petra is on her knees in front of him. He tries to think about *Petra*, her kinky blonde hair pulled back into a ponytail, her lanky body and tiny soft breasts, her head pumping like a pigeon or an oil derrick. He tries not to think about Maggie because he's standing here in the darkness with *Petra*. It's *Petra* kneeling in front of him. But he thinks of Maggie, and now it's Maggie—barefoot, sweaty in the heat, an old black band t-shirt, and her legs in tiny jean shorts, and now Joey's knees are giving out and he doubles forward and holds onto Petra's skinny, naked shoulders for support and grits his teeth and loses himself for a quick, dizzy stream of seconds into her mouth as her head continues to jerk back and forth in his lap and knock against his stomach.

It's New Year's Eve. Four p.m. and Joey has no plans.

Petra spits in the mop sink and rinses her mouth under the tap and they sit cross-legged on the floor of the broom closet and talk while she holds a cigarette lighter between them so they can see.

Petra wants a rating. She wants to know how she did, what was good, what wasn't. "This," she tells Joey whenever *this* happens, "is *practicing*." She calls it "practicing" and she says things like, "We're just friends, Joey." "I'm practicing." "This means nothing." That has been established—earlier, weeks ago.

"Well," she says. "Be honest."

"A scale from one to ten?"

"Details. I want details."

Joey looks at her in the flickering glow of the lighter, warm orange skin from the flame, the heavy bottom lip of her frown, the lazy way she leans forward, slouching, the pink tips of her breasts as she holds the lighter and talks to him—and she means nothing.

"Is it bad that I spit it out?"

"I don't know, Petra."

"Do guys want girls to swallow?"

"I guess it depends."

"There was a lot. I would've thrown up. There was a *gross* amount."

"Sorry."

"Well. Come on. *Info*. Tell me what was good, what you liked, what was bad. You know, *constructive*."

Joey tells Petra what was good and what he liked best and he makes up something minor for the bad and he says it constructively. Petra listens and nods her head and holds her lighter and stares at him and he can see she's getting impatient.

"Alright," she says. "Thursday? Same Bat-Time?"

"Okay."

The lighter goes out and it's dark in the broom closet.

"Oh . . . Happy New Year, Carr."

"Happy New Year." Joey helps himself up with the edge of the sink. He can see the dim outline of Petra pulling her shirt back on. Petra the friend, the co-worker, the nothing, just like his nothing; she turns on the light and steps into her shoes and picks up her sweater and her backpack and puts them both over her shoulder.

Joey leans in to kiss her.

She moves away and he gets the side of her head.

THE EMPLOYEE LOCKER ROOM, FOUR HOURS LATER

Joey: "Tyler, check it out. You know what you need?"

Tyler: (shrugs)

Joey: "Vegas."

Tyler: "Las Vegas?"

Joey: "Totally."

Tyler: "You think so?"

Joey: "You, my friend, need a cheer-me-up road-trip. You need to stop obsessing about where she is and what she's doing and who she's with. It's not healthy. It's creepy. You need to head on out to the desert with me and go totally nuts. Just like *Fear and Loathing*. Hunter S. Tyler. Joey S. Thompson."

Tyler: "I know but—"

Joey: "But nothing. We're going to Las Vegas, just me and you, and it'll be like the coolest, funniest buddy cop movie without any of the cop parts. A room at the Circus Circus jerkus berkus, hangin' out on the Strip, people watching, swimming in the gawdamn *pool,* horrible food, tequila, speed, pills, 24-hour dumbness."

Tyler: "I've never been to Vegas."

Joey: "Even better."

Tyler: "Where is it?"

Joey: "What do you mean where is it, it's like four hours away on the I-15."

Tyler: "Oh. In California?"

Joey: "Nevada. You need to get out of the house."

Tyler: "That's probably true."

Joey: "You study too much."

Tyler: "I do. I study too much." (breaking into a shaky grin)

Joey: "Vegas, I'm telling you. It'll work wonders in the you-feeling-better department."

Tyler: "Okay, we could do that. That sounds great actually. That sounds . . . yeah, let's do it!"

Joey: "Good! I'll drive. You concentrate on the not-thinking-about-Maggie. Your life will be nothing but getting stupid and crazy with your best friend on Earth."

Tyler: "And who would that be?"

Joey: "Batman."

1978

FEBRUARY 1ST

My big news is that I'm back in school. It's night school and it's unaccredited, but it's good to be in the rhythm of tests and lectures and course work and deadlines again. This fall I hope to start up at State, but right now I'm taking night classes at the junior high building. I keep telling myself this is just a stepping stone, and that gets me through the work and keeps me excited. It's good to be back.

FEBRUARY 2ND

How weird to be taking quote-unquote college—or maybe "adult education"—classes in a room that junior high kids use by day. Makes you feel a little less than legit. The construction paper art pieces on the wall. A poster about the Mayflower. These little chair-desks and a tiny black ski coat left behind on the coat hooks by the door. Perched on the chalkboard railing, a bathroom hall pass—an oversized wooden key with "Room 2" written on it in black marker.

FEBRUARY 3RD

I met a girl. She missed the first few sessions but tonight she was there before everyone and I got a seat next to her and we hit it off immediately. Her name is Channy Morning Greene. (Morning, she said, is a family middle name.) Channy is twenty-three, a few years older than I am, and she works at a hospital during the day and takes classes at night (mostly writing classes: She wants to write novels). I've never met anyone like her (other than myself). Like me, she studies hard and she doesn't drink or socialize all that much or go out at night. She moved out of her parents' place when she was sixteen and she's lived alone since then and worked to support herself. She reads and she makes plans and she wants something better than what she has. We're perfect for each other.

FEBRUARY 4TH

Channy is beautiful. She's tall and willowy thin and she has pale-blonde hair to her shoulders and snow-white skin and this (how to describe it?) angular, teardrop face. (If I could draw like Jake I'd draw her right here.)

FEBRUARY 9TH

At first I figured she was Russian or German or Scandinavian but she told me her family is "Irish, Irish, and nothing but Irish." She's a mystery in that sense. There's a trace of an accent to her voice, something vaguely High North European, but she was born in Oceanside and so were her parents, who now live in Toronto.

FEBRUARY 10TH

My brain's exploding. I need a plan.

FEBRUARY 15TH

Channy likes Ed Distler too. Something else to talk about. I'm gonna need to re-read his stuff. That and books on Ireland.

FEBRUARY 29TH

This morning I went to the P.B. library and checked out a stack of books on Irish history so I'd have something to talk to her about if I ran out of things to say.

MARCH 1ST

I've been reading all afternoon. The Cambro-Norman mercenaries and Richard de Clare. Catholic Emancipation. The Home Rule Act of 1914.

MARCH 2ND

Fianna Fail and Fine Gael! De Valera and Michael Collins, Ne Temere, the Celtic Tiger, James Craig.

MARCH 10TH

The NICRA! The Battle of Bogside! Patrick Galvin! It's silly but I have to do something.

MARCH 14TH

Okay. Alright. Let's start at the beginning. After class last night, Channy and I went for a walk in the neighborhood to get soft serve at Mr. Frostie's and we kept walking (eating our cones) until we were at the beach at the foot of Law Street. It was dark and cold and we sat on a bench on the cliff-side and talked. I told her about the shooting and she told me that she was mugged in the eucalyptus groves on the UCSD campus, walking to the dorms from a night class.

"He had a knife and . . . god, I still can't believe what he *said* to me. He said somethin' like, 'If you tell anyone about this I'll find you wherever you are . . . and I'll take you somewhere that no one can find you and I'll *burn* you to death.' Can you *believe* that? How could someone *say that* to someone else? Like that's all I am, evidence to destroy if I don't let him get away with taking my purse with a *hairbrush* and my student *ID* and my *Elements of Style* and a bag of M&Ms and . . . what . . . *twenty bucks*? Jeez. It made me feel so *disposable*."

After that she dropped out of school and had a hard time getting her life back on track. She wandered for a while. Took buses across the country then turned back west again. Hitchhiked. Slept with an ex-boyfriend. Slept with a bartender. Couldn't focus. Made a lot of mistakes. Walked around like a zombie. It was just like me: The man's face, she kept seeing it wherever she went.

Who kissed who first I couldn't tell you. We were sitting close and I was looking down at her and the moon was on her face and the light pooled up and shimmered in her eyes and her lips were parted and then we were kissing. She was chewing spearmint gum. At one point it went into my mouth but then it went back and she laughed and spit it out into her hand and we kept kissing.

After a while we stopped and I put my arm around her and she cried a little then fell asleep with her head on my shoulder.

The sun came up. It rose over the hills behind us and the ocean was calm and smooth and pink-red and the whole coast was dead silent and serene. I could hear her breathing and I could smell her hair and it was the most perfect moment of my life.

When she woke up I walked her home. I wasn't planning on going in, but she opened the door and left it open and I could smell her perfume trailing behind her and then she was gone and I couldn't smell it anymore but—this is weird, maybe it's weird, maybe not—I felt like it was still in the *air*, a rope that I could—should—pull myself along with. I don't know what it was—rose?—but, god, it smelled like a girl and I felt crazy. ("Hungry and lonely and crazy for something warm and close and giving," wrote Distler.) From inside I heard her laughing and then she said, "Well?"

I went in and she made us breakfast and then put a kettle on and before our tea was cool enough to drink she took my hand and she led me into the bedroom.

MARCH 15TH

Channy Morning Greene. Her long white legs and her soft feet—the nails unpainted, she doesn't believe in it. Her beautiful hips (small and wide at the same time) and her flat perfect stomach and its dip of a bellybutton and her tiny breasts with the squared nub on the end. Everything about her—the perfect white pillows of her ass, her pointed chin and her long, graceful neck and her lips—without lipstick, always—and her white-blonde hair that smells like pine needles, like a forest.

MARCH 19TH

Channy in the big claw-foot tub. Her pale white hand on the edge (steaming), drumming her nails, and her pretty feet on the tap, crossing, uncrossing, rubbing themselves, then crossing again. Her feet and her hand, all you can see. I'm lying on a towel on the floor (in her bathrobe) looking through a copy of *The Reader* while we talk. The window high above the bath, a solid block of darkening blue. Hours pass. Then black glass, steamed gray. We're getting to know each other. (I think. I'm not sure how this works. How do you get to know someone?) I know this: Her bathrobe smells like her and sometimes I forget I'm me and I listen to her talk and it's like it's me doing the talking. Then I see my ugly, hairy legs poking out of the bathrobe, feet crossed like hers, and I know it's me again.

Channy: "My grandpa was my hero. He was this . . . this . . . *Old West* figure to me growing up. Classic American. World War I vet. Total war hero, from what my grandma would say. Serious American man. Marlboro Man. The kind you don't see anymore. Stoic, but gentle, moral . . . like, *firm* in his belief in God, but never preachy. He just *knew.* Knew God was . . . was out there and keeping things together and he knew without doubt or worry. It was part of his makeup, who he *was*, how he . . . how he made *sense* of the world and gave it order. I was *sure* he was a cowboy. Just *sure* of it. I always . . . I tried to get him to admit it when I was little. '*Just admit it, Grandpa*, you were a cowboy when you were young.' He was in the first World War at the very end and then he worked construction up until the sixties. It was . . . I'm not sure what it's called . . . deep-earth construction, deep-earth moving? Digging shopping mall foundations and big parking lots and that sort of thing. He worked every day, never sick, never had money but . . . but he was there with his hard-hat and his black mailbox-lookin' lunchbox ready to punch in. He was a worker in . . . in the classic sense, a worker for the good of his family, for . . . for the betterment of . . . of . . . because he knew as a *man* you work or you're not a man. His fists were *square*," her left arm rising steaming above the bath edge, making a fist, sinking back down again. "Totally square, like blocks of stone. And he wasn't . . . he wasn't death-white-blonde-Irish like the rest of the family. He was red, red as clay, blood red, dark kinda like you and his hair was as black as yours, *blacker*, made your hair look *brown*. My first story . . . the first short story I wrote was about him. I got second place in this writing contest my school held. My eighth grade English teacher Mr. Hughes turned it in without me knowing. Pulled it out of the trashcan after class . . . read it, entered it in the contest. At first they didn't believe I wrote it because I used a lot of technical terms about war stuff. There was a meeting with my parents and the principal and the English department, the full deal. I was like, 'Look, it's called *research*.' I was pretty snotty back then to adults. Didn't take any shit from them. 'What're *you* lookin' at?' Like that. I still have the twenty-dollar savings bond. Maybe it's worth something now. I keep it . . . like how a business keeps its . . . you know how businesses keep their first dollar? In a frame? Once I sell my first book, I'll spend it. It's ceremonial."

Me: "I was always jealous . . . if that's the right word, jealous? . . . of kids whose dads were around. I didn't have anyone looking out for me besides my brother and he was never around either, you know, with football and after-school clubs and all that jocky high-achiever stuff. My mom was a ghost, even when she was still with it. I spent a lot of time watching TV."

Channy: (singing) "'Splish splash, I was taking a bath.' No one writes songs about taking *baths* anymore."

Me: "My brother called me a 'shit puppet' a couple days ago. What does that even *mean*? A puppet made out of shit? Would that even *work*?"

Channy: "I *love* taking the bus. There's nothing like riding the Greyhound cross-country and just . . . *droning* away with the engines and . . . and watching the world go by. If I had my way, I'd ride the Greyhound back and forth across the country full-time. When I . . . you remember I told you about leaving school after I was robbed—when I quit school, I spent three months crossing the country by bus, back and forth, reading books, writing postcards, taking showers in motels when I had layovers. I even slept with a trucker. Three months. Nonstop. It seems crazy now to think I did that once. I feel so much *older* now."

Me: "You wanna try me? I remember 'em all. *I Love Lucy*, of course, which my brother loved. *Abe Burrows Almanac, House of Shock, Foodini the Great, Roy Doty, Meet Millie, Ozark Jubilee, Ricki & Copper, Wanted, It's a Business, Police Call,* maybe *Black Saddle, Voice of Firestone, Circus Boy* (what a stupid show), *Rocky Jones, I'm the Law, Kids and Company, Hotel de Paree, From These Roots, I Married Joan, Action in the Afternoon, Markham, Igor Cassini, Zoo Parade, Mama Rosa, Leave it to Larry, Mantovani, Portia Faces Life, Imogene Coca, Lamp Unto My Feet, Lash of the West, Willy, Victory at Sea* (my favorite, still my favorite), *Village Barn, The Web, Night Editor, Law of the Plainsman, The Mail Story, Wagon Train, It's Polka Time, Marge and Jeff, It Could Be You, Yancy Derringer, Whirlybirds, Make Me Laugh, The Vise, West Point Story, Adventures of Ellery Queen, The Lawless Years, The Ford Show, Maverick, Al Morgan, Hitchcock* (love *Hitchcock*), *The World is Yours, Answers for Americans, Hopalong Cassidy, Juvenile Jury, Sam and Friends, Zorro, Witchita Town, Armed Forces Hour, Big Town* . . . I can keep going if you want. Seriously, I'm like a machine."

Channy: "I saw a dog get killed by a car once. It was terrible. I wish I could unsee it. I'll never forget it. Never. It was running across the intersection on Grand and Ingraham and the car hit it and it rolled up over the hood and up the window then fell off to the side and just *lay* there. The guy got out of his car and just stood there forever looking down at it. I was like, Why doesn't he do something, why doesn't he move, call the cops, look at the collar, *something*. But then I realized I'd been standing there just as long watching him watch the dog. God, I missed that dog for *weeks*, like I'd actually *known* it. I'm tearing up thinking about it. *Fuck*."

Me: "You know those trees all over P.B? With the big brown seed-pods that smell like dry salami? Or like how trees at playgrounds always smell stronger when you're a kid. Trees are less . . . less a part of the *background* when you're young. They're present, tangible. They smell like things and they have sap that gets on you and their bark scrapes your skin and you pick up pieces of them and make games from the things they drop; you hear the sounds they make. Sometimes you hear the sounds they make at night and they scare you . . . or thrill you, excite you, take you to somewhere else. These days I go months without even *noticing* the trees. One of the first things that caught my attention out here was the smell of the eucalyptus trees. It's strong. Bitter, sharp? It's a very . . . *dark green* smell. Does that make any sense?"

Channy: "I lost my virginity in this condo up in Del Mar. It was so embarrassing. My boyfriend at the time . . . Keith Martin, I think I mentioned him . . . my cousins and I called him K.M. . . . used to housesit for a living. He was older. Eighteen or nineteen . . . I was sixteen, no, fifteen . . . and he took me up to this place in Del Mar that he was supposed to be taking care of and we watched a baseball game on TV of all things and I pretended to drink vodka and orange juice while he got drunker and drunker and . . . it was bad. He was nervous and drunk and he didn't know what he was doing but he acted like he did and it went on for . . . *hours* and he never came and I got drier and drier until it started hurting like crazy. I finally faked an orgasm to make him stop. It got better. After that, the sex was good. Sex without . . . you know, without any love or attachment, but fun . . . fun sex, silly, y'know, in the back of cars and in his brother's dorm in the middle of the day, on the beach at night . . . just wherever we could. We'd hitchhike all day and find a field and go at it under the moon. Felt so free. We hitchhiked from San Diego to Denver once, took a week. Slept on park benches, in farm fields, ditches. He was terrible at giving head, but he liked it, so I'd let him go down on me for what felt like weeks. He used to say the lamest, most embarrassing shit, 'God, I love the way your pussy tastes.' 'You're so wet that it's driving me insane.' I'd make up songs in my head. Give pretend interviews about my 'writing.' He owns a bunch of farms now up in Central Cal. Makes like six billion trillion bucks a year. He calls me every once in a while. He's that . . . that kind of ex-something you have that whenever you're single again after a relationship you end up getting together with, even if it isn't what you want. I think K.M. and I have been on again and off again since, like, 1492. It's kind of boring but it's easy and it happens again and again and again."

Me: "The first week I was here, I got lost in a parking lot at the mall."

Channy: "Preachers are creepy. I think it's like a rule. White male preachers, anyway, they look like pedophiles. I think it's the *hair.* When we were still going to the North Park Adventist church, we had this . . . this exchange program thing with Balboa Seventh Day, the black church down in Logan. Every month they'd send a group of their kids to us for the day and we'd send a group of ours there. I went a couple times and it was incredible. Everyone was up and clapping and singing and there was none of the . . . the *gross, sad* decrepitude of our church, what with the beige paint and bad lighting and the old ladies nodding off asleep in the pews, the pastor phoning it in, the damp smell when you'd walk in, *ugh*. There was *spirit* and *energy* in that room. Big choir in their robes and a band and the preacher dancing all around and speaking . . . well, singing half the time, then speaking the most beautiful words, guy was a *speaker*, a real honest-to-goodness orator. Brilliant man. Reverend Charles Rontom. I'd go to his church in a second if it were still around. You could feel God behind you like this big, strong *wall* holding you up. You felt God's hand, his benevolence . . . this *heat* and strength, firmness. After Balboa, the North Park church felt like a cold, clammy *tomb*. The North Park church told me one thing: God is dead. Up at Balboa, God was in the *room* with you."

Me: "This is gross. Don't laugh. Come on, you can't start laughing yet. You're laughing. Come on. Okay. Peanut butter and cheese rolls. A slice of American cheese . . . cheese from the plastic wrap . . . peanut butter inside, rolled up. I still crave 'em sometimes. My family was into fine dining . . . before we lost everything. Maids, seven courses, alot of boring soups you had to sip really slow. Because of that, maybe in spite of that, trashy American delicacies were *huge* with me. Spam, which I'd never eat now in a million years, ugh, you know Spam and scrambled eggs, yuck, Chef Boyardee, mac and cheese, White Castle, Twinkies, Kool-Aid, Kool-Aid *especially*. My teeth hurt just thinking about it."

Channy: "I like the idea of it but watermelon makes me *vohhhhhhmit*." (Pretends to vomit over the side of the tub, then looks up and smiles at me, wet-faced, hair plastered back and dripping.) "Why are you looking at me like that? Oh, don't be crude! You stay right there, Mercander!"

Me: "I think I've had . . . maybe a *dozen* beers in my life. Drinking's boring. It's okay for a sip or two, but I don't get it. I've been drunk once and it felt like having the flu. Anyway, people are so sad and embarrassing when they're drunk. Slurry, not funny, off-balance. Just this . . . *reduced* version of themselves. Why would you *do* that to yourself? For me, life's about being the best possible version of you, the strongest, smartest . . . the you that'll live long and enjoy things as much as possible. I don't get sabotaging yourself. Why be your own enemy? It just seems *stupid*."

Channy: "My mom was in Dallas the day that Jack Kennedy was shot. She couldn't see from where she was standing, but when the crowd started to move, she saw the motorcade for a second and Jackie Kennedy in the car reaching back for the Secret Service guy. Then the crowd closed up again and she fell and was nearly trampled. That's how she tells it, anyway. I don't know about the trampled part. She's dramatic. It still chokes me up thinking about him and his poor brother, *gaahd*. We'll never have a president like that again. He was beautiful. Just a beautiful, good guy."

Me: "I make lists. My dad did, too. I think that's the only thing he passed down. In this? No, it's a journal. No, you can't read it. Someday."

Channy: "Yeah, fuck lying to kids about Santa Claus. Total loss of illusions. You find out he's fake and suddenly magic is dead. Because if Santa Claus and the Easter Bunny and the Tooth Fairy aren't real, what *else* isn't? That's how it went with me. I began looking at all these things I believed in and realized they were lies. Anything is possible if someone like Santa Claus is real. Without that . . . I don't know, without the *belief* that magic things can happen you die a little and a hopeful part of you that's in all kids gets snuffed out. I stopped believing in God for a while after that. It's a long story but my belief came back.

Not in the same way, and maybe not even in the . . . the same kind of *God*, but it did come back."

Me: "War history calms me down. Just dropping yourself into the minutiæ of details is . . . it's *satisfying*. Getting lost in it, crawling through the . . . the *tunnels* and the passageways and secret doors. I think I'll probably teach. Or . . . I don't know. What else do you do with all this . . . this big ol' garbage bag of *facts* and *theory*? Maybe I could be a consultant to films. That'd be cool. I don't know, I don't know. I need to make a living but I'm not sure how. I had a journalism minor, but I didn't get much from it. I guess I could do that. I don't know, I read a lot and I remember everything . . . there's got to be some kind of real-world application for that. I don't want to be rich. I just don't want to *worry* about money all the time like I am now. Being a tour guide in a museum would be cool. I'd love to be a lighthouse keeper. You wanna go live in a lighthouse with me? We'll eat clam chowder and sourdough bread all day and drink black coffee, sit up in the lookout and stare at the sea, read books, I'll grow a big beard, what do you think? Sure, you can have a beard, too, if you want."

Channy: "Perfect baked potato à *la* Channy Morning Greene. Preheat the oven to 425. Wash the potato, stick a fork in it a couple times, rub it with extra virgin olive oil and sea salt, like really work it in, give it a shake of pepper, then set it directly on the baking pan, no foil, and give it sixty minutes. Sour cream, cheddar cheese, mozzarella, salt, diced Roma tomatoes, diced black olives. I'll make you one tonight. Two? Okay. Two it is."

Me: "We should go to Mexico. Deep down. I'd love to see Mexico City. Spend all day in the libraries. Go see where Frida and Diego lived."

Channy: "When I was a little girl and we were living in the trailer park out by the I-5, my dad used to tell me stories to make me sleep. It was this big endless story called "Caveworld". Adventures starring me. All of it inside this mountain out in the desert. The mountain was hollow and you got into it . . . you got inside it through this one cave. Inside it were 'an infinite amount of caves,' he would tell me, and I'd say, 'What's infinite?' and he'd explain it but I never really got it. He'd . . . he'd start the stories by saying, 'Well, ma'am, once upon a *time*,' and I'd just *sigh* with happiness. I had bad night terrors when I was little. I always knew they were coming on because I felt this . . . it's hard to explain, jeez, I don't know . . . I had this feeling like my bare feet were walking on a tightrope but the tightrope was thin, like wire, and I could feel the wire pressing into the soles of my feet. Whenever I'd have a rough night of night terrors, before it happened I got that feeling. This uneasy, *shaky* feeling in the pit of my stomach of my bare feet pressing into the wire and bending around it. I get it every now and again but I can think it away these days. It comes on and I get up and take a walk outside or something. Ride my bike in the neighborhood. Do some . . . some aerobics. Sweat a little. I always imagine this inner drill sergeant that says something along the lines of, 'Walk it *off,* Greene, walk it off.' That sort of thing. It helps. "

Me: "The first time I went to see my mom out here, she just sat there in bed looking at the wall. Nothing. Nothing at all. I went a couple weeks ago and she would look at me but I could tell she didn't see me. Her eyes were blank and then they weren't. They'd . . . they would flicker back to her again and I could see my mom in there and she'd start to stir, but then she'd go blank again. It was awful. I can tell she's in there but she's far off . . . buried, wandering or looking for something or . . . I don't know. It's like she's lost in a big house and she's walking around the rooms looking for us, her family, but she . . . but she can't find us. She hears our voices and she knows we're there and she calls for us but she never finds us. I remember calling for her as a little kid, 'Mom, Mom!' and really, *really* needing her, and the thought of her doing it for us and us not being able to find her . . . *argh.* The truest thing my mom ever told me was, 'If you have a friend who's gossiping about someone else, you can be sure they're gossiping about you as well.' She also told me, 'Mercander, only boring people get bored,' which is kind of reductive but it works. I'm never bored. I'm . . . maybe . . . restless or nervous or even morose, but there's always something to occupy yourself with. Those . . . those little bits of wisdom your parents give you are priceless. They stick with you forever. I wish I had more of them."

APRIL 12TH

Today was a perfect day. Channy and I got up early and I made her breakfast (waffles with fresh strawberries and whipped cream; she wants to quit eating meat) and then we took a shower together and went back to bed. (In the shower she gave me a blowjob and I had a hard time standing up when I came. After that, I went down on her while she stood against the stall but she stopped before she came because she wanted to wait until we were actually fucking.) Channy's sitting up against the headboard with the sheet pulled around her (it's cold in her apartment even when it's warm outside) and she's reading my bootleg translation of Aksakov's *Years of Childhood*.

She says: "I've always wanted to write a memoir of my childhood," closing the book and setting it on the mattress between us, "Always wanted to."

"You should."

"I've been writing a lot of short stories lately about childhood stuff. Sending them to journals. A few months ago Miracle Press accepted one for their *25 Under 25* anthology."

"That's cool."

"But I think I'm ready. Ready to write something bigger. The memoir . . . I don't know . . . I feel like it would write itself."

"What would you call it?"

"I have a title already, but it's a secret."

"You can tell me. I'm good at secrets."

Smiling: "You'll tell everyone. You'll *ruin* me."

"No way. Scout's honor."

Serious: "Nope. I don't trust Boy Scouts. I was a Brownie. We were at *war* with you."

"C'mon. I'm the most honest person you'll ever meet."

Pretending to be suspicious: "I don't believe that for a *second. Who are you?* What happened to that sweet boy with the funny name?"

"I'm honest. I'm the *most* honest. I've won *awards* for it."

Pretending to be dismissive: "That's nice. What kind of awards?"

"Trophies."

"Lovely. Where are they? I don't see them anywhere."

"I had so many that I threw them in the ocean."

"Prove it. Go jump off a boat and find 'em."

"I've won honesty medals, too."

"I don't see any medals." She rolls over to me and smiles and taps a finger on my chest, and then her hand slides under the sheet to my lap. "Are they down here? Oh, I think I found one. It's getting bigger. How strange."

"I have medals. Thousands of them. I'm decorated."

"Oh yeah?"

"Yeah. I'm a four-star general of honesty."

"Four-star?"

"*Seven.*"

"Seven-star, *wow. Impressive.*"

"It is."

"I didn't know there were seven-star generals."

"I know. I didn't either."

"I think you're making this up. Take off your mask."

"Channy, I hate to tell you this but . . . but I'm a *spy.*"

"So am I."

"I *thought* I knew you from somewhere."

"Merc, I'm a spy and I'm your boss, so give up now or you're fired. You'll never work in this town again. You can do what you want to me . . . torture me all you want; I'll never tell."

APRIL 15TH

Channy's pregnant.

1999

PACIFIC BEACH, NOON

On New Year's Day, Joey gets up late and nukes a slice of leftover Domino's and sits down at the dining room table by himself and stares at his plate. Hangover food. Sausage and olive pizza instead of toast. Dr. Pepper instead of orange juice. No family breakfasts. Joey's aunt at the bank in the drive-up window all day. His uncle working on his car in the garage and drinking beer and listening to tapes. (In order of play: 1) Starship's *Knee Deep in the Hoopla* (twice, singing along, loud), 2) the first half of Hendrix's *Axis Bold as Love*, and 3) the Yes album *Tormato.*)

As Joey eats, he imagines a dream family—a mom and a dad on the couch, the TV loud, the dog watching them eat potato chips from a big yellow and white bag. The mom talking to the dog, doing both voices herself. Her own voice reasonable, authoritative, serious. In the persona she assigns herself, she's goodhearted and loving but wary of the dog's tricks. The dog's voice is irrational and excited but, above all, adoring. "Well, hi, Mom, I'd like a potato chip now," she says in the dog's high, wobbly voice. "No, these are *my* potato chips, doggy," she says in her own voice (firm, in command). "But I'm *such* a good dog." "You *are* a good dog." "I am. I really am." "I know you are. Do you love me?" "Oh yes, oh yes, of course I love you, Mommy." "Here's a potato chip, good dog." (She throws a chip to the dog, who jumps up to snatch it in the air. Snatch. Done. Sitting again. Tail wagging against the carpet.) "Thank you, Mommy. I love you." "I love you, too, good dog." Joey's never had a pet and he smiles at the idea and then it makes him feel sad and small and he decides to take a walk down to the boardwalk. He gets up and goes into the kitchen and opens the fridge and squeezes the bottle of Hershey's Syrup into his mouth.

Last night was stupid. He and Tyler doing GHB and smoking speed then going to all the fratty beach bars to be ironic. Moondoggies, P.B. Bar and Grill, Margarita Rocks. Tyler was in heaven. Laughing and happy with his fake ID ("Peter Fillanimore," twenty-three, from San Clemente, wide, dark-haired, cow-eyed, goateed, clearly not the white-blonde, elfin Tyler). And Tyler into the spectacle of being douchy Peter. Loving the it's-cool-because-it's-not of it. Joey bored out of his mind, sitting at the high table, stabbing the lime slice in his cocktail with his straw until it's pulpy. Tyler talking to girls with fake breasts and orange tans, high-fiving drunk guys and yelling "New Year's Eve '98!" and then "Wooooo!" Tyler off dancing to all the shitty club music to be funny. Throwing himself down in the middle of the dance floor, doing the worm, getting up to poplock and everyone in a circle around him clapping. "Go Peter! Go Peter! It's your birthday! It's your birthday!" Joey, in on it but too embedded to like the joke, too close. He's never lived anywhere but here; it's all he knows and it's hard to find the irony and fun. (It's not what he loves but it is who he is.) Tyler's further removed.

In his room he smokes a bowl of cheap Mexican weed and stares out the window at the bright lawn and the pink apartments across the way, and he tries not to cry. "Men don't cry," his uncle would say. "Don't be such a little *bitch* all the time, Joey."

THE BOARDWALK

It's a cool, breezy day at the beach and Joey tight-rope walks along the seawall and looks down at the sand—the wind blowing in off the ocean, a lifeguard truck rolling slow along the shoreline, a plane in the sky towing an advertising banner reading, 'Advertise on high! Call about rates! We Are Cheap!'

At the amusement park by the public pool, the roller coaster clacks up and then races down its track and the people scream happily with arms above their heads and a trio of red balloons floats in the sky, tied together, racing up and out and away. Joey stands by the ice cream shop and stares into the sky—perfect blue, the balloons moving fast, and soon they'll be over the sea, and then gone. All week he's been planning to take his own life. His uncle's handgun. In the living room, where they'll find him when they get home. Fast. Easy. Showy. Make them feel what he feels.

A blonde girl his age walks past him talking loud on her cellphone, saying, "My New Year's resolution was to not cry when I get drunk. Oh, and to visit another city." He can see her underwear peaking up above the waistband of her jeans. Light pink. Tag showing.

The crowd moving past. Triplet babies in a three-piece stroller and Joey smiles and makes faces at them and one of them laughs and kicks its feet (its two siblings asleep). Tourists walk with cameras and straw hats. A group of Japanese men with matching polo shirts and backpacks and ball caps, talking, excited. (Joey smiles at them.) Teenage girls carrying waffle-cones or smoking cigarettes, walking slow, acting cool. A pair of old people looking at the bumper cars and Joey watches them and he loves them all. *So nice*, he thinks.

Joey looks up. The balloons are gone. And now the breeze blows through the amusement park and an old man loses his cowboy hat. Joey starts to run to fetch it but the man chases after it and it rolls across the pavement, past the sunglass shack and the shaved ice stand. Finally it comes to rest up against the chainlink fence surrounding the Tilt-a-Whirl ride. The man jogs up to it in the bowlegged clopping way you run when you're wearing healed boots. He picks it up, mashes it down on his head and smiles big and waves to his family, then heads back to them, holding the hat down on his head with one hand as he walks.

1978

APRIL 18TH

My brother's been screaming at his wife all night. She came back this morning and now they're quote-unquote reconciling. As for Channy and I, we're done. When she found out she was pregnant, she locked herself in the bathroom and I stood at the door, feeling useless. I tried to talk to her through the door but she wouldn't answer. An hour later she came out, pushed past me, eyes down, went into the bedroom, and came out ten minutes later, calm and composed. She had my books and clothes in a stack and she handed them to me and said, "Please leave. I never want to see you again." And here I am.

APRIL 19TH

My brother's in jail. Last night he and Sorel took the fight out into the front yard and someone called the cops. Why am I lying in my own notebook? It was me. I called the cops. It's not something I'd normally do, but I was at my wit's end. *Something* had to happen. I feel bad about it but what's done is done. If I hadn't have done it, someone else would've I'm sure. Forget it: I'm not feeling guilty about this.

When the squad car arrived, Jacob went crazy and hit Sorel in front of them. After that, all hell broke loose. Jake pushed one of the cops into the hedges and Sorel punched the other cop and that cop hit Jake over the head with his nightstick and knocked him unconscious.

This morning, I went outside and Jake's biker neighbor Mel was watering his front lawn.

"Hey kid, you see what happened with your brother last night?"

I shrugged. "Were you home?" I dug the toe of my sneaker into the grass and squinted at him. It was bright. A bright, hot, sunny day.

"I was, yeah. Me and Patty saw the whole thing from the window. Cops showed up and your brother *smacked her one*. Right across the mouth and that was *it*. You ask me, she *deserved* it. Kid, your brother's wife is *foul*. I've thought about hitting her *myself*."

The cops took Jake but they also took Sorel. Jake's going to be in for a while because there's no money for bail, but Sorel was released this afternoon. She's in the kitchen frying bacon, the radio blasting some awful hippie song about someone called "Cosmic Charlie" and how he's "truckin' in style along the avenue."

Fuck Cosmic Charlie.

APRIL 20TH

Jake's still in jail and it's just me and Sorel in the house. As much of a screw-up as Jake is, I think he was the one that kept the place together. Sorel's a monster. The dishes are piled up in the sink and her clothes are all over the living-room floor. The coffee table is covered in beer cans and McDonald's bags and a thousand coffee cups for ashtrays, and Sorel's on the couch, slumped low, legs spread in short-shorts, staring at the television, smoking a joint, dead-eyed.

Now, here's where it gets bad, and if you've found this notebook and you're reading this, please, I repeat, *please*: Put it down and respect my privacy.

See, Mel was right, Sorel's foul but there's something about her . . . something that makes me want her and I hate myself for it. She's terrible—loud, small and wide and big-legged, pink as a pig, filthy red hair snaking all over, sweaty pink cleavage spilling out of her tank-top, bangs cut right at eye level and her eyes done up in thick, black Cleopatra makeup.

Sorel doesn't wash and the place smells like her feet and her tomatoey sweat, and as gross as it is, it makes me want her even more. She's not beautiful and ice-sculpture perfect like Channy but she's got this raw animal thing and when I see it or . . . I don't know, smell it, sense it . . . I want to grab her and throw her down and fuck her brains out. This is not me. Channy and I was me. I'm not like this.

The dreams are the worst part. I haven't had sex dreams since junior high school, but every night Sorel's there and something new and disgusting is happening. I need to get out of this house but I'm out of money. The only other person I know in town is Channy and she won't answer my calls. It's just me and Sorel and her filthy short-shorts and tank-tops and her horrible red hair in her eyes and her stinking body that's so pink she looks like she has a fresh sunburn all the time. My god, and the stupid things she says in her white-trash twang. "Hey Merc, do you think black people like to *travel*?" "Hey, Merc, you think Mickey Mouse ever takes a shit?"

Sorel and Jake got together four years ago when she came out to San Diego on vacation with her parents. Sorel Marie Bushmill was fifteen. She and Jake met at the beach and Jake got her high under the pier and they did acid that night at a bonfire on Fiesta Island and fucked back in the dunes and then it was quote-unquote love. She hid out with Jake, and her parents filed a missing person's report and after a few weeks they gave up and went back to Alabama. Last year, the day Sorel turned eighteen, she wrote her parents to tell them that she and Jake were getting married, that she'd been safe all along, and that she was afraid they'd try to take her home. The letter came back, opened and Scotch-taped shut, marked 'Return to Sender' in her mother's handwriting.

APRIL 21ST

Sorel's screwing some random guy she met earlier tonight. She brought him home a couple hours ago and told me to stay in my room, and now they're going at it in the kitchen. Sorel's loud and they keep knocking things over and she's shouting the grossest, most perverted things you could ever imagine: what parts of her body she wants him to come into (or onto). Where she wants him to stick his "fucking cock." How those parts of her body feel with his "fucking cock" in them. The worst part is hearing her makes me want her more, and the more I want her, the more I hate myself.

I never went through the reckless self-loathing stage everyone goes through as a young teenager. While kids in high school drank and went to parties and did drugs and got into trouble, I studied and exercised in order to be the strongest, best possible version of myself. I'm no jock, but I can do two hundred push-ups without breaking a sweat. In school, I ran track and played baseball and lettered in both and since then I've just gotten faster and stronger. Yet here I am, crawling out of the muck to shower once a week. Lying in bed all day trying not to touch myself to the thought of this horrible girl in the next room. I stopped going to night school and I've stopped reading and I haven't done so much as a sit-up in days. All the places I wanted to visit when I first got here—Fort Rosecrans, the museums, Shelter Island, the Whaley House, the Mission—I haven't been to one of them. I'm stuck here in this ugly, low-class house that smells like marijuana and peppery, fried food and Sorel's stale, rancid body. I'm ashamed and I know where I'm at and I know how I got here, but I don't know how to get out. For the first time in my life I have no plan.

APRIL 25TH

I slept with Sorel last night.

1999

HOME, 10 A.M.

At the end of winter break, Tyler starts his next semester at San Diego State. Maggie turns eighteen and takes a road trip up to San Francisco where she does crystal and goes to a rave and kisses her childhood friend Joel Campbell. Joey has done nothing.

It's a mild winter even for San Diego—warm days, cool nights, fog in the mornings. A week after Valentine's Day, the phone rings from Joey's bedside table and wakes him up.

"Carr? It's Nicole! I've got good news!"

From July 13rd, 1996 (1:12 a.m.) to September 9th, 1998 (3:29 p.m.), Nicole Alexandra Hale was the one. Now without Nicole, Joey was rebuilding his social group. Of course in the early part of a new love, isolating yourself as a couple seems like a fine idea. You think about a future together; a future when one person is enough. This is *the one*, like it's always the one. Six months ago, Nicole left Joey for an Internet tech. David Horowitz. (Middle name "Uriah," but a secret known only to a select few, because the initials for David Uriah Horowitz are "DUH.")

In the first of two photos Joey's seen of Horowitz, he's dressed in black and yellow, riding his bicycle in a pack of cyclists who look just like him—spandex and helmets, little slipper shoes, razor sunglasses, the whole group of them leaning into the turn. The photo was printed off the Internet but it was as clear as a TV image. The second photo—also printed off the Internet, this one badly pixilated—is Horowitz at an office party dressed up in a Santa Claus suit, without the beard. He has a patchy goatee, expensive-looking glasses, and big flat smiling fish lips. Joey used to dream of shooting him in the face with his uncle's gun, blowing that smile from the photo out the back of his skull. He doesn't anymore. Horowitz is twenty-six years older than Nicole and that alone is revenge enough. Most of the time.

"Hey Nicole."

"Guess what!"

"What?"

"No, *guess*."

"*Nicole*."

"Don't Nicole-me. C'mon, Carr!"

"I'm not guessing. Hale . . . just tell me."

"Guess! Don't be such a *grump*."

"I'm not guessing. Just tell me."

"I'm Mrs. David Horowitz! We got married! In Vegas! Last night! We just, y'know, *drove up there on a whim* and did it! It was soooo crazy! We stayed at the effing *Bellagio* and ate *room service* all night and went out to all the famous casinos and walked around and we kept spending all this *money* and I called my mom and my brother and my sister from our room and told them about it and they were all super, *super* happy and I called my dad and he *totally cried*! He was *so happy*! My dad's *never* cried! Not even when Burkley died! Oh! You *have* to see the ring. You have to! It's *so* big! No, wait, check it, listen, are you listening? Listen, check it, I'm knocking the diamond on the receiver right now. Hear that? Dude, that's the effing *rock*. Doesn't it sound *huge*? I'm totally emailing you a picture. I'll send it right now. What's your email? Oh here. It's still mister-(uh, like spelled out, not 'M' and 'R')-dot-joey-dot-carr-at-hotmail, right? Oh wait, there's another one. Joeyette-underscore-the-underscore-spy-at-worldview-dot-net, is that one old?"

"Nicole. You don't have to."

"*Dude*, aren't you *happy* for me?!"

"Yeah, I'm—"

"You're *happy*, right?! Say you're happy."

"I'm really, really . . . yeah."

"Good! I'm glad! Check it, we're moving to a new housing thingamajig. One of those, like, those new subdivision . . . subdivision things they're putting up in the hills above the freeway in Rancho Bernardo near Gummy's old place. A gated effing *community*! Giant *heated pool*! Huge workout room! *Sauna. Saaaaauna,* Carr. You should see the *picture* of the sauna on their website! It's so effing *huge*. I'll send it to you. Okay, I sent it. The place . . . it's called Manzanita Ridge. You get to drive golf carts around if you want. Golf carts! How cool is that? I'm totally getting my own golf cart! I'm gonna be straight *buzzin'* around the neighborhood, just smokin' a cigarette and wavin' to the neighbors. Just me and my trusty golf cart. Imagine me with a *golf cart*. How weird is that? Isn't that *great*?"

"Yeah. Weird. And great. Look, Nicole—"

"What? *C'mon*."

"I need to go."

"No, *c'mon*. Let me tell you about the diner we went to on the drive back. The Mad—"

"No, no, I reeeally have to go. It's just . . . I've got a lot . . . there's a lot I need to, like . . . I dunno, *do* today and I'm supposed to . . . I'm actually just . . . *just right now* stepping out the door. *So*, like—"

"Call me later, then?"

"Yeah. Okay."

"Alright, bye, Carr. Don't forget! Call me. Okay? Don't forget the us-being-friends-now thing."

"Yeah. Bye."

In bed, holding the phone to his cheek, Joey stares up at the ceiling.

2 P.M.

Joey's still in bed when the phone rings again. The caller ID says 'Vicente Ramirez' and he picks it up. "Hey, Chente." The breeze from the window and sun flickering through the curtains. A fly buzzing around the screen. Outside the calliope sound as the ice cream man drives by and Joey thinks about Neapolitan ice cream sandwiches and red, white, and blue Bomb-Pops, and he starts to cry.

"Joey Carr!"

"Hey, Chente."

"You alright?"

"Huh?"

"Nothing. Look, *ese*, what are you doing right now?"

Joey sits up in bed, the phone held to his face. "Sitting around."

"Joey, hey, *carnalito*, what's wrong? You sound funny."

"Nothing . . . I'm . . . Nicole got married."

"*What*? Married? To *who*? *Married*?"

"The Internet manager, like, office guy or whatever. The one, y'know, the one from back in September?"

"The *old* fuck?"

"Right. The old fuck."

"*Fuck* the Internet manager." Chente makes a sound like he's spitting on the floor and when he does that Joey feels better. "Fuck Martha." (Martha is Chente's name for Nicole. Martha Stewart. The whitest of white. Chente's last five girlfriends were all given nicknames too. Simone Reyes, (used positively; Chente only dates big women) "Baby Shamu." Jennifer Morrison the budding country singer, (also positive) "Fatsy Cline." Melody Nobels, (negative) "Melody No Balls." ("Joey, Melody No Balls was a girl who couldn't say 'Fuck it.' You need a girl who can say 'fuck it.'") Adia Morena, (neither positive or negative but rather, passionless, a reflection of their arrangement and her job at the Hillcrest Taco Bell) "Adia Tortilla.") Chente clears his throat. "Joey, you're better than that shit. You been over that drama for *months*. Fuck Martha."

"I know, but—"

"But nothing. You know what, Joey? You know what, we're going to Tijuana tonight and we're getting some *whores*."

"What do you mean? What does that . . . what does that mean?" Joey—a blank sheet of paper, a white wall with nothing on it but paint.

"What that means is *you* and *me*—" (Chente says this slowly, like he's talking to a child) "and Javier (who you *know*, fat Javier from work) and my uncle's friend Fernando are going to the *Coahuila* and we're going to get some nice Mexican girls and we're gonna get—"

"Oh." In his head, Joey sees Nicole, ice cream trucks, huge golf carts, manzanita trees, huge workout rooms, yellow-brown hills, saunas the size of ballrooms and a thousand fat Javiers in towels waltzing across the floor clutched tight to each other.

"*Sonofa*! I *knew* you'd be down! *Simón*! Listen, I'll be at your aunt's at nine *sharp*. You better be *ready, maricón*. Tell them you're going to a tennis match or camping or something else white people do, okay?"

Outside, the ice cream man's song fades down the block until the notes begin to drag and warp on the breeze. Then silence—quiet. Birds singing. Joey forgets about Chente on the other end of the line. He thinks about green grass, clear water from the hose, an ice cream bar shaped like a blue foot. And on the big toe? A pink gumball for the nail. Nicole's favorite.

TIJUANA, NIGHT

In Tijuana, the sidewalks are lit by club neons and the small licking fires of rotisserie stands. Further up, groups of tourists eat at the cafe tables of outdoor bars and file in and out of tiny, brightly lit seafood restaurants. Joey and Chente (in front) and Javier and Fernando (trailing behind) cross the street and walk past a line of carts selling tiny fish tacos and foot-long *churros* and bacon-wrapped hotdogs. Javier stops to buy a hotdog. After that, they stop again in the plaza square so Javier can tie his shoe. Every stop is a relief for Joey. Postponement.

The vendors in the plaza have closed up shop for the night and the courtyard of the market is empty. Javier lights a cigarette and gives one to Fernando, then holds the pack out to Chente and Joey.

"You know I quit those things," says Chente.

"Thanks." Joey takes a cigarette and Javier lights it for him as a rangy, gray dog lopes across the square. "Thanks, I'll get you back." The dog sees them then ducks into a dark passageway between storefronts.

"That's how I feel right now," Joey tells Chente as they walk. They pass the dry, pit-scarred fountain and the mechanical bull-stand.

"The bull?"

"The dog."

"Oh, don't be so dramatic. You don't even *remember* Nicole. Nicole who? Nicole Brown *Simpson*? You're moving on. Don't dwell so much. You dwell on that shit and it snowballs. It gets worse, and it wasn't anything to begin with. You and Martha broke up because it was time to break up and it was *good* for you. It's in the past."

"I guess."

"Get over it. It's *healthy, carnalito*. We'll find you some . . . like, some big ol' *culona* down here and you'll never think of Nicole ever *again*. What you need is a *fat girl*. After Fatsy Cline I'll never date a little skinny girl again. Fat girls will fuck your shit *up*. Fat girls will change your life, *carnal*. Big ol' legs and a big ass all slow-down-wide-load bumping out behind you like you got a couple couch cushions. Nicole . . . her ass was all *bone*. That ass was *bone*. You need somebody big like Fatsy Cline who knows what she's doing and knows how to make shit *happen*. Fat girls for *life*. Fat girls *forever*. That's my next tattoo. Big girls forever ever ever."

"I just wish—"

"No more wishing. Wishing's for people who are too afraid to *act*. You're *better* than this. Like in *Lonesome Dove, carnal*, 'ride away from it.'" (Chente—a collector of Western novels. *Lonesome Dove*, his sixth favorite after Leigh Brackett's *Follow the Free Wind*, Owen Wister's *The Virginian*, Zane

Gray's *Riders of the Purple Sage*, Elmer Kelton's *The Far Canyon*, and George G. Gilman's *The Godforsaken*. Gilman's book a dead-tie with the first Sackett novel—for sentimental reasons.)

Javier, a fat Mexican teenager with greased-back hair like Chente's, catches up to them and throws his big arm around Joey's shoulder as they walk. "Joey, *carnalito*, Chente tol' me about that *puta*."

"Yeah, it's—"

"Look, homes, what you need is some *good Mexican pussy*. Only the best and you never go back to the rest or whatever-something-*I-dunno*. Doan you worry about *nothing* tonight. We got your back, *cabrón*. You're with *friends*."

Chente stops walking and grins at Javier and shakes his head. "Who's *this guy* all swaggering and macho like Keith Sweat and shit? *Listen*, Joey, *carnal*, the other time we did this, Javy, Mr. Good Mexican Pussy here, couldn't even get his shit up enough to bust."

"Chente, you doan know—"

"Homeboy told me he had the girl *chupa su pito por cinquenta minutos* and even then he couldn't bust. Even *then*."

"Chente, you weren't there. You doan know *nothing*." Javier frowns and shakes his head, a battered look on his big, kind, flat face. "You doan know what," he whispers.

"Hey, *tranquilo*," says Fernando. "I don't wanna hear nothing about who couldn't bust or who *could* or what." Javier shrugs and starts to talk but Fernando puts his hand up to silence him. "No. Stop. *Sabes que*, there's *enough* people gonna be assholes to you who *aren't* your friends."

"*Simón*," says Chente, nodding. "'Nando's right."

"*Ay*, 'Nando," says Javier, grinning again, shrugging sweetly, "You know iss all gooood. Me and Chente, we *good* like that."

Fernando grew up with Chente's uncle, Baby, in El Centro. After a coke deal went bad, Fernando took the blame for Baby and spent six years and twenty-seven days in a Central California prison. He came out stacked with muscle and covered in tattoos and spent the next six years selling weed in Seal Beach. Now he goes to NA meetings and takes night classes at City and works two part-time jobs to support his girlfriend Lupe and their baby son, Minos. To Chente, Fernando's word is final. (A week earlier, Chente told Joey the following facts about Fernando. 1) Fernando was so calm and sensitive (and as a result, successful) with the opposite sex that Chente's uncle Baby nicknamed him Ferdinando the Bull. 2) Fernando's son Minos took his first steps at an astounding six months and by twenty-eight months already knew how to rap the first two verses from "California Love" with perfect pronunciation and a worldly sneer. 3) Fernando once (intentionally) crashed a pickup truck into a hipster Greek restaurant [Zorba the Freak's Deli and Dine-In] and set the truck on fire because the white [non-Greek] owner said "No way, José" to him in jest. 4) Fernando was the first person to string a pair of sneakers over the telephone wires to denote a place to buy drugs. 5) Fernando's nickname in high school was "the F Word" because he never swore. 6) Fernando once kicked a mailman so hard between the legs that the mailman shat himself and cried for fifteen minutes. 7) Fernando robbed a Denny's where his cousin was the manager and everyone knew him but he got away with it regardless. 8) Fernando once met the actor John Candy in Laguna Beach and told him to "lose some fucking *weight, cabrón*.")

They leave the plaza and take the pedestrian bridge over the Tijuana River, Javier straggling behind, dragging a stick along the guardrail, singing softly to himself.

"Hold up, *maricónes*, I'm taking a leak," says Chente.

They stop in the middle of the bridge and Joey looks out over the side at the dry cement reservoir—yellow-lit, a trail of water down the center, graffiti up the sides, old car batteries and shopping carts rusting where the river once was. The low cityscape of Tijuana sprawling out in the distance below them—a black, hilly mass with countless tiny lights sprinkled across its shapeless hump.

Chente stands along the guardrail and pisses over the side. He turns and looks back at Joey. "What I like best about pissing off tall things like this is your piss goes straight down to the ground in . . . in, like, this massive . . . unending stream and it's like one big extension of you. Like your dick is a hundred-fifty feet long."

"That must be *nice* for you, *carnal*," says Javier, smiling, "since it's really just one point five *inches*. *Como un* little brown *golf* tee." Javier holds his fingers apart and shows Joey and Fernando and giggles happily.

After Chente's done, Javier pisses over the side and Chente makes like he's going to push him off.

"Ay! *Ssstop* it, Chente." Javier steps down, fumbling with his zipper and Chente jumps around him, laughing and shadowboxing. "Chente, you *scared* me. You know that?"

At the end of the bridge it's the tourist district and they walk past bars and busy restaurants and all-night pharmacies.

"No offense, Joey," says Chente as they walk, "but here's where you get to see how much white people are ruining TJ."

"None taken."

"Look over there, look at those . . . those fucking . . . those college kids on the corner, and over there, by the taco stand, bunch of rich white shitheads acting like . . . like little kings and queens. Little kings and queens on safari. The ugly American. Fuck that shit. Fuck those people."

"Yeah, I—"

"Don't worry. You're not like that."

"I hope so."

"You're not. You hang out with me enough and you'll turn Mexican."

"How's that work?"

"It just does. Javier used to be white when he and I started hanging out. He was from Sweden. His name was Kaarl, like with two a's and an umlat or some shit."

"Kaarl Vanderhooven?"

"Vinderlanderlaiden. I'm playing but you know . . . you don't . . . you don't have to be like them."

"Deal."

"Stick with me, *carnal*. I'll turn you into Edward James *Olmos* and shit. *A la verga*. You need to get tough if you're gonna hang out with us."

"That sounds okay."

"Whenever you're afraid to do something, you just tell yourself, 'Do it for rock 'n' roll,' and you do it."

"Do it for rock 'n' roll?"

"Do it for rock 'n' roll. That's what Mexicans do. Even if they don't like rock 'n' roll, they have that shit in their *blood*. We're born tougher than white people. But I guess everyone's born tougher than white people. That doesn't mean you have to accept it. You can be tough if you want."

Further up they pass by a dance club with a two-story inflatable Corona bottle out front.

"Big John's beer," says Chente as they walk.

"Noooo, I was *jus' about to say that*," says Javier, laughing.

"Who's Big John?" asks Joey.

"Oh, nothing, *carnalito*," says Chente. "In school we had this friend Big John who's—"

"Big John was *big*," says Javier smiling, reaching his fat hands high above his head and standing on his toes as he walks. "Big-big!"

"He was big," nods Chente. "He was like six-and-a-half feet tall, five-hundred pounds, all muscle, so whenever we see something really big we say Big John's whatever. Like you see a big . . . uh . . . like, like, one of those extra-size Whoopi Goldberg *Jumpin' Jack Flash* novelty toothbrushes that are like four feet tall and you say 'Big John's toothbrush.' Like that. It's dumb but it's been going on—"

"Like for *years*," says Javier, smiling.

"For years."

"So—" Joey points at a mural on the side of a building of a massive hand with 'Stop Here for Beer, Gringos!' painted across the palm in Old English letters.

"Right, Big John's hand, exactly," says Chente.

"And 'Stop Here for Beer' was typed by Big John's *typewriter*," says Javier.

"It doesn't work that way," says Chente.

"But still. Like, like, 'He's so Mexican, his *typewriter* is in Old English!'"

"Javy, you know the joke isn't how *Mexican* he is."

"Whatever, Chente. There's no rules."

Joey laughs and Fernando grumbles under his breath.

"Javy, I started the Big John game and that's how it works. This isn't Jeff *Foxworthy*. Joey, Javy and his family love Jeff Foxworthy. They love that shit. 'Uh, you know you're a redneck if . . . ,' you know, 'if you do something stupid and white trash, whatever.' That kinda bullshit. They watch that shit all the *time*. They all get together and eat popcorn from big pink bowls and drink milk and go all Jeff Foxworthy *crazy*. That's why Javier isn't a real Mexican. Javier's typewriter's in *cursive*. It's in little bubble font letters and shit."

Javier throws the stick he was carrying into the street. "Forget it, then," he says under his breath.

They cut through the neighborhood and pass strip clubs with blinking signs and men standing in doorways smoking and talking in Spanish. It's begun to rain—a light sprinkle and then harder until the shoulders of their jackets are wet and the awnings drip and the streets shine black.

"Up there, *carnales*. We'll drink there until the rain stops." Fernando points to a bar at the end of the street, its neon sign dim-red in the drizzle. *Duenas' Cerveza y Comida*.

10:19 P.M.

Fernando buys a round of tequila shots and Coronas.

10:35 P.M.

The next round is on Javier, who orders a plate of pork tacos (*carnitas*, extra cilantro, fresh onion, and lime slices) with the drinks.

10:54 P.M.

Chente has the one after that and then it's Joey's turn and he buys a round of Cuervo shots and four chicken *tortas*. They eat the *tortas* with hot sauce and fresh lime juice and then Fernando orders a plate of *carne asada sopes* to share. The bar is empty and when the owner leaves, his daughter Rosa sits with them and then they're drinking for free.

11:34 P.M.

Javier is dancing with Rosa to a slow, tender *ranchera* ballad, and Fernando, Chente, and Joey sit at a table by the dance floor nursing their beers. The tabletop is covered in Tecate and Modelo bottles and shotglasses and empty plates and toothpicks and crumpled-up napkins. Fernando is sitting in his chair backwards, slumped forward, drunk and relaxed and smiling at Javier and Rosa. Chente is bent over the table writing something on a placemat with one hand and rolling the empty hot sauce bottle on its side with the other.

Above the bar, a TV set glows with a soccer game on mute, the field bright green and tiny men running across it in a blue and white pack. From outside, the rain runs soundlessly down the window, the glass lit up red by the neon signs.

"Jus' *leave me here*, alright," Javier yells, happily. "I'm in Javier *heaven*. Leave me *here, carnales*." He holds the girl close. His eyes are shut, his round face smiling and sweating. "Me and Rosita, we're getting *married*. I *live here* now. This is my *bar*. This is my *street*. I doan need none of this *pinche Coahuila* business."

"*Ay, Coahuila*?" Rosa makes a playful show of pushing him away.

"I'm only kidding, *mija*, you know, you know. Rosy," singing now, "dahhhhn worryyy about *naaaathing* / *Weeee are in Javier heaven*."

"It's okay, it's cool," she whispers, blushing. "I don't worry about *shit*, man. Never ever." She pulls Javier back to her and rests her head on his big chest. "It's cool. You okay? You happy? You got enough to drink? To eat?"

"*Baaaastante, mijita*," Javier says, drunk and content, singing now, "*Estoy bieeeeen pedo, guey*."

12:03 A.M.

Outside the bar it's sprinkling and they stand on the sidewalk in the rain. Chente pulls the back and shoulders of his jacket up over his head and then Javier does the same and the four of them turn the corner and walk down a dark street.

"It's just up here a ways," says Chente. "We're almost there."

A rowdy group of Mexican cowboys bursts out through the swinging doors of a bar as they pass, laughing and singing and knocking each other over. A short, feisty, curly-haired girl with them waves at Javier and shouts, "Hey, fats!" She thrusts her hips at him. "Hey *guapo*, come *drrrink* with us!"

Up the block they pass a gay club with pounding house music beating through the walls and then a night service church with singing coming from it ("*Dios, mi Diiiiios* / *Mi Jesuuuuu Chriiisto*"). Javier stops in front of the church to cross himself. ("Jus' in case, *carnales*. Can't hurt to have the *jefe* on your side when you're in the *Coahuila*." Fernando does the same. Chente spits on the church steps and says, "Satan.")

Further up, a park full of teenage boys kicking a soccer ball on a wet field, the water spraying up around their heels, silver in the light. Then nothing. Apartments with high fencing and no lights. (A radio playing a rumba, tinny and distant, humid, a voice from decades ago, an island country, burning banana trees, a dark night and a murder over jilted love in the cane fields.) Then houses with stone walls and barbwire. Everything dark, the sliver of moon behind clouds. Then busy again. Along the street under the awnings of closed-up shops are groups of young girls in short dresses and high heels. A few of them shout and wave at Joey and Chente while Javier and Fernando walk ahead, and one laughs and pulls her friend aside to whisper that (translated) "the white boy's friend looks just like Lou Diamond Phillips from *La Bamba*. Can you believe it?"

Chente stops walking. "See anything you like, Joey?"

"I've never—I mean, ugh, whoa—how does this work? This is freakin' me out."

"You pick one. Remember: Do it for rock 'n' roll."

"You just *pick one*? Just like *that*, you pick one?"

"Just like that." Chente laughs. "Now listen, Joey, this is *important*. The *most* important. Listen."

Joey looks past Chente. Javier and Fernando are up the street talking to girls. A barefoot kid in white shorts and a ratty black sweater runs across the street, jumping the puddles like a ballet dancer. Somewhere in the neighborhood behind them a car backfires and Joey startles.

Chente laughs. "Whoa. It's cool. Don't worry. It was a car. Okay, listen, alright? Right, this is important. The plan is only *one* of us goes upstairs at a time. Okay? *One of us*," he shows Joey his forefinger. "The girl will give you twenty minutes for twenty dollars, and she'll *time it*, so twenty minutes is twenty minutes. When it's done, it's done. Even if *you* aren't. Got that?"

"Yeah, okay."

"Now, we need to make sure there's *always* three of us down on the street, all three of us, right?" he shows Joey three fingers, "and we need to make sure we know where the other guy is at all times and which girl he went up with."

"But this is legal, right?"

"Don't be so *nervous*. Of *course* it's legal. But that doesn't mean—"

And then a hand is tugging the sleeve of Joey's jacket and he turns and it's a girl in a short black dress and tall purple boots. She smiles at him and looks him up and down. "You wan' to fuck me tonight, you think?"

"Go ahead. *Talk* to her," says Chente, pushing Joey in her direction. "Tell her you're shy," he says and then turns to the girl, "*Lo siento, mija, mi amigo es un poquito tímido*. Look, Joey, I just told her you were a little shy. It's cool.

Talk to her. *Lo . . . lo siento, mija, momento. Él se llama Joey . . . como . . . como José.*"

The girl laughs and covers her mouth with her hand. "Joey . . . maybe you wan' to fuck me tonight?"

"Go, go on," says Chente, taking his comb out of his front pocket to slick back his hair. "Talk to her."

Joey turns back to the girl. "Yeah, sure. *Is that okay*?"

"Is okay. Come with me, alright, buddy?"

"Joey, remember, relax and be cool and have a good time. I'll see you back down here. Right here. *Twenty minutes*." He taps his finger on his wrist and Joey looks down at his watch.

The girl takes Joey's hand and they walk up the street past Fernando leaning against a storefront window talking with a tall, horse-faced girl in a black cocktail dress. Fernando's girl laughs and leans forward and puts her hand on Fernando's chest as they pass and Fernando looks down at his shoes and laughs and shakes his head.

Joey follows the girl up a flight of stairs and down a white-washed hallway lit by a single bulb, and up to the desk clerk, a short heavyset man with a drooping mustache and tired, pouchy eyes. The man sits at a small wooden table covered in loose papers and takeout boxes and stapled-together receipts. He hits the stapler and sets a new receipt on the pile.

"Okay, buddy, you give him your moaney now," she whispers, arm wrapped in Joey's. "Give him your moaney and we go to the room. Okay?"

Joey hands the clerk his twenty-dollar bill and the man takes it without looking up from his paperwork and folds it into his front pocket and waves them on.

"Less go, buddy." The girl takes Joey's arm and leads him down another hallway and into an open doorway. "Heeere is the room, buddy!" She locks the door behind them and sits on the twin-size bed and crosses her legs. "Is okay, this room?"

Joey's knees shake but he walks around the room to play it off. "Totally, it's fine. It's great."

The bed has white sheets and two pillows and no blankets. Next to the bed is a small nightstand and a gray trashcan with a clear plastic trashbag. On the wall, a painting of a beach scene with a gold plastic frame—Mediterranean cliffs, bright blue sky with streaks of yellow and orange clouds, people on canvas chairs under colorful umbrellas.

"My name, it is Angelica. Thank you for choosing with me." She sticks her small hand out for him to shake and smiles big and Joey sees she has braces with red rubber bands.

He shakes her hand. "I'm Joey. I . . . I mean—"

"Is alright. You doan need to be shy, okay?" She stands again and reaches up under her skirt and yanks her panties down to her hips and then pulls them down the rest of the way and steps out of them. They're neon green mesh and padded like a swimsuit. She picks them up off the floor and smiles and sets them on the bedside table.

"Now buddy, you get to pick." She snaps open her tiny black purse and pulls out a strip of condoms. "Pick one you like for you."

"I guess this." Joey points to the strip without looking.

"Is nice choice." The girl tears the condom off the strip and then rips open the corner with her teeth. "The *best* choice, buddy." She hands Joey the open package and sits back on the edge of the bed and smiles up at him. "I am ready for you, okay?"

He pulls the condom out of the wrapper. It's huge. A Magnum. The girl giggles behind her hand. He holds the condom by the base, bright pink and shiny, and he knows all is lost.

When twenty minutes is finished, the girl does her makeup in the mirror by the bed. From the room next door a set of bedsprings creaks softly and then a headboard begins to smack against the wall and someone yells "*Dios! Dios! Dios!*" followed by a great crash, and then it's silent. The girl looks back at Joey and giggles and covers her mouth with her hand and then leans close to the mirror and opens her eyes wide.

Joey stands by the window. Down on the street it's raining and the cars and blacktop reflect the light from the streetlamps.

"Whatchu do?" the girl asks, with her back to him. She draws a black line around her mouth with a short makeup pencil, then sets it on the bureau, and digs in her purse for lipstick.

"Huh?"

"Whatchu do for your . . . you know for your . . . *job*."

"Oh, for my job. I'm a waiter at a retirement home." He sits on the edge of the bed and ties his shoes. Double knots. Triple.

"Oh. That sounds . . . cool?"

"I guess. I don't know. What about you, what do you . . . I mean, besides . . . like . . . I'm sorry. I shouldn't even—"

The girl sits down on the bed next to him and kisses his cheek. "Thank you for asking. What I do *also* is go to school to be *enfermera* . . . you know . . . to be *nurse*. I have a husband and a daughter, too. Her name is Marlena like my *abuela* . . . my . . . grand*mawther*. My sister, she watch Marlena when I am working. You have brother, sister?"

"I have a sister but we weren't raised together."

"'Raised together' is how?"

"I grew up in San Diego with my aunt and uncle and—"

"Oh, I know how you mean 'raised together.'"

"Yeah, and she, my sister Macey, she was raised out in the Midwest. We see each other . . . I don't know, like, once or twice a year. My family's kind of . . . *divided*. Macey's cool, though. She's . . . I don't know. She's into sports. She's . . . she's like a school sports superstar or something, so even though her grades suck she'll go to any college she wants. Anywhere. She played water polo and swam for the first two years. High dive or whatever that's called. Girl's soccer. She's kind of . . . she's a total redneck."

"Redneck?"

"You know, 'yee haw, howdy, y'all.'"

"Oh, like a cowboy."

"Kind of. What about yours? Your family."

"My family come here from Bogotá—you know, from Columbia?—two years ago. My daughter, she is four and a half. I have her when I was . . . no so many years old. Now I am *diecinueve*. Nineteen. *Quantos años tienes*?"

"I'm twenty-one."

"Oh, you know some *español*?" she smiles, then covers her mouth.

"*Un poquito*. Just a little. I can follow along when people talk unless . . . y'know, unless they talk fast, and I can read it but I can't really . . . y'know, *talk*."

"Where you learn?"

"In college."

"You go to college?"

"I dropped out."

"Why you dropped out?"

"I don't . . . I don't know."

"For me, I would *never* drop out. I would—" she stops and sighs. "What is this for?" She squints at the pin on his jacket collar.

"It's a button for my friend's band. My friend I came down here with."

"Your friend he is *famous*?"

"No. I mean, to some people maybe."

"Is nice. Can I have?" she puts her finger on the button and taps it twice.

"Yeah, sure, of course."

"Put it on me?"

Joey unclasps the button and pins it on the front of her dress like a corsage.

"You are very nice boy, Joey. And thank you for the . . . *band button*." The girl kisses his cheek. "Is time to go. We go now, okay?"

They leave the room and she leads him past the man at the desk and back down the stairs and out the front door, and she smiles at him one last time, and then walks off in the rain toward the line of girls.

"Hey, Joey, homey!" Chente calls, jogging up to him.

"Hey." Joey gives a halfhearted wave.

"So how *was* it?! I was up at the other place." He jerks his head in the direction he just came and Joey looks—nothing but darkened street, more girls, cars at the intersection, their wipers clicking back and forth.

"I thought we were all watching out for each other." Joey tries to say it sarcastic but it comes out flat. "Wasn't that the . . . that was the plan, right?" His voice breaks and he feels the tears welling up in his eyes. He wipes the water off his forehead with his jacket sleeve. The rain is letting up but the air is still wet and the gutters are flooding over the curbs.

"Yeaaah, *I know* but I met this girl and she was . . . oh, Big John's Tonka," Chente says nodding as a raised pickup with big tires turns the corner. "Uh, but, yeah, this girl up there. You know how I like big girls. I had to. It's alright. We're here. It was good, though? It was good?"

"Yeah. It was good. Where we going now? We should get some food." Joey tries to change the subject. He can't tell Chente the truth. How there was nothing good about it. How he barely got hard and how she lay there grimacing while he did it and how he couldn't get excited enough to finish by the time twenty minutes was up.

"Yeah, food. Let's go someplace back on Revolución. The bars down here get a little crazy this late. Ohhhh, wait, shhh, listen, Javier was behind me coming down the stairs. Don't say anything but I talked to him and he said he couldn't get it up enough to bust. Again! Don't tell him I said that. Here he comes."

Javier struts toward them, smiling and zipping up his jacket. "That was gooood, *carnales*! How was yours, Joey?"

"Mine was . . . she was good."

"*This* girl," says Javier, grinning and pointing back with his thumb, "I was like bam bam bam, like, doggy style, like, uhn uhn uhn, and I—" but a siren rings out and cuts him off. They turn to see a flatbed military police truck with two men in the back under armed guard. The truck stops behind a red taxi cab and honks its horn.

"Wait, hold on," says Chente, squinting. "Is that . . . is that *Fernando*? It's Fernando! Holy sh—hey! Fernando! Over here!"

Fernando sits in the back of the *Federale* truck, head bowed, hands cuffed in his lap.

"*Ay 'Nando! Mira! Qué onda*?!" yells Javier, jumping up and down and waving his arms over his head. "*Mira! Fernando!*" Javier turns to Chente. "*Do* something! Chente, help Fernando! You need to *help him*!"

"Over here!" shouts Chente. "Fernando! Hey! Look!"

Fernando looks up and tries to stand but one of the *Federales* puts his hand on his shoulder and sits him back down.

"It's okay, *carnales*!" he yells. "Go home without me! They're jus' taking me to jail for tonight!"

"Fernando!" shouts Javier. "What do we *do*?!"

"I'll be out tomorrow morning! I spit on some guy's cousin and there was a fight. Thas all."

Chente shakes his head. "Should we call Lupe?! Where should we—"

"Go back to the bar! Get drunk with Rosa for me! I'll call you laaaater." His voice trails off as the truck turns at the stoplight.

"Ferdinando the Bull," says Chente. "There he goes."

PARKING LOT, THE NEXT MORNING

Joey's eyes blink open. Blue sky. A plane flying overhead so high up he can barely see it. He's on his back in the bed of his truck. A cloud now—thin and ragged and panning west to east. He pulls himself up and climbs over the side and drops onto the asphalt. Impact—pain through his feet and ankles and knees, rippling upwards, coursing down then gone. And nausea, the hangover hits and he drops to his knees in the shade of the truck and vomits onto the blacktop. Yellow on gray. Flecks of cilantro and strings of chicken, undigested. He gags and does it again and then it's done and he feels better.

Joey pulls himself up with the truck's side-mirror and wipes his nose with the neck of his t-shirt and walks around to the driver's side. Chente—curled up on the seat, smiling in his sleep. His hair greased back. It's perfect. A swoop of black with lines like the groove of a record.

The window is down and Joey's reaching in and shaking Chente's shoulder. "*Chente*." His voice comes out raspy and thin and he tastes bile. "Chente." He clears his throat and swallows and his voice is back. "Chente. It's *tomorrow*."

NOON

On the freeway, cars weave in and out of the lanes. An empty yellow school bus, then a carload of teenagers, tough and serious in a battered red Toyota, the dark blonde hair of the girl in the backseat blowing around her face, bare arm out the window surfing on the breeze. Joey thinks about Maggie, quiet and tough. Calm and strong. The red Toyota drives past them and takes the exit and then a woman in a gray business suit driving an SUV with one hand on the wheel and the other holding a breakfast sandwich wrapped in yellow paper takes a reckless bite and swerves to the left and nearly hits them without looking up. Joey honks the horn and Chente waves at her when she looks and gives her the finger with both hands.

"Hey Joe Fro, you know the ancient Aztec magic trick to avoiding hangovers?"

"There's no trick."

"There is a trick. The trick is always drink so much that when you wake up you're still drunk. Then deal with the hangover later. Things are always worse now than they are later. They're also better now . . . I mean, when they *are* better. It's like being on Mexico Time. Oh hey, Joey, *carnal*, what's relative humidity?"

"It's a weather thing. Right? Something about weather?"

"No, it's a joke."

"Oh."

"I heard it last night. What's relative humidity?"

Joey shrugs and shakes his head. "I don't know."

"The sweat on your balls when you're fucking your sister."

"That's horrible."

"It's great. The girl I was with last night told me. I love girls who can tell a dirty joke."

The radio cuts from station identification to the surf report: "This is Smokin' Sam Kines with your Pyramid Beachware 101.7 surf report. There's a solid west swell in today. Eight to ten and closin' out at the beachbreaks in Mission and P.B., head-high but choppy at the Shores. Big Wave Dave from Bird Rock Glass is callin' double overhead and better at Windan and Blacks, and I'm hearin' good things about the Cliffs and O.B. It's a nasty one and the waves are *super* close together, so make sure your leash is in good shape and don't paddle out without a buddy. A drive up to North County'll pay off. Pipes, Seaside, Cardiff Proper, Swami's, all lookin' nice and hollow with some intermittent offshores. But be careful, it's gonna be *hella* crowded because the word is OUT. This is Smokin' Sam Kines from Pyramid Beachware, your go-to spot for all things surf and sand in mighty, mighty South Mission, and that was your 101.7 surf report! Peace out, and as always, *mahalo*."

"*Mahalo*," says Chente. "*Fuck* that guy." Chente has his shoes on the dash, his knees bent up to his chest. "Look at this." He laughs, scratching at a brown food stain on the thigh of his pants. "It's refried beans," he says. "What a cliché."

12:45 P.M.

Joey drops Chente off at his apartment and takes the I-8 to Ocean Beach to avoid his aunt and uncle until the hangover's passed.

In O.B. he drives down Newport past the Mexican restaurants and beach bars and antique stores. As the sunny, crowded streets pass by, Joey hears the voice of his fifth-grade teacher Mr. Lewis listing off the former names of Ocean Beach and giving the kids a trick to remember them with. "Mussel Beach, Mussel Beds, Medanos: The three M's, remember them as the three M's. Like Mmm, like you're eating something good." And all of the kids went, "Mmm."

In the parking lot at the foot of Newport, Joey pulls into a spot facing the ocean and cuts the engine. Stillness. Then silence. The boardwalk and pier and white expanse of sand. The ocean sparkling under the sun and thick lines of waves rolling in; the whole coastline alive and busy and people standing on the boardwalk watching the waves and taking pictures with cameras on tripods, and surfers in black wetsuits jogging down the sand, boards under arm.

Joey rolls down the window and the sea air is clean and salty and cool and the sound of the surf booms wildly. *"Mussel Beach, Mussel Beds, Medanos." Maggie, Nicole, Angelina. No. Was that it? Angelica. "I have a husband and a daughter, too. Her name is Marlena, like my* abuela *. . . my . . . grand*mawther*."* Joey unbuckles his seatbelt and leans forward against the steering wheel with his arms resting on top of it and stares out past the surfers and the waves to the hazy point where the sea meets the sky. Out of the corner of his eye, he sees a surfer to the right of the pier paddle into a wave. It picks him up and he gets to his feet, angling his board across the blue wall of water. *Don't do it. Cry now and you won't stop.* The wave begins to curl over the surfer and he squats down and disappears behind the curtain and Joey sees his blurry image passing through the tube. *What was that last night? This isn't you.* The wave breaks on the sandbar into a wall of whitewash and the man is gone. When Joey wakes up, it's night and the moon hangs high and pale yellow over the ocean.

1978

MAY 2ND

It's been a week since Sorel and I got together. The first time took me by surprise. I was sitting in the easy chair looking at a *National Geographic* photo of Tutankhamen's sarcophagus (Sorel loves anything Egyptian) and she was lying on the couch smoking a cigarette, digging a finger into one of her little pink ears, and she said, "Hey man. Know what? Come over here a sec." I got up (as if on autopilot) and stood next to the couch and she looked up at me with the mess of her red bangs in her eyes and the Cleopatra makeup around them and gave me this mean, dark snarl, and then reached up and pulled down my zipper.

The next thing I knew, I was sitting on the couch with my pants around my ankles and she was tugging down her shorts and climbing onto me and then I was inside her and her arms were around my neck and she was smacking up and down in my lap. I came fast. It was over before I knew it. Two minutes, three, tops.

After I came, Sorel climbed off me and wiped between her legs with a sock from the floor. "Well, then," she said and pulled her tanktop over her head and walked, slow and naked, into her room. I followed her and we didn't leave until morning.

1999

MISSION BAY, 2:34 A.M.

It's a warm, breezy night on Fiesta Island and the bay has a raw and coppery smell—sewer, brackish water, oyster mud. Tyler and Joey drive over the paved land-bridge then circle the island looking for the bonfire. They see nothing—the shapes of sand dunes to the left of the car leading into the island's palmy interior; the black bay-waters to the right, inky and flat and featureless as far as you can see. Somewhere off on the water are the blinking lights of the *Lindsey Marie*, a three-mast sailcruiser up from the Aegean Sea, thirty-two people on board, a party with Greek wine, red potatoes, and roasted lamb (dill, fennel, rosemary) to celebrate the crossing. Beyond that, the dark bayshore cove at the Campland trailer park and its half-ring of lights in the blackness.

"There. Yeah." Joey points at the bonfire through the windshield and Tyler turns the radio off and slows down.

"Huh? Where?"

"There."

"Out there?"

"The fire."

"Oh yeah. You sure?"

"Yeah, yeah, yeah. Park up, bud."

"I see it. Okay."

A dot of flame strains left in the breeze down by the water—rising, falling back low, bending flat and whipping in a long, orange tail, the black stick-figures of bodies moving around it like something primordial.

They park on the road along the dunes and walk across the sand to the water to find a roaring, gushing, smoky fire and a big group of kids sitting on pallets, drinking wine and beer, bored, the boombox playing a blaring loud pop song.

"Oh shiiiiit! I *love* this song," says Tyler as they near the fire. He does a little dance in-step and sings along. The woman on the radio is singing about fellas leaving your girl with a friend and ladies leaving your men at home because it's eleven-thirty and the club is jumping jumping, but Tyler sings "jumping" as "bumping."

"Hey Ty, where's Maggie? She's not here."

"Huh. Weird. You wanna go home?"

"Let's wait and see if she shows."

"Okay."

"There's a keg."

"There *is* a keg."

Joey takes two plastic cups from a stack next to the keg bucket and hands one to Tyler and pours himself a beer from the spout while Tyler pumps the handle. Someone turns the radio off. Quiet. Low conversation. Darkness all around. A girl laughing, but a quiet, mean laugh. No one says hello. The fire crackling and popping—releasing clusters of sparks that drift up to the sky before dying out.

Tyler taps the empty beer cup on his chest then puts it over his mouth like a red plastic beak. "Maybe . . . maybe she was already here and left," he says, muffled by the cup. "Maybe she left."

"You're up, bud."

"Okay." Tyler holds the keg spout over his cup and Joey pulls the handle up and pushes it down until his shoulder hurts. The nozzle sputters and coughs foam into Tyler's cup and then flows evenly until the cup is full.

They walk away from the keg and stand off to the side of the fire and Joey takes a sip of beer and it makes him feel worse. He takes another sip and his hangover is gone.

"Man, Tyler, I've got a *story to tell* about last night. Fuckin' Tijuana."

"Oh yeah?"

"Not here. I need to be . . . I need to get drunk to tell this one."

"Craziness? Bad craziness?"

"The worst. I think I'm done with TJ for a while. You won't *believe* this shit. Seriously."

"J.C., I don't think she's coming." Tyler gives the people around the fire a wary look. "Yeah, she's probably, like . . . I don't know, not coming or something. It's hard to . . . pin her down to showing up somewhere. Like . . . *anywhere*."

"She's on Mexico Time."

"Huh?"

"Nothing. Something Chente said this morning. Maybe we should . . . Tyler, maybe we should wait around and see if she shows. Let's chill out and wait for a while. It's early. Don't you . . . don't you love the smell of campfires? And the . . . like, the *red glow*. It's relaxing and—"

"It's like *3 a.m.*"

"Huh?"

"You said, 'It's early.' It's not." He holds his watch up for Joey to see. "I have school. It's hella late."

"True. I guess. Let's give it a minute then split. Is that cool?"

"A minute."

"Counting down." Joey squints through the flames at the faces in the crowd. Strangers. Twelve of them. Three more down by the waterline, one of them running away from the other two, shouting drunkenly. A few more in parked cars on the road. Joey's eyes stop at a tall, awkward-looking kid in a filthy brown suit. The kid has thick glasses and an uneven bowl of black hair.

Someone familiar. Someone he's seen with *Maggie*. Right, with Maggie. Maggie from afar, walking down 6th in Hillcrest before he knew her well enough to say hi; Maggie with the kid in glasses, laughing in a big group of people, all of them with backpacks and shoulder bags, happy, relaxed and confident. "Hey Tyler," talking low, "who is that guy? I see him *everywhere*."

"I don't remember this name. Ben Something-or-other. He used to go to school with Maggie but I think he dropped out. He's one of her friends."

"Do you know him?"

But Tyler doesn't hear Joey. He's staring at something behind them in the dark and Joey tries to see what Tyler sees but there's nothing—black, the dim line of sand-dunes, shadowy parked cars, a couple kids lying on the hood of a pickup, one of them pointing up at the sky, a jug of wine between them. They're talking about making Thanksgiving turkey hand paintings in preschool. Joey and Tyler don't hear this and the kids themselves won't remember talking about it. (What they [the kids] will remember: 1) Earlier, the blonde girl by the fire, Kellie Roman, twenty, UCSD feminist lit major, talking about anime cartoons featuring underage rape scenes between Japanese schoolgirls and tentacled beasts; 2) The cops pulling them over on Sports Arena Blvd, an hour into the future, the wild windmill of lights; 3) The arrest and the DUI and the subsequent fallout and the end of their friendship.)

Joey looks back. The kid is sitting cross-legged in the sand between two girls who are bickering at each other. The kid sits quietly and drinks wine from a dark bottle and stares down at the sand. As Joey watches, the kid takes off his suit jacket and tie and filthy white-and-red-striped shirt. Underneath he's wearing an ancient, faded, green Ninja Turtles t-shirt, the Turtles standing around a table with happy open mouths and smiling eyes before a giant pizza, the ends of the crust drooping over the side.

"Oh wait. I remember," says Tyler.

"You remember what?"

"Frank. His name's Ben Frank."

"Oh. That sounds familiar."

"Joey, let's bounce. Fiesta Island is boring. The bay's stupid and lame anyway. It smells like poop."

"Poop?"

"P-O-O-P. Poop."

The kid on the sand lights a cigarette and pulls up his green t-shirt sleeve and snubs the cigarette out on the flesh of his shoulder. Then he lights it again, takes a drag, and does the same thing, calm, expressionless.

Tyler turns back around. "Whoa. What is he *doing*?" he whispers. "Why would anyone . . . like, *do* that?"

One of the girls sitting with the boy shouts, "No, it's *you,* Becca. You just don't know it's you. Which is, like . . . *super, super* deluded." The girl gets up and stomps off into the darkness toward the water, the sand kicking up behind her feet. She's enveloped by the wall of black, and the other girl stands up, embarrassed, and follows her friend until she's just a pale non-color moving along the shore. Her friend, dressed all in black, has become invisible and the non-color argues with no one.

The boy turns to watch them go then shoves his thick, black-framed glasses up along the bridge of his nose. He sets the cigarette's cherry to the skin on his shoulder and the cigarette sinks in and he holds it in place, the fire reflected hot orange on the front of his glasses.

Tyler frowns and turns away and laughs. "I can't watch this."

A tall, acne-scarred boy with a choppy, black, pixie haircut drops a new pallet on the fire and the sparks jump up and catch in the breeze. He stands next to a rosy-faced blonde warming herself by the fire. (Kellie Roman, the object of affection of the kids lying on the car hood.) The girl lights up a joint and the tall kid tries to take it from her but she moves it from one hand to the next and sits down in the sand. She pulls the front of her red sweatshirt over her knees and its hood up around her face and hits the joint. She smokes and stares at the fire, her gaze inward (thinking, "Am I the kind of person I think I am?")

The tall kid walks off toward the cars, hands shoved in his pockets.

"Hey, Joey, this party's not even a party. Let's go. I have class early." Tyler pours the rest of his beer on the sand and winds up like a baseball pitcher and throws the cup back toward the road. It spirals, arcs up and back in the breeze and drops at his feet. "Joey, did you *see* that?" He bends down to pick up his cup and shakes the sand off it and laughs. "Did you see what I just *did*? I should join the fucking Padres. They keep asking. Like every day. 'We need you, Tyler. We need to stop sucking so much dick.' I think I'd be one of the greats. I should get some tight white pants. Can you see me in tight white pants?"

"Huh?"

"Nothing . . . I was just . . . I don't know."

Joey takes the cup from Tyler and stacks it inside his. "We should maybe . . . I mean, we *could* stay a little longer in case she shows up. That would suck (for her) if she showed up and we weren't here."

"No, I think we should go. Joey, *these people*? People like this? Hipsters? Pretentious assholes? Butthole hipsters? This is lame. You want to leave, right?"

"Sure." Joey lies. "Yeah. Definitely. I could eat the hell out of some El Cotixan. Let's bounce." He drinks the rest of his beer, crumples the plastic cups as one, and drops them in the trash drum.

1978

MAY 4TH

My brother came home yesterday and found Sorel and I together. Nothing was happening but it just had. I was lying on the couch wearing Sorel's fake kimono bathrobe and Sorel was sitting on the floor, topless, rolling a joint on one of her *National Geographics*. She was sweaty and high and in a good mood. We'd just fucked. In the kitchen, and before that in the backyard on a beach towel. The plan was dinner. Fish tacos.

Jacob came in smiling with a bag of groceries under each arm. He'd gotten a haircut in jail and shaved his mustache and beard and he looked younger and healthier. He was the old square-jawed Superman Jake, only heavier, darker around the eyes. "What did you—" was all he got out and then his groceries were on the floor and Sorel was running into the bathroom with her arms crossed over her chest and I heard the bathroom door slam shut and Jake was on top of me, hitting me over and over again.

When I woke up I was on the floor and one of my teeth was rolling around—*clicking* around—in my mouth. I sat up and spat the tooth into my hand and the room swayed and my vision doubled and I was out again.

I guess one of them brought me to the hospital, because here I am with an IV in my arm.

Sorel came to visit a few hours ago and stood by the bed for a while without saying anything. Finally, she said, "I brought your car. It's in the parking lot."

"Thanks. Sorel, I need to—"

"No, Merc . . . Jake's starting over. I can't do this anymore. *We* can't."

"Yeah. I . . . yeah. I'm sorry. I don't know. I'm . . . sorry." That was all I had.

"Here, for when you get out." She set my notebook and some wadded-up twenties on the end-table. "Merc . . . don't come back, okay?" And then she was crying and she leaned over my bed and held her hair back with one hand and kissed my forehead and walked out.

MAY 6TH

Today I checked out of the hospital and drove downtown. With the money Sorel left I got a hotel room by the bus station and dropped my stuff on the floor and drank three glasses of water from the tap and went straight to bed. After a few hours of hard, deep sleep and tsunami dreams, I took a shower and changed my clothes and went out for a walk.

It was getting dark and the streets were full of people. Sailors and rough-looking kids my age smoking cigarettes and walking in packs. Loud, yacking, sunken-mouthed women and sinister hippies and more homeless men than I've ever seen in my life. It was like half the city was homeless—bearded and shuffling, wearing packs, in coats or shirtless, drinking beers from brown-paper bags, pushing shopping carts, talking in groups, sleeping in empty lots, playing acoustic guitars, smoking in doorways.

Back in the hospital, Sorel gave me sixty dollars. Sixty is a week's stay in the hotel and a week's food and gas for the car, but after that I'm out of options.

I walked from my hotel down to the harbor and watched the sun go down over the dock-yards. The air had a good smell—salty, mellowed, tarry like new asphalt. I sat on the dock's edge and looked down. The water was dark with an oily sheen, colored, swirling. It was a quiet dusk and you could hear the water hitting the dockside, lapping. It was slow and rhythmic, a heartbeat of something calm and huge and motionless. Something that doesn't talk. Never talks. Some great universal heart.

A job will be a new start and an end to all this bad luck, I told myself. *You're a new man, Mercander. It's time to step up and start living life the way you used to. No, better. You need to be better. Push forward. Always be better than yesterday. Get out of this slump.*

I left the harbor and went straight to the Chinese diner on the corner and treated myself to a big bowl of *won ton* soup. It was cheap and gluey but good and hot and filling and it gave me energy to sketch out the next phase of my life: 1) Get a job, 2) Get Channy back, 3) Make things right with Jacob and Sorel, and, 4) The final step, move Channy and yourself back to New York City and start your life again.

MAY 7TH

Sat all day in the Chinese diner going through the cheap, newsprint want ads. People came and went. Mostly bums and sullen Navy guys and a lot of grizzled old men with missing teeth and rheumy eyes. It was a sad, gray, blustery day—the windows steamed-up and rain speckling the glass and everyone coming in damp and no one talking to anyone else, heads down over plates of noodles and rice, bluesy.

My options as I see them:

1) The service. Pros: Quick, easy. I'm the right age and the war is over. I think I'd be happy in the Army. Do my part. Support my country. Be a man, and be honorable. I've studied war history since I was eight. Proud traditions and all. Why not? Cons: I'd get stationed somewhere stupid like Okinawa or Frankfurt and that would make getting Channy back next to impossible.

2) Manual labor. Pros: I'm strong and getting a construction job would be a breeze. Nothing like physical labor to clear your head. Cons: I've never worked a physical job in my life. Who am I kidding? Don't romanticize this

stuff, buddy.

3) Restaurant work. Pros: I could learn. Not glamorous but it would be easy. Cons: I'm way too much of an eater. I'd be the Goodyear Blimp in a month. Maybe I wouldn't. Keep that as an option.

4) Go back to Weston and work on Roy's farm. Pros: I could (legitimately and in good conscience) call myself a cowboy and that would be cool. Riding horses. Working with cattle. Living with Roy and Clara, who are about the best people you'd ever want to meet. Fresh beef for dinner. Big sky. Country air. Living on the FRONTIER. All my Old West dreams come true. Cons: Same as the service: Too far away. I'd lose Channy. Or . . . [underlined emphatically] or, unless I got back together with her *first* and took her out to Missouri afterward. No, that doesn't work. Money first, then Channy.

5) Astronaut, knight, pirate, movie star, samurai, hot air balloon adventurer, Lawrence of Arabia, Robin Hood, James Bond, Jack London.

6) Hari-kari.

When I left the diner, I went to a payphone and shut the door and called Channy.

She picked up on the first ring and her voice was hoarse.

"Hello? Hello, who's . . . somebody there?"

And I hung up.

Soon. Not yet.

MAY 8TH

Nothing. No leads. Spent tonight in the hotel common room with the rest of the bums watching TV. (*Police Woman* then *Johnny Carson.* The guests were Joan Rivers, Gabriel Kaplan [from *Welcome Back Kotter,* the guest host], some country singer with a nice voice, and some comedian with stupid hair.) Warm, quiet, a clock ticking somewhere. A great humid, boozy reek coming off the people around me. We watched in silence. Now and then a fart. A cough or a laugh (or both, indistinguishable). The sound of clothes settling and creaking floorboards.

The place I'm staying must have been pretty fancy in its day. My room is a tiny box with a kid-size bed and a shaky wooden table but the lobby is all gold paint and gilded mirrors and dark red carpeting and carved fixtures. Of course all of that is rotten and faded and mildewed and water-stained. Metaphor?

MAY 10TH

Nothing makes you feel so low as being turned down for a dozen shitty jobs in a row. Tried to read myself to sleep but I can't concentrate. I keep coming back to that. *A dozen jobs.* My *god.*

It's storming outside and the thunder shakes the window pane and the man in the next room is shouting, "Hello, Jesus! *Goodbye*, Jesus!" over and over and over again.

A dozen jobs? Fuck California. I hate this place.

MAY 11TH

Rained all day today so I stayed in. Nothing to report, other than the fact that I'm starting to feel at home. Who am I to complain about those dozen jobs? Why am I so much better because I'm (almost) college educated? Looking back on what I wrote yesterday, I feel like a prick. The truth is that I'm no better or more entitled to greatness or ease or "a break" than anyone else. I need to put my ego in check. I'll get a job if I deserve one. Same with anyone else. I'm not special.

Sat up in bed with Ed Distler's last book in my lap and listened to the rain come down and felt a million miles from home and from my life as it once was back in New York City.

The hotel is called "California Palace." Metaphor.

1999

NORTH PARK, NIGHT

In June, Nicole leaves a three-minute-and-thirty-two second voicemail on Joey's machine to tell him she's filed for divorce from David Horowitz. They meet at Denny's for coffee (two cups for her, five for him) and they talk and share a plate of onion rings and a Moons Over My Hammy (no ham), and Joey tells Nicole it's good to see her and she tells him she's glad he's here.

Later, in her new apartment, they sit on the couch surrounded by moving boxes and smoke weed from a metal pipe and watch a PBS documentary about phosphorescent insects.

On the screen, the film crew sets up a camera in the woods at dusk. It's Virginia. Deep-green woods, tall trees hanging in the heat, and a dark purple sky. The sound is cicadas and crickets, a washing drone of swampy bug noise.

Joey hits the pipe, coughs, and hands it to Nicole. "That was harsh. My *lungs*. God. I hate weed."

"You hungry?"

"Yes. Always. Always hungry."

Nicole gets up and comes back with a shiny black bag of Smartfood popcorn and a red plastic bowl. She rips open the bag and dumps it in the bowl and sets it on the coffee table. "Popcorn party. Dinner is served."

Joey stuffs a handful of popcorn in his mouth. "I love this stuff. I could eat this shit all day."

"I bet you *could* eat shit all day."

"Yeah, yeah."

"Hey Joey, did you ever . . . *whoa*, look at that firefly they're filming, it's *so* big. Holy shit, dude."

"Hand me the pipe."

"Here."

"Thanks."

"Oh, wait, that firefly's the *moon*. Never mind. Argh, effing PBS. I'm too stoned for this."

"I wouldn't mind being a firefly."

"Being a firefly how?"

"If someone was like, 'Joey Carr, you now have to be an insect. Pick one now or suffer the consequences!' I would be like, 'Firefly, please.' No question. 'Firefly, make me a firefly.' Done and done."

"I always forget how dorky you are. You know that? You're a dork. A huge, awkward dork. That's a weird word . . . dork, say it: dork, dork, dork. Doesn't it sound, like, *wrong* or something?"

"No, really, Nicole, I bet they lead a pretty decent life. Look at them . . . look at that."

Nicole squints at the screen. "Yeah, until some shitty little kid comes along and kills them and rubs the . . . whatever, the, like, *glow juice* all over their hands."

"I'm way too stoned for you to say shit like that right now. Keep it positive, Nicole. You're breakin' the rules."

"C'mon, you're tellin' me you never did that? *All* kids do that. Kids don't care."

"For one, I've never been anywhere that has fireflies. And two, no, no, I couldn't kill a firefly. No way. That's evil. I couldn't kill *anything*."

"For one, whatever, I *know you,* Carr, you're not as nice as you pretend to be."

"I can't smoke weed these days. Makes me a social cripple."

"And that's a new thing?"

"You sure this's just—?"

"Just weed? *Yeah*, it's just weed. It's the same stuff I always get from Curt."

"Strong."

She laughs. "Whatever, caveman. *Strong. Weed strong. Am stoned.*"

"I'm a caveman . . . because I'm from the *stoned age*."

"Oh, man. Just don't, okay?"

"It sounded good in my head."

"*Yeah*, don't talk anymore, alright? The *stoned age.* Really? You used to be a lot funnier."

"Whatever. I'm funnier than you are."

"Hey, how's your aunt and uncle? You know I kind of miss your uncle sometimes. I miss, like, wakin' up in the morning and goin' out to the front yard to smoke a cigarette and there he is working on his big ol' honkin' seventies car."

"Ugh, the El Camino. I hated that car. He sold it, finally. It never ran. He had it for years. I never once got a ride in that piece of crap."

"Aw, no, I liked it. It was cool. It was totally bad-ass. He'd be working on his car and he'd kinda grunt at me and I'd smile and be, like, 'Good mmmmmorning, Mr. Carr!' I think he thought I was crazy."

"No way, they liked you. Especially my aunt."

"They're okay, though?"

"My uncle's been at home a lot. Injured at work. He has workman's comp but it's his back and he might end up retiring. It's pretty bad."

"That sucks."

"Yeah, he's home all the time watching TV for hours and hours and hours. Watches any kind of war movie you can imagine. My aunt's the same as always. Works all day. Listens to really terrible eighties music. Drinks white wine at night and pretends she's not drunk. She's trying to lose weight again but you wouldn't be able to tell by looking at her. She's like completely round now. Like a grapefruit with pretzel sticks for legs. Her and my uncle look like two gray-haired beachballs sitting next to each other on the couch. Fat. As. Fuck."

"That's mean, Carr."

"I'd be nicer if they weren't such fucking fuckfaces about everything."

"How's your sister?"

"Macey? I haven't seen her in forever."

"Doesn't she graduate high school this year?"

"I can't keep track. I think she's on her first year of college now. She's supposed to be coming out this summer to stay with my aunt and uncle and take some kind of intern position thing at SeaWorld, which sounds like the lamest shit ever."

"SeaWorld's great. You're on crack."

"Your mom's on crack."

"Whatever. You seein' anybody new?" She leans forward to knock the ash from her pipe onto the glass tabletop.

"Not really."

"What's not really?"

"There's somebody I like but it's . . . it's bad. She's Tyler's ex-girlfriend and he's still in love with her."

"That girl Maggie?"

"You know Maggie?"

"No, but I remember Tyler talking about her that time . . . that time I went to your work's holiday party and he and I smoked a cigarette outside and he drunk-talked me."

"When did you go to one of my work parties?"

"The Del? You know, the night he danced with that tall woman who kept saying, 'Haaaated it!' about everything and kept yelling 'Kick this party *up* a notch!' She was a *monster*."

"That was my old boss, Deana."

"What's she like?"

"My old boss?"

"No, c'mon, retardathon. *Maggie*."

"Maggie? She's like . . . she's the kind of girl I'm not even going to *think* about anymore because I'm not an evil person and I don't want to kill my best friend."

"Oh, whatever, just *do* it, Carr." Nicole leans back into the couch and brings the pipe to her lips. She flicks the lighter on, but lets the flame die out. "If there's anything I've learned from this stuff with Dave, it's that you better take a chance when it comes to you because there's a reason they call it a *chance* and not, like . . . not a normal . . . consistent . . . like, *predictable* part of your everyday reality."

"Who's stoned *now*?"

"Naw, for *reals*, Carr. Just because you're doing something for yourself doesn't mean it's selfish. It's not a *sin* to want a better life." She takes a hit and holds it in and hands the pipe to Joey, pointing at the bowl with her thumb to let him know it's still burning.

"Thanks. No, I'm good. Hey Nicky, do you really think I should . . . like, go after Maggie or whatever? I mean the moment I saw her it was just . . . I can't stop *thinking* about her. There's just something . . . she seems so *brave* and *tough* and smart and . . . and combine that with how she looks . . . old-worldly . . . like out of place in 1999 . . . she's like some kind of little Greek island warrior girl fighting the Nazis when they, like, when they occupy her village or something. Running around in the woods with a rifle and—"

"What are you *talking* about?"

"I don't know. I mean . . . I think about her *all fucking day*, like seventeen hundred thousand times a day."

"That's a lot."

"You know what I mean. Don't be a dick, Nicole."

Nicole takes a hit and lets it out with a cough. "Whoa, my lungs felt that. Yeah, totally. I mean, *yeah* you should. Tyler'll be fine. Boy needs to get over it anyway. Even if he finds out and it breaks his heart, it'll do him good. Breakups are healthy, but if you hold on obsessing about the person you broke up with, you're not doing yourself any favors. You remember my grandma, right?"

"Big Bepa, of course. Big Bepa loved me."

"She still does. She always asks about you whenever I see her. It's always, 'How's Joey Carr? Have you seen Joey Carr lately? How's that dog of his?'"

"I've never had a dog."

"I know. She loves her dog Mickey Mouse so much she thinks everyone has a dog."

"Oh I remember Mickey! He was a *great* dog! He always wrestled with me when I came over and he was . . . he was cute. Mickey! How's he doing?"

"He got married. Joey, who *cares* how the dog is doing? Listen, check it, whenever I was going through some stupid lame breakup, Big Bepa used to tell me that teenage relationships are doomed from the start, no matter how much you think you love the other person. Nobody stays with the person they dated that young and if they do they're going to regret it later. Teenage relationships . . . it's just playing house."

"Same old Hale, always quoting your grandmother in an argument."

"Okay, first off, this isn't an argument."

"A *discussion*."

"And second, I always hated when you called me by my last name. Like we were on the same *football* team or something. *Girls* can do that to guys. *Guys* can't do that to girls. And, *eff yeah* I quote Bepa all the time because that shit's *gospel*. She knows what she's *talking* about. Look at us back then. I think that's why everybody's so horny when they're seventeen or eighteen. You need the motivation to mess around as much as possible so you can be with a lot of people and find the one that works best for you. You need to weed out the bad combinations."

"No pun intended."

"What?"

"Nothing, go on."

"Oh right, weed, haw haw. But, I don't know, it's true, it wasn't me for you and it wasn't you for me. If you settle with the first person you get together with chances are you're going to be disappointed with your life. That's what happened with my mom and dad. And look at them. Living on two different coasts. Haven't spoken in forever. And at one time they loved each other more than anything in the *world*. Enough to have me and my brother and my sister. Now they're total *strangers*. I don't know about you, but to me that's *heartbreaking*. That makes me wanna *cry*."

"Please don't."

"I'm just saying."

The TV on mute. Foreign news. Smoke pouring from a burned-out bus as seen from above and the body of a man face-down, blue work-shirt dark with blood, tan pants, legs splayed out wrong, and then he moves. His arm moves. Reaching out at something.

Nicole shudders and turns the channel to a cartoon duck beating on a cartoon dog's head with a tennis racket. She laughs and sets the remote on the arm of the couch. "You okay, Carr?"

"Huh? Yeah, I was just thinking. About what you said."

"Don't take my advice if you don't want to but I feel like I've learned some stuff these past few months. I've been through some B.S., you know, total effing B.S. that's opened my eyes to—" she stops talking and looks down at the pipe in her hands. "You know David used to hit me?"

"Nicole—"

"No, it's okay. It's okay. He'd get really . . . like, *angry.* Like really, really, super possessive if I hung out with Rory—you know, my *best friend*, who I *should* have been hanging out with because it's *healthy* to have friends outside a relationship. But he'd work 'til six at TalCorp and he'd expect me to be home and waiting for him, and when I wasn't, when I'd go to Twiggs for effing *coffee* with Rory or see a movie with my mom and my brother, he'd come home and he'd push me around."

"Jesus, Nicole. I'm so sorry. Is that why—"

"Why he and I split up? It's part of it. But what I'm trying to say is . . . I'm trying to say I've been through some lame effing shit lately and I feel like I know what I'm talking about. I don't think I'm the same stupid, frivolous person who messed things up and was crazy and screwed around on you last year."

"I'm sorry about you and Dave. I mean, the other stuff . . . I had no idea."

"Nobody does. Not even Rory. I think she'd kill him. Like for reals. She'd find him and torture him for a week and cut him up in a million pieces while he was still alive. She'd kill him *slow.*"

"She totally would."

"She would," Nicole says quietly.

"You know if you ever need to talk or just hang out—"

"I know. It's cool. Don't worry. You know me. I can handle it. Maggie's not the only tough . . . what was it you said? Tough Greek island warrior girl in your life."

After the cartoon ends, they change the channel to a TV movie about slavery.

"Joey, I've got six million channels now. How did that happen? Remember when we had, like, *nine*?"

"My aunt and uncle've had cable for as long as I can remember. TV's like their main reason for living. My aunt would kill herself if she missed an episode of *Friends.*"

"I like *Friends.*"

"I'm leaving."

"Haw haw. Everybody likes *Friends.* It's okay to admit it, Joey. You care what happens to Ross and Rachel. Everybody does. They're the glue that holds us all together."

"I said I was leaving, right?"

In the movie a famous NFL quarterback/actor from the eighties is talking to a plantation owner. "No sah," says the football player, shaking his head emphatically, "No *sah.*" The overseer's eyes narrow to mean, dark slits and he says, "You dihnt see who stohl them hogs and Miss Nancy Alexander's roostis?" "No sah." "And you was heeuh the *whole time.*" "Yass, suh," he nods. "*Yes*?" "Yass suh, I's here the *ho time* and I dihnt see *nobody* steal no roostahs and no ho-ags."

"Wow, Joey, TV used to be so *bad.* Ugh. Thank god for Ross and Rachel."

"You're so lame that it makes me want to tear my own head off."

"I was kidding."

"Nicole, you know a kid named Ben Frank?"

"Doesn't sound familiar. Why?"

"Nothing. Just some kid I saw at a party. Seemed like somebody I'd want to be friends with."

"That's creepy. You're not getting weird on me, are you, Carr?"

"No, I don't know. I can't explain it. I'm *bored.* I'm sick of having, like, *two friends.* I feel like I'm the new kid in school ever since we broke up."

"Totally. I don't think I would've married David if I had more friends."

"I don't remember how to *do* this. How do you make new friends? It gets so *hard* once you're out of school."

"I know what you mean. We kind of effed up that one for ourselves, didn't we? It seems like everyone I used to know is either married or in school or totally out of the picture. You might have two friends but all I've got anymore is Rory, and Rory's too popular to spend time with me." Nicole picks up the remote and hits power and the screen goes from a bustling farm scene to black with Joey and her reflection in it, sitting together on the couch, smaller and shorter than they imagine themselves. Nicole sets the pipe down on the table, pulls her legs up under her, and sits cross-legged on the couch. "Two friends beats one friend." She trains her yellow-brown cat eyes on Joey. "Do you, like, want to *stay* here tonight, Joey?"

"Nicole, no, we can't. Not after everyth—"

"Not to *do* anything. *God.* I'm just saying, it's been *forever* since I've hung out with anybody my *age*, with anybody who *knows* me. We'll sleep in our clothes."

"Yeah, yeah, I'll stay over."

"And no sleeping with that stupid *switchblade* in your pocket. I don't want that shit to go off and stab me."

Joey laughs. "Of course."

"And if you spoon me, you better not get an erection."

"Nicole! Jesus! Don't be so . . . *crude*."

"Kidding! I'm kidding. Look at your face! *God*, lighten up, Little Boy Blue!"

"Little Boy Blue?"

"*You got the blues,* dude. I can *tell*. I think you're lonelier than you're letting on. You need to figure your shit out, stat."

"Whatever. Everybody's lonely. It doesn't matter."

"That's the spirit. One day we'll be dead and that's worse than all this . . . all this effing *Dave* stuff and *Tyler* stuff and Maggie stuff and boyfriend-girlfriend stuff. I'm gonna go take a dump. Pack us another bowl."

1978

MAY 19TH

You are now talking to the new front-page reporter for *The Midtown Times,* a tiny weekly paper with a staff of six. They wanted a writing sample and I had to promise I wasn't a druggy and that my car was dependable—both of which are true. (I did lie and tell them I was twenty-three and they bought that without question. Newly broken nose. Scars where Jake hit me and his big stupid skull ring ripped my face open. It works in my favor. Silver linings, and all.) After the interview, *Midtown*'s publisher said, "Now . . . since we're a brand-new publication, we don't have space here in the office, so you get to work from home. Until we can . . . you know, move on up to a bigger place . . . which is in the works . . . bigger staff, higher circulation, office closer to downtown . . . six-month plan . . . for now we're workin' with what we've got. So . . . so, as long as you're getting the work done and showing up for meetings, we'll be friends."

The paper's been around for a month but it looks like they've got a good business plan. The publisher: He's an okay guy, older, a little hot and cold and pretty moody but when he's on he makes it happen. He's also got a temper, a bad one. Regardless, I feel *great*. If I knew *anyone* in this city, I'd go out and celebrate. Big seafood dinner, cake, something. Everyone I know in San Diego hates me. How stupid is that? I wasn't expecting this at all. You always think people are going to like you when you go to a new place. Sometimes that doesn't pan out.

Anyway, work is good and when I'm not working, I read in the motel or walk around Downtown or go sit in the Chinese diner and look through the *New York Times*. Work is crazy—deadlines, long days, a good fast pace—but my off time is quiet and lonely. Alone in a city you don't like to begin with. And when you *feel* alone no one wants anything to do with you. They smell it on you. No one wants to be lonely and no one wants to be with you when you're lonely. After all this I've vowed to start treating people different, *better*.

MAY 24TH

Not much to report. The job's going well and I'm making money. With my first paycheck, I found a studio apartment in the neighborhood just above Downtown (it's either Golden Hill or Golden Hills, depending who you ask). I'm sleeping on a foam pad but at least I have a place to get my thoughts in order and level out. As far as Channy goes, I haven't called her. The problem is, I'm afraid to let her see what I've become. When Channy and I were together, I was starting from scratch in a new city but I had a plan and I was confident and full of purpose. I was *excited*. Fire inside. Ambition for a better life. Now I've got a job and I'm out of the hotel but I still feel like a deadbeat. Every time I look in the mirror and see the scars where Jake hit me and my crooked nose, it all comes back. It's worse when I brush my teeth. That missing back molar . . . it feels like pure darkness, a downward slide; it's the sum of all my failure and everything I've done wrong since I got to San Diego. Maybe if this job goes well, I'll get a replacement. We'll see.

Anyway, my studio sits in the shade of a giant eucalyptus tree and it's sandwiched between two abandoned old Victorian homes on a back street. Beautiful Victorians, stately old gabled mansions given over to rot. I imagine all the life they once held and it breaks my heart—kids running down the halls shouting happily, a good woman on the porch looking out over the treetops to the sea, babies sleeping in cribs, studious teenagers and men back from work, men worrying, women talking about their kids, men eating with their elbows on the table, women laughing in the front room. All of them gone. Bones in some graveyard gone to seed. Goddamn. I need to get out of my head for a while. Jesus Christ, Mercander. Okay, shifting gears, right . . . the neighborhood. The neighborhood's fine. It's quiet. Wide streets and a lot of big, three-story houses—most of them condemned and boarded up. Great old houses. Empty. C'mon, buddy. No more. Fuck it. Okay. Alright. Driving from my apartment to downtown, you take Broadway and as soon as you start down the hill, the whole harbor and bay and cityscape opens up in front of you. The ocean silver and endless in a westward arc, the city clean and busy and construction cranes and big Navy ships in the bay . . . on a clear day it's nothing short of breathtaking. I don't think I'll ever get over that view.

Okay, the room. One of the perks of my job is they gave me a nice, new (used) typewriter for work. It sits in one corner on an old wooden orange crate ("Fresh Valencia Oranges! Santa, California!") next to the phone. Above the crate I've tacked a picturebooth photo of Channy and I for inspiration. In the first frame, we're looking at the camera, cheek-to-cheek, dead serious, frowning, mean. In the next one, we're kissing and her hands are on my face. We look very young. (We are very young, but we look younger). In the final frame, we're cheek-to-cheek again and we're smiling the happiest smiles you've ever seen in your life. My eyes are closed, hers are open.

That photo and the typewriter are the only good things about the room. Besides that, it's a hole. The door opens and you're a foot from where I sleep. There's a shower and a toilet and the bathroom has a door, but the kitchen is nothing but a hotplate, a tiny sink, and a dead fridge. (I'm using it as a dresser. Top shelf: pants, second one down: shirts, etc. My socks are in the vegetable crisper with the money I'm saving up.) The floors of the room are slanted and the electricity is bad but the landlord won't send anyone out to check the wiring. When the lights go out, I use candles. (I guess there are worse things.) Oh: the grapefruit tree in the front yard. Not a bad thing. My whole block is vacant so no one takes the fruit and I eat a half dozen of them a day. There's a one-step porch and I sit out there with a knife and cut grapefruits open and eat them and watch the sun go down after a day's work, and that's pretty nice. Beyond that, the place is a dive. Sometimes I think of moving into one of the old abandoned houses. Living without power in someone's old mothballed dream. Joining the ghosts. "Hi, I'm Mercander. I'm as dead as you. I love it." Since moving in, I haven't seen any of my neighbors. There are no cars on my block and you never hear kids or TVs or anything but the breeze in the big eucalyptus trees. When I can't sleep, I trick myself into believing that the world has ended and that I'm the only one left. Channy, Sorel, Jake, gone. Mom out of her misery (if she can feel misery to begin with). Nothing left to do but grow old and get quieter and quieter until I'm a piece of the landscape. A moving stick-figure on the horizon. Lying in bed, I can pretend that's the case and I get okay with it and my heart slows to a crawl and I fall asleep and have dreams where everything is safe because there's nothing left to threaten me. No one knows I'm here because there's no one left. Of course, when you're as lonely as I am, you can only indulge that sort of fantasy for so long until it starts to get to you. Sometimes I want to open my door and stand on the stoop and scream, "Hello?! Is anyone out there? Where did you all *go*? Why did you leave me here alone?!" Just me in that weird violet dusk-light. Tropical. Silent. So still.

JUNE 1ST

Now: Sorel. Sorel and Sorel and Sorel. Last week, she showed up on my doorstep with a copy of the paper. Said she'd tracked me down through my editor. Of course I was lonely, and she looked good squeezed into a pair of blue jeans and a Mexican top, and I let her in and she was hardly through the door before I was pulling her shirt off.

I feel worse now than I did the first time around. Sorel will come by and I'll tell myself, "Yes, now, *today*. Today is the day you're going to be a good person and break things off and set this straight." But then she'll be kissing my neck and grabbing my hand and shoving it down the front of her jeans and there I'll be, stuck.

Last night, Sorel came by drunk and we fought over "what the two of us together *means*." At the end of the fight, Sorel told me she'd leave Jacob if I asked her to. I said I didn't want to come between their marriage and she said, "You already have," and she wrapped her arms around me and I held her and looked out the window over her shoulder and it was nothing but black and our own reflection.

The story I'm working on right now is about the "mysterious palm tree arsonist." He's been setting fire to palm trees for a month now—thirty-seven trees in all. I've done three stories on him so far and we've got a lot of positive feedback about it from the readers. My publisher wants to make it a column: says it's "provocative." But is it news? I don't think so. His line of thinking: "Make their *jaws* drop! If you can't do that, you've got *nothing*! We're too small to be boring, kid! Don't give me writing: Give me *juice*! These stories should be like bad sex; you get *in* and you get *out* . . . quick as possible."

Last night after Sorel left, I got a call from the arsonist. He introduced himself as "the palm tree guy" and said he got my number through the paper and told me that if I drove to Fiesta Island right now I'd get a good photo for my next story.

First I called the fire department and then I drove down there.

Three tall palm trees in a row on the empty sand-flats near the bayshore.

It was pitch dark and windy and their tops were burning and the fires licked off to the side in wild trails. It was the most beautiful thing I've ever seen and seeing it alone broke my heart. I kept thinking about how Channy would see this. Before we broke up, she was writing a short story about a murderer. A man who killed women he met at clubs. But it wasn't as dark as it sounds. After each killing, the story would follow the woman's spirit as she rose up from her body and went to be with the people she'd lost. It was graceful and strange and wonderful in its own way. I could see Channy taking the burning trees and bringing them into a story. That's how she did things. Everything went in. Whatever she did and whatever she saw made its way into stories and the stories weren't about her but because they had pieces of her they felt true. What would Channy do with this?

The fire department was a no-show.

I took a few pictures and watched them burn, then got in my car, and drove back home as the sun rose over the hills to the east.

1999

LINDA VISTA, 6:31 P.M.

At the Fourth of July carnival, Joey and Tyler and Tyler's kid-cousin Natalie pay their admission at the gate then stop at the concessions, and Joey buys a hotdog and covers it in relish and mustard and ketchup. It's sundown and the carnival grounds are dusty and crowded. Packs of kids stream past mothers pushing shaded strollers and around lines of people waiting to play games and teenagers smoking and walking in bored, sullen groups.

The smell of pears. The sound of a radio somewhere, fuzzy and distant-loud. A big woman with round, opaque eyeglasses rides an electric wheelchair past Joey and Tyler and Natalie with two plastic American flags duct-taped to the back bars of the seat. (Tyler says, "Code word TFTW," and Natalie says, "What's that?" "Too fat to *walk*," and Natalie says, "That's mean.") The heat comes in waves and Joey feels off-balance and feverish and he shuts his eyes as they walk and lets it pass all around him; the warble of carousel music (distorted, stretching); the smell of the hotdog in his hand and cigar smoke and fresh-cut grass and dust and (pears again and) kettle-corn. He opens his eyes—a flash of sun overhead against pale sky and the sound of a flag snapping in the breeze, the rope's clasp clanking against the pole, slow and dry and plaintive.

Joey buys a churro and a lemonade and Tyler and Natalie wait in line for the Ferris wheel while he sits on a bench under an orange tree. He eats the churro then sets the paper plate on the bench next to him as a tall black girl jogs past, heavily pregnant in a low-cut top and brown shorts. Her light-skinned, blonde daughter runs ahead, zigzagging through the crowd, a white balloon with red and blue splatters jerking in the air behind her on a string tied to her wrist. "Danielle Marie!" the woman shouts, hands on her hips. "Dani Marie, *you come back here.*" The girl racing up to her mother. Stops before she gets there. Won't come any closer. Shaking her curls. *No, no.* The woman sticks out her arm and opens and closes her hand at her. Fast. Impatient. "*C'mon, Dani.*" The girl backs up, the balloon straining away from her in the breeze. (A plane overhead, droning, a slow and dragging sound.) The girl smiles and then the smile is gone and she frowns and rubs her left eye and her lower lip juts out like a little shelf and she shakes her head side to side. "Danielle *Marie,*" the mother warns. "Don't make me count at you. One . . . two . . . *three* . . . Danimariehoney, you better come to mama . . . *four*," and with that the girl runs to her mother and throws her arms around her leg. "Awright, Dani, alright, sweetsy petesy," she says, petting the girl's springy hair, "Awright, Dani baby." Joey turns in time to see Tyler and Natalie climbing out of their Ferris wheel car, jogging up to him, holding hands.

"You bored?" Tyler says, smiling, out of breath.

"No, I'm good. I'm fine. Why?" Joey cocks his head and squints at gangly Tyler and short Natalie, the sun in rays all around them.

"I mean, because—" Tyler looks down at Natalie and she smiles and nods up at him, "—because I think we're gonna ride it again."

"Yeah, no worries."

"But *only* if you're not bored. *Only*. We can totally do something else. If you want to do something else we can do something else, no problem."

"Go ahead. Do the ride again."

"Sure?"

"Course. Yeah. I'm sure."

"Thanks! Okay. Good!" and Tyler and Natalie run back to the Ferris wheel and get in line.

7 P.M.

Sitting on the bench watching Tyler and Natalie do the rides Joey has the following seven conversations with himself. Topics: 1) Am I an unhappy person and does that mean I've failed? 2) Am I a bad person because I lie so often? 3) Why did my aunt and uncle keep me if I'm such an imposition? 4) Why does Chente hate people who do drugs? 5) What changes do I need to make in order to enjoy my life? 6) Should I give up on Maggie and go after Nicole again? 7) Natalie is twelve but her boyfriend is fourteen. Is that weird? Sub-topics, related/connected and not: 1) Should I get up and get a corndog? 2) What would it be like to have sex with the tall girl working the Hotdog on a Stick stand? 3) Does Nicole want me to try again? 4) What would Chente say if he found out I do drugs? 5) What do the bodies look like when a car burns to the ground? 6) What do my aunt and uncle say about me when I'm not there? 7) Where's Maggie? 8) Will I go bald? 9) Why haven't I ever thought of asking Rory out? 10) Why do I hate the name Don but like the name Dawn? 11) Who was it that played Colombo? 12) Should I try the hamburger place in O.B. that Petra's always raving about? 13) Am I white trash because my family is? 14) What's the difference between purple and violet? Is there a difference?

8:58 P.M.

When the sun goes down, they stretch out in the empty field behind the rows of houses to watch the fireworks. There's a twig poking Joey's back and he pulls himself up onto his elbows and finds it and tosses it aside and looks at Tyler.

Tyler, staring up at the black sky, waiting. Not smiling, but content, happy.

And then the first one—a golden umbrella of light that breaks open above them and drizzles back down like the branches of a willow tree.

Another one, dark red, a shower of sparks.

"Ooh!" shouts Natalie. "Aw!"

As the fireworks die out in trails of sparks and dust, burning pieces land in the dark patches of field and start fires and a group of Mexican men in black Dickies and oversized 'EVENT STAFF' t-shirts rush out from behind them and scatter across the field and stomp on the fires.

"Where did *they* come from?" asks Natalie. "Is this even *safe*?"

"Definitely not," Joey says, sitting up. "My cousin (she was your age) she lost her whole family like this. Ten of them and their cats on the Fourth. They were hit by a firecracker and they just up and caught fire where they were sitting, and that was that." He lowers his voice. "*We could be killed any minute now.*"

"*No, we couldn't,*" says Natalie, rolling over onto her side, glaring at Joey. She gives him a menacing kid-frown and shows him her fist and he laughs.

Tyler laughs. "He's just kidding, Nat. Don't worry. You're totally safe. Joey, tell her you're kidding."

"I am. We're totally safe. Hey, Ty . . . what's Maggie doing tonight?" This comes unprompted but it comes before Joey can push it back.

"Oh. She's way down somewhere in Mexico." Tyler sits up and points in the direction of the border. "Somewhere down there."

"She's way down in Mexico, no, really." Joey wraps his arms around his knees. "Where is she?"

"She went down with the Ben Frank kids. Milla, Charlie, Kirk, Nate, May, Byron, those kids. They're going to some beach to do a thousand drugs and get arrested and murdered and killed by the Burrito Bandito. What about Nicole?"

"Something with Rory somewhere. I guess I don't know."

And then the opening strains of the national anthem on a radio from one of the houses behind them.

"This is my *jay*-am," says Tyler. "I think I'm going to sing."

"Please don't."

"You know you want it." Clearing his throat. "Ho-oh-zaay, can you seeeeee," he sings in a high-pitched voice, plugging his ears for dramatic effect.

"By the dawzurly liiiiiight!"

Natalie giggles. "That's not the *words*!"

"What so prowwwwwdly we hailed by the twi-light's last glea-ming. Whose broad striiiipes and bright staaaaaaaaaaaaaars! Through the pare-uh-liss frigh—*fight*. Oh, the raaaaaaaamparts we watched were so gall-unt-ly streaming," pause, holding back a laugh. "And the rawwhh-ckets' red glaaaaaaaare, the bombs bursting in aaaaaaair, gave prooof to the niiight that the flag was still there!" A pair of blue fireworks pop out and expand in the blackness, followed by a green one. "Ho-zay does tha-at star spangled ba-ah-nner-er yeh-et waaaaay-aaaaaaave? Oh, the laaah-and of the freeeeeee and the hhhhome of thuhhhhhhh braaave!"

"*America!*" shouts Natalie, fists raised to the sky.

The grand finale comes and all of the fireworks popping around each other, the black sky full of flowering light. And it's done. And quiet. Somewhere off in the neighborhood behind them a string of firecrackers snaps off in rapid succession like a machine gun. They lie in the grass and watch the smoke clear.

THE NEXT DAY, 4 P.M.

The next day, Nicole and Joey sit on the boardwalk by the hostel drinking Slurpees. The ocean is flat and stormy and the wind is hot and dry and it comes in whipping gusts.

Joey takes his Ray-Bans off and cleans them on the front of his red t-shirt. "Tyler's ironic thing really bums me out sometimes." He puts them back on.

"How so?"

"I don't know. Last night . . . last night him getting all sarcastic when the fireworks were going off . . . it felt really mean-spirited and he's not that way. That's not Tyler."

"Everybody gets sarcastic sometimes."

"He's like that a lot now."

"He's just having fun. It's innocent, Joey."

"It felt really dark, him singing the national anthem all silly and dismissive like that. It felt mean."

"You need to lighten up. People like to have a good time and even if they're making jokes, that doesn't mean they're doing it to tear something down. Half the time, jokes are more about . . . about . . . like about getting the laugh than the subject. The subject's just the means to get to the punchline."

"That's stupid. What a . . . it's a waste of time. I hate that people are always looking for the joke in everything."

"You're that way too sometimes."

"No, I'm not."

"Sometimes."

"Well, I'm gonna stop."

"Be careful how seriously you start taking things. That's the road to being . . . like, to being a grumpy, colorless old man. Don't get *old* before your time, Carr."

"I'm not."

"No, I can see it happening. You've got a scary kind of judgmentalness . . . is judgmentalness even a word? Anyway, it's really unbecoming. You need to watch that. No one likes bitter people. They're awful to have around. No one wants to sit and listen to you complain about everyone else. Life isn't so bad."

"I don't know. I don't know what to think anymore."

"Just relax."

"Easier said than done. Hey, how you doing, Nicole . . . with all the Dave stuff."

"Fine."

"No, for reals."

"You really wanna know?"

"Yeah. I do."

"He keeps showing up at my apartment drunk and he begs me to let him in."

"Agh, jeez, I'm sorry."

"It's my fault. The first time I let him and we talked and it was alright. We even had sex and it was really, *really* good. I came like three times that night. Whoa. I'm sorry. Too much information. Too much everything. *Anyway*, yeah . . . anyway, the next morning . . . it was the same ol' thing. We talked a bunch and then we fought and he hit me and this time he hit me really effing *hard*. He hit me so hard that I fell off the arm of the couch where I was sitting and I smacked my head on the bookcase and blacked out and when I woke up he was sitting there looking down at me, drinking the good expensive vodka I bought for my birthday. The lame part is I still love him. It's bullshit. I don't know what to do. I feel like I'm on *Cops* half the time. Shit is getting *hella* white trash. We used to be so much *classier*, me and him. How do you go from squared away and kinda cool to trashy so quick?"

"I had no idea it was that bad."

"He told me he bought a gun."

"A gun? Wait. *What?*"

"It was super late one night and he called and left a message and I could tell he was really drunk and it was somethin' like, 'Nic, this is Dave. I want you to know I bought a gun today.' And that was it. Click. Dial tone." She makes the sound of the dial tone and then laughs, but it's a tired laugh, and Joey feels the world pressing in around him.

"That's really scary, Nicole."

"*Right?* I think I need to get a restraining order against him."

"You should."

"I might. Here, try mine. It's perfect." Nicole hands Joey her Slurpee and he sips it.

"I don't like the Coke ones. Cherry all the way." He hands it back.

"You didn't do anything weird when we broke up, did you, Carr?"

"I threw a party and invited Ben Affleck and George Clooney and, like, and Jennifer Lopez."

"*Carr*," she smiles and shoves his shoulder.

"Nicole, really . . . be careful. Don't . . . don't let anything *happen* to you. It would . . . that would be bad."

"Yeah. I hate how *easy* it is for men to make women scared. I was looking back at these emails I wrote Rory last year and I was super, like, *spirited*. In the emails, I was talking shit and saying all this crazy, wild, excited stuff and making plans and telling her how I was going to do this and do that and take over the world. I was quoting rap lyrics at her and using slang I would never in a *million* years use now. It was all just so, I don't know, filled with *personality* and *youth* and ego or something. Now I feel like a meek, quiet . . . little *mouse* hiding in the corner without any ideas of my own. I feel like somebody's boring-ass normal *mom* who's been stuck in the suburbs for a decade and has, like, given *up*. Like *seriously*, Carr, *I* should be the one buying a gun. The me from last year would straight roll up to Dave's condo and blow his ass *away*."

They don't say anything for a while. They sit and they watch the sea and the wind blows and the gulls drift overhead and when Joey looks at Nicole again, her face is wet but she's stopped crying.

1978

JULY 3RD

It's been a while since my last entry. The only time I write in this thing these days is when life slows down. The important stuff, the real living, gets left out. Which is a shame, but what's more important: *life* or documentation of life? The former, I think. Lately, life is work and work and work. Work is all-consuming. In the middle of June, *Midtown* folded and I started at one of the big dailies here in town. With a little bit of résumé under my belt, I was able to score an in-office editing job on the City page. No more late-night drives to make a story. No more being on-call all day. It's been nice, but stressful. With a daily paper, there's no downtime. News happens around the clock, as they say, and you're there until you put the issue to bed. It's a lot of work, but there's a different energy with a daily. The people here are hardwired and they rattle through the day, and then they're out drinking and raising hell until last call. Journalists are a hard-living breed and the result is a very raw, honest social interaction. Of course, most of the guys here are twice my age, but being around this kind of environment might be good for me. Still, as much as I like it here, I'm not sure if they accept me yet. If I go out for drinks after work, it's a beer or two and then I'm headed home. As far as they know, I'm twenty-six (another lie) but these guys are lifers. They have stories about the trenches. A whole career under the deadline, first-hand accounts of the big news events they covered: the Bay of Pigs or the fall of Saigon or Kent State, MLK, Manson, Atlamont, Watergate—and half of them have novels that they're finishing (whether quote-unquote finishing or otherwise, I imagine it varies). It is, to put it lightly, intimidating. And inspiring. I guess that's an okay mix.

On weekends, I stay at home and Sorel sneaks over to see me. It's good. She's changed. She listens now and when she talks, she has a lot more to say. Most of it is about how unhappy she is with my brother, which is hard to hear, but she's also figuring things out. I forget sometimes that Sorel is my age. She's nineteen, and she's not so much of a screw-up as half her friends. These days, Sorel's working full-time and taking jazz dance classes and aerobics at night over at Kate Sessions. "The Egyptian phase is over," she told me last week. "I'm done with silly raccoon eye makeup and the stupid pyramids and pharaohs. I've been into Egypt since my awkward stage in junior high back when I looked like some ugly, fat little boy. Too much *baggage*. It's time to grow out my bangs and get real." Now she's into 'earthiness and being a natural woman.' Whatever that means, it's nice to see her change and it's good to be around someone my age after the hard days in the newsroom. Still, it's not love and stringing her along feels terrible. For all her faults, Sorel's a good person; she deserves more than this.

Tomorrow's the Fourth of July. My brother's out of town riding three-wheelers with his friend Herman in Borego, and Sorel and I are spending the day together. We're going down to the bay to watch the fireworks and then we're coming back to my apartment to make dinner. She's learning to cook. "Baby, wait until you taste my recipe for linguine with garlic butter sauce and clams. I know you, you'll go crazy. You'll *love* it." What she doesn't know is, after the night's over, I'm going to break it off with her. I feel like I've done what I can to make my life presentable to Channy. I've come a long way; it's time to call her and start our life together. My only concern is how I'll tell Sorel. I hate that it has to be this way, but this is what I've worked for all these months. Still, I can't shrug off the fact that I'm keeping something away from Sorel.

1999

NORTH PARK, LATE AFTERNOON

The sun comes through the white curtains in the living room and casts a dusty beam on Nicole in her ratty brown bathrobe. 'The Bear' she used to call it, when she and Joey were together. It was, "Where'd I put the Bear?" or "Do you think I should wash the Bear? Does it stink?" or "The Bear's getting old but I'd never *dream* of replacing it. You can't just get another *Bear.*" And now Nicole's on acid, wrapped up in the Bear, staring straight ahead past Joey, her eyes glassed over and high, nodding her head, saying, "In this new, advanced, *evolved* state, mothers pass consciousness onto their babies." Smoke curling up from her cigarette. She waves it away like a fly. "But it's not happening yet. It'll happen, but not for thousands . . . *millions* of years. First, our brains need to grow into our big empty heads." Nicole's voice is low and droning. "Millions of years, Carr, after we've evolved from where we are now, which is nowhere, the desert . . . a camel with a cigarette standing next to . . . like, a giant . . . a giant cartoon Arab who lived ten thousand years ago and knew Jesus and Nostradamus and Dracula—the *real* Dracula. Dracula and The Wolfman. *Versus* The Wolfman."

"You took the words right out of my mouth."

"Carr, you know how some people say 'woof' instead of 'wolf'? I've always liked that."

"Oh, me too. For sure."

"Carr, do you know if you say 'fuck you' into a harmonica it comes out sounding like 'fuck you' said by a robot? But kinda musical. Like a robot singing? Fuhhhhhhhck youuuuuuuuuu."

Joey laughs under his hand like a cough. "Nicole."

"Yeah?"

"Don't forget you're on acid. Alright? Just, like . . . don't forget."

"Carr?"

"Yeah?"

"Suck it."

"Nicole . . . hey Nicole, I'm gonna get a Coke from the fridge. Just keep talking. You're great. This is great."

"Talking, okay, I can do that. And I'm on acid. I am. I won't forget." The front of Nicole's robe has fallen open and one of her breasts is out, small and freckled in the light, the tiny blonde hairs around the nipple iridescent in the sun. "The babies," she says, taking a drag off her cigarette and blowing the smoke to the ceiling, "the babies will be able to access not only the consciousness of their *mothers*—their memories, their *personalities*—they'll be able to *live* as their mothers."

Joey comes back in the room and cracks open his Coke can and sits on the couch. "Go on. Sorry."

"Look at you sitting there, Carr," she laughs, shaking her hand. "I keep seeing you on the moon in an astronaut suit with an American flag and a Coke in your hand."

"You see me on the moon?"

"Don't laugh. I see you on the moon with 'MTV' written below your feet. 'MTV' in block letters flashing on and off. 'MTV News'. You. Hear it . . . doot dah doot doot doot . . . *first*.'"

"I should be filming this. *Nicole On Acid*, coming soon to a theater near you. Rated I for insa—"

"Carr, you laugh, but you only see . . . you only see me and the Bear and the couch and the TV and the wall and that painting of sunflowers and my Gerontology 101 book . . . I'm on page ninety-six . . . I mean not right now . . . in general, I'm on page ninety-six . . . you . . . you see . . . the ashtray, see it? And my bike hanging on the wall . . . look at the wheels . . . the wheels, they're turning aren't they? A little? And those boxes over there and that sandal on the floor and that Diet Pepsi my mom left over there when she was here last weekend. It's warm. The Diet Pepsi . . . what's worse than warm diet soda? Carr . . . you see this *room*, Carr. I see this room and a thousand layers of the room all stacked up together: Joey, meet Joey, meet slightly different Joey, meet vastly different Joey . . . well, have fun with that." Nicole shuts her eyes and sinks into the chair. "The babies . . . the babies will download their mother: That is that crux. *But*. But, they'll download their father, uncles, aunts, brothers, sisters, cousins, grandparents and great-grandparents and great-great grandparents, great-great-great, etc., etc., ancestors and on and on until they're cavemen and apes and single cell thingies or protozoa or whatever shit that came . . . like that came on a meteor, shit from space. Did you know all the gold in the world came from space?"

"No."

"From meteors. Makes it seem . . . I don't know, cooler."

"Gold's lame. Silver all the way. Silver's rock 'n' roll. Gold's for . . . it's for old people."

"Shut up."

"Sorry."

"Shut up and listen to my . . . to my grand, genius, drug-addled ideas. Okay. Of course, the further removed by blood, the more diffused the downloads will be. Now, the *stronger* the connection—placenta, blood, sperm, eggs—the clearer the download. The baby will be able to access each personality and live as them, as the ancestor, snatching their soul up from the darkness where you find when . . . when you flip the light over and catch its underside before it sneaks away like a tiny . . . little . . . slippery . . . *snake*. They will reboot their soul from the point of whenever the mother severs the umbilical connection. Cut, like that, Carr." She makes her fingers into scissors and cuts the air in front of her. "Snip, snip, *cut.* The moment that begins, *life* begins," she lets her hands fly out like birds. "Carr, have you read any García Márquez?"

"Who?"

"It's like the scene with the vampire bats in *Of Love and Other Demons*; the reason I'm so tired and pale all the time is that slippery little snake comes under my door and drinks my blood at night. The woman next-door keeps him in a tube sock tied with a big knot and lets him out at midnight to feed on me. García Márquez talked about the bats that drank the copper-haired girl's father's blood while he slept. For me, it's a snake. And in my bed while I sleep. Look. Right here, the tip of my finger. See the marks? There's nothing I can do. I'm okay with it now. I'm beginning to like it."

"I'm sorry, Nicole. That sounds awful. Snakes are assholes. Fuckin' *dicks*. Too much *attitude*."

"Carr, you eat too many tomato sandwiches. I've always wanted to tell you that and now I am. It's gross."

Joey laughs. "Oh yeah?"

"You have a little head and your skin is shiny and tight like a tomato. If I cut you, seeds would come gushing out."

"I don't think that's true at all."

"Carr, tomato sandwiches are disgusting. Why do you eat so many of them? Why don't you put some cheese in there? Put some *ham* in that shit."

"I'll stick with tomato. Ham's gross. I want to quit eating meat."

"Why *tomato* of all things? Ew. Squishy. Squishy and grainy and slick. Like eating some rotten old *dog* tongue you found in a ditch."

"Because when I was a kid, my favorite book was *Harriet the Spy* and she always had tomato sandwiches and I wanted to be like her, so I ate them, too."

"That's beautiful, Carr. You know, you should get a job somewhere where they let you talk about eating tomato sandwiches all day. You deserve it, Carr. I think you like Maggie because she's Harriet the Spy grown-up. That's so sweet. You're spies. You're both spies. Carr, I think I'm gonna cry."

"Nic, don't. Please, don't."

"I'm gonna cry, okay? Just for a second? I'm not sad. It's pressure. The tears just want to . . . to go out into the world and live and get jobs . . . and get married and have baby tears and be nice to other tears and smile. Oh, god. The little tears with their lives and their jobs and their cars and their—"

"No, no, no, Nicole! Hey, stop, stop, stop. Nicole, tell me more about the babies and the DNA. The *happy* parts."

Nicole's grandmother's Jack Russell terrier Mickey Mouse struts in from the bedroom. He springs up onto the couch and rolls over on his back and stares at Joey upside-down with his tiny, black, squirrel eyes. His lip droops down, the miniature white teeth fixed in a snarl.

"Okay, Carr. Okay, so the babies and the DNA. Your DNA code (down, Mickey, *down*) is carried in genetic matter, like file storage. DNA holds the basic building blocks for who you are, but, deeper in, deeper than scientists have gone yet, it also holds individual memory which is what makes up the entire spectrum of your personality. You, your dreams, your pain, your secrets, the things you like to eat, the people you admire most, the way you react to problems, I don't know . . . the way you say your 'R's and 'W's, your very impulses: It's all in that memory code and you can plug the code into someone else and you'd wake up in their body. Of course a lot of genetic matter is passed from baby to mother during the nine months of gestation. The baby is getting (Mickey, *down*! Leave Joey *alone*!), the baby is getting pumped with the DNA of his whole genetic line for nine months. When the child accesses the DNA code and downloads the consciousness of the ancestor, the ancestor is *jolted* awake and they're *aware* of being alive in that body. The child knows the ancestor is part of them, too. Your memory and personality becomes this co-dependent thing and both personalities collaborate to make decisions, like two men driving the same truck, one with the steering wheel, one working the pedals. Now, if the person being downloaded is *dead* then they *restart* and their last memory is of dying, but not of death. If they're still alive, then they realize they're inside somebody else but they also know they're still in their *own* body, which is horribly confusing for them. They'll have laws against downloading the living. It's kidnapping and you know people, bad people will do it for money but the penalties will be . . . oh, they'll be *horrible*. Carr, it'll be terrible. Oh, Carr, you don't want to see this. You don't want to know the punishments that will be put in place. Carr, just stay in the present with your tomato sandwiches. You're a nice boy, Carr. You're a liar and a hypocrite and you're . . . I think you're getting uglier right in front of me . . . but you're a nice, sweet, kind boy. I wish you were my son. I wish you were Jewish. I wish I was Jewish, too. We should all be Jews. Joey . . . Joey, your aunt and uncle, I love 'em to death, but as non-Jews they don't have the means to protect you; they're gray and dying, they're done. They're wilted lettuce and nobody'll eat wilted lettuce, not even dogs. I don't want you to know what's coming. I really don't. Oh, Carr. It's so beautiful outside with the grass and the trees and playgrounds and the sun shining but . . . you're not going to heaven. I'm sorry, Carr. I am. I'm—"

"Nothing's happened yet. Nicole . . . you're on acid, don't forget."

"I am. I'm on acid. I forgot. Carr . . . I was getting dark there. Jesus Christ, Carr. Sorry."

"Listen, Nicole, tell me . . . I want to hear the happy parts . . . the babies.

The happy parts about the babies and the downloading and all that stuff."

"The happy parts. Right. Okay. So, like I said, the ideal situation is to download dead people. Since there's no afterlife, it gives them another chance at living and does so for as long as their genetic line continues. When they're not being downloaded it's like they're on pause."

"So nobody really dies unless the genetic line is cut off completely."

"Right. Nobody dies." She says this calm and satisfied and then snubs her cigarette out in a cereal bowl on the coffee table. "Nobody."

"I like that."

"Hold that thought, Carr." Nicole gets up and walks down the hall with Mickey chasing her feet and nipping at her ankles. Joey hears the bathroom door shut and the shower turn on and then he hears her retching. She's gone twenty minutes. He sits and stares at the empty couch, the dust moving in the light. Dust motes, green tweed couch, scratchy. He picks up the *People Magazine* on the coffee table and flips through it but he doesn't see any of the pictures. It's from Nicole's grandmother's subscription. Her name on the front. January Alice Hale. Not "Bepa." January Alice, a name she lost when she became Mom and then Grandma and then Big Bepa. Two weeks ago, Bepa passed away suddenly. A stroke. Nicole has been drunk or high since she heard the news. Joey sets the magazine back on the table and thinks of Bepa . . . half-blind Bepa, sarcastic, happy, quiet, white curls and sunken mouth, brown-tint glasses with lenses the size of drink coasters. Bepa watching soaps on TV but only hearing the stories. Afraid of "the *goddamn* Orientals." Glenn Miller records on repeat. Don Ho. Pearl Bailey. *Hee-Haw* and *Lawrence Welk*. Potato salad and deviled eggs and Ruffles on Memorial Day. Sticky jar of sweet pickles, untouched. Maraschino cherries that Joey ate greedily. Pepsi cans with movie ads. Endless cigarettes. Pall Malls. Chips and French onion dip. Glass table. Giant decorative keys over the mantle and a dozen ticking clocks. A casserole with cheddar cheese and broccoli, steaming, and Bepa at the sink washing her hands, saying, "Dig in. Don't let it get cold. No leftovers allowed in this house." Bepa, her husband long dead. Her family scattered across the country.

Nicole comes back in the room and sits down on the couch and her face is pale and sweaty and her hair is wet. "I frew up," she says, her eyes tired, her lips swollen and bloodless. Mickey jumps into her lap and Nicole pulls her robe closed and smiles sadly and tugs at the dog's tiny ears, one white and the other brown. "Mick-Mick, *who's a big little man*?"

"I like that."

"You like 'who's a big little man'?"

"I like your theory."

"Huh?"

"The babies . . . the downloads, no one dies . . . ."

"Carr, I'm on acid. Don't listen to me."

"I know, but—"

"But I'm on acid."

NORTH PARK, NIGHT

In August, Chente plays a show at the club across the street from his new apartment. It's a big one for the band: the owner of a record label flying out from New York to watch, the weekly paper running a cover story previewing the event. Chente tells Joey it's no big deal, but it is—something's happening. Something. A minor shock, a tremor. But something.

To make sure it's a packed house, Chente calls everyone he knows and six carloads of his friends drive out from El Centro to support him. Riding in the backseat of a red 1985 Corolla-Tercel (right taillight out, strawberry air freshener, overdue June tags) is Isabel "Chavela" Zevella Martínez, a pale, violet-eyed Mexican girl who Chente was in love with in high school but never had the courage to ask out. ("The guts," he says, never had "the guts" to ask out and Joey thinks of viscera, gut piles, blue tubes of intestines, flies buzzing around them, a disemboweled horse his uncle saw on a road in Baja and told him all about when he was six to scare him. "The goddamn thing was exploded all over the goddamn highway. Its guts were like a buncha fucking . . . a bunch hoses, firehoses.") Chente takes Joey aside before the show and what Joey is left with are the following facts: 1) When Chavela filled out her first passport application, she wrote "Santería witch" on the line stating occupation. 2) Chavela carries a butterfly knife and once pulled it on a teacher and the teacher was too scared to report the incident. Mr. Yates, "Mr. Masturbates," "Yaterbation," "Mr. Yaterbates," nine fingers, sweaty, a terrible comb-over, pariah. 3) When she was only eight, Chavela took her uncle's Savage/Stevens .22/.410 over-and-under from above the front door and shot a coyote that had been terrorizing her aunt's chickens all week. It was the first time she'd used a gun and she put a .22 rimfire through the coyote's right eye. (A clean shot, beautiful—death without knowledge of death.) She and her cousin Pokey buried the body in the desert and Chavela dug it up three years later and saved the skull. 4) Chavela brought the same lunch to school every day before she stopped eating meat at the age of seveteen: Three chorizo tacos wrapped in yellow paper (chorizo fried with egg; additional cilantro, sour cream, rice), a thermos full of Ocean Spray cranberry and Malibu rum, and a lemon from her grandmother's tree—her grandmother's lemons, freakishly large, grapefruit-size, the envy of her neighbors, and also a strong point against her, distrust, resentment, superstition. The myth, unfounded: The secret ingredient was semen in the potting soil. 5) Chavela has three tattoos Chente knows about (and one he doesn't). a) entire shoulder, left, growling [or yawning] cat face. b) wrist, left, "Seis Seis Seis" c) wrist, right, "MexyCaly." d) the unknown tattoo, breast, left, upper corner, tiny crucifix, self-done at the age of twelve, faded to blue.

After the show, Chente and Chavela are nowhere to be seen. In the backseat of his car, everything goes well until—accidentally, a slip in the moment—Chente butts his forehead against Chavela's mouth just as she starts to come and splits her lip. But that doesn't matter; she comes and that makes him come and all is right and good.

In the backseat of the car, in the afterglow, Chente fingerpaints "*C.R. y C.M.*" across Chavela's chest in her blood (pausing to kiss the fading cross) and in that instant he's in love.

The next morning, the three of them drive down to Tijuana in Chente's drummer's van for a late breakfast. They cross the border and park in a pay lot and find an open-air cafe near the plaza. Chente orders three plates of *chile rellenos* and an ice bucket of Coronas and tells Joey and Chavela that whatever they want is on him. "Anything, you guys. You name it. My treat."

"Good," says Joey, "I'll have lobster and *filet mignon* and a nice single malt scotch."

Chente laughs. "Do you even know what single malt scotch is, because I don't."

"No," says Joey, happily, "I guess . . . I guess I don't."

"Even better."

"Together in ignorance."

And they knock their beers together.

Joey takes his first sip of beer and then cuts through the breading of the *relleno* with his knife and fork and white cheese melts out the side and the steam hits his face and it's a revelation—he smells Spanish rice (garlic, pepper, cayenne, lime, onion) and he smells refried beans and cilantro and he knows he's somewhere new and all his spirit comes back and he feels strong and ready for anything. Across the table, Chente and Chavela look just as capable and it makes Joey feel safe and dangerous at the same time and it's a good feeling, the noise of the city swarming all around them, the hot gray grind of sky overhead. They eat then order more drinks and soon their hangovers are gone and they're in charge of their lives again. After breakfast, they get up from the table and Chente tips the price of the meal. In his pocket, a roll of hundreds, part of a six-grand signing bonus from the record label, paid in cash, an act of good faith. ("This is an act of good faith, Chente. You make me a record I can sell to all these hipsters . . . here and . . . all of them out there and present, future, etc, and Red Patent Records will bend over backwards for you. I saw you up there. Those kids . . . those kids *wanted* it. Whatever it was you had to sell them they were waiting for it. Look. What you . . . what you need in this business . . . and it is a business . . . is to make your shit worthwhile enough that kids'll pay the fifteen dollars to have access to your world for a while. That fifteen dollars doesn't come cheap to people, they work for it and they don't wanna part with it and they don't have . . . they don't have a lot of time but if you give them . . . if you *give* them what you had up there tonight, they'll buy into your world. You keep that up, year after year, and that's . . . it's damn near impossible, but you'll have a *career.* An act of good faith . . . now, go talk to her, but call me in the morning. First thing. Don't forget. An act of good faith! My flight's at nine. Don't flake on me, buddy.")

On the way out of the courtyard, Chente tips the *mariachi* band that played for them, then tips the waiter and the girl who brought the beer and then turns and goes back and tips the band again, happy and in love, dancing around the place, confident, proud, delirious; things are working; life is happening now; this is good; this is what you wanted.

It's a warm, overcast afternoon and all of Tijuana is out shopping and sitting in cafes and walking through markets with parrots in wooden cages and flies on slabs of pink meat and great bins of mangoes and misshapen, shriveled papayas. Walking past a boombox at a fruit stand, the singer singing (distant, staticky), *"Ay esa vieja tan rechismosa / Como le gusta chismografiar."* There are *vaqueros* in boots and straw ranch hats. Old men in white slacks and long, embroidered wedding shirts. The singer of a *narco* band (*Los Animales de Tijuana*) wanders through the stands, drunk and high, sweating, tired, looking for his drummer, singing along with the radio he's just passed, "*Y hay va enseguida todo a agrandar.*" Joey and Chavela and Chente walk past a table of watermelons and Chente says, "Big John's jellybeans" under his breath, pleased with himself, but pleased without ego, content and quiet in his place. Traffic rolls by (gridlocked), the smell of exhaust and bus fumes. A hotrod, classic car, low and red, the engine rumbling the ground all around them, revving, slow, but ready to peal out at a moment's notice. "Look," says Chente and he and Joey nod respectfully as it passes. "Bad ass," says Joey. Chente: "Bad fucking *ass.*" Kids hustle in the streets selling fake silver necklaces and pukka shell bracelets and boxes of Canel's gum, shouting, "*Chiclet!*" Tourist couples walk arm-in-arm with cameras around their necks, short pants, all-terrain sandals with Velcro straps, big Reebok sneakers from the '80s, t-shirts that say stubborn things, fanny-packs with an American flag and Hawaiian flower print, saggy necks like turkeys, big thighs, skinny white legs, sunburns, fake breasts, potbellies, big women, small men. Chente and Chavela pass right through them. Joey floats along in their wake. Drunk. All things good. In his mind, Joey says *Fuck you* to each person he walks past, joyous, *Fuck you*, harmless, *fuck you* without anger, a celebratory *fuck you*, full of love, *fuck you, fuck you, fuck you, and fuck you.* He imagines patting their heads as he walks past, *fuck you, fuck you*, bopping their heads, but nice, *fuck you, fuck you, fuck you.*

3:05 P.M.

They cut across the plaza and go into the wax museum. In the back rooms, the walls are built like catacombs—rows of stone skulls grinning out from cavern aches and the frowning mouths of tunnels. The wax statues—posed in cave rock alcoves lit with hidden bulb lights like lanterns—dark, sooty orange. "It's just like the Natural History Museum," says Chente happily. "I'll take you there, Chavy. Sometimes as part of . . . of, like, of one of the Meso-American exhibits, there's this old woman who sits in the lobby and makes corn tortillas."

"The tortilla lady," says Joey. "Totally! Do they still have her? I love her tortillas."

"Yeah, see, Joey knows. The tortilla lady. She makes them the old-fashioned way with a stone grinding bowl and you can buy them for a donation. They're tiny with a little bit of butter and maybe some lime juice."

Chavela smiles and snaps a Polaroid of Chente telling the story, grinning, hands in front of his face, patting out corn tortillas in the air.

They take more Polaroids. Picture #2 (3:35 p.m.): Joey posing with a frowning Cabrillo, holding Chavela's butterfly knife to the *conquistador's* wax throat. Picture #4: a family photo (taken by the museum janitor, Reni Duenas, forty-five, an ex-Federale) with Chente, Chavela, Joey, wax Cortés, and wax La Malinche (beautiful, braided) all in a proud, stern line. Picture #5 (3:48 p.m.): Chente stands in front of a frowning Ayatollah Kolmeni in a low boxer's stance, ready to knock his turban off if he says one word about Chavela.

It's dark and cool in the back rooms and soon Tijuana is no longer there. The caves are real caves. The wax bodies are ghosts, but they're ghosts frozen in time, and Chente and Chavela and Joey walk among them without trouble.

Before they leave, Chente and Chavela pose for one last picture (#8, 4:12 p.m.) standing in front of a witch. "A *bruja*," says Chavela. "My great-grandmother Morena, she was one but she wasn't all . . . all, like, *ugly* and fake *scary* like this. She was a woman of the *earth*, beautiful, and an eloquent letter writer. Chente, I should read you her letters. I have all of them in a box back home at my aunt's. Morena's husband Gustav, he fought in the Revolution. One day, the fight came to his own village and they rode in to defend it and Gustav was with Morena one last time, one last night, and that's when my grandmother and her twin sister were conceived. Huerta's troops . . . Victoriano Huerta, *El Chacal* . . . rode in the next morning and beat back the resistance. They hung the leaders and then they stood Gustav and his fellow soldiers up against the wall of the church and they shot them and made Morena and the rest of the women watch. After that they burned the whole village and raped and killed the women and took the children. Morena and the town potter were the only ones who survived. The potter lived by hiding inside his kiln as soon as the fighting started. He was a coward and one night someone walked into his new shop in the next town and shot him through the forehead and they found him the next morning, facedown in his clay. (He had made his own death mask.) Morena, she lived because she was so beautiful they refused to shoot her. That's what my grandma says anyway and I believe it." (The real story, long since lost: Gustav, Juan Rey Riviera (the baker) [the potter, Rudolfo de Nigris Guajardo, was killed in the skirmish], and Morena survived the battle by hiding in the kiln. Gustav was impotent and Rey Riviera was the true father of Morena's twins. Gustav killed Riviera when he found out a month later [facedown like the story, but in his dough] then died the next day in a shootout with Huerta's men. Shot through the cheek, left thigh, groin, and neck. Ears and genitalia cut off in celebratory desecration. Left in the desert, eaten by coyotes, only his skull and pieces of his left hand recovered, a decade later, a town mystery for weeks until the mystery was forgotten. Secrets die with the secret keepers.) The final picture: The wax *bruja* grinning terribly and stirring her cauldron with a gnarled, roped-together stick, and Chente and Chavela holding hands in front of her. Chente, his head tossed back and to the side, serious, fiercely proud. Chavela, her lip bruised and puffy, radiant and smiling.

5:30 P.M.

Driving back to the border they share a plastic bag of mango slices flavored with chili powder and lemon juice and they listen to a cassette tape Chente bought at the *Ramón, Ramón y Ramona* bootleg stand. "Vicente Fernandez is the king of *ranchera* music," Chente says. "When you're a kid like me without a dad, you need to look for men who you respect and then base yourself on the things they do well. This guy's the Mexican Johnny Cash. His music: You just have to listen."

Chente hits play on the car stereo and the music begins with a dramatic flourish of acoustic guitars and the singer half-singing, half-laughing, "*Hahai yai yia y-aaiiiiiiiiiii!*"

His voice is a deep opera tenor over trumpets and trombones, punctuated by bold, defiant guitar strums. "See, in this song he's beat down but *he's alive.* He's living and trying things out and . . . he's making mistakes. He's not . . . he's not, like, *sitting on the sofa* watching TV all day or playing around on the Internet. He's putting himself out there. He's living as . . . as an *antidote* to all the boredom and sadness and general class warfare bullshit they throw down on him. Listen to this line."

"Soy borrrrracho y trobador / Pero cuantos millonarios quisieran vivir mi vida?"

"What he's saying here is he's a drunk singer, a poor old vagabond . . . kinda Bukowski, Tom Waits, Miller, John Fante, hobo-deadbeat-sorta guy, but all the millionaires are jealous of him and want to live his life. Of course they can't, they *couldn't*. The rich men don't see how hard it is. They see the romance and that's all. Being poor's only . . . it's only romantic to people who . . . maybe they've been *broke* but they haven't been *poor*. There's a difference. If I could write a song this good . . . *agh* . . . just listen. Where's the tequila, Chavy?"

In the long line of cars waiting to cross the border, they pass a bottle of tequila that Chente picked up at a duty-free shop. Men walk past the van selling black and gold *sombreros* in stacks and *piñatas* and glass sailing ships with fishing line rigging. Chente and Chavela hold hands in the front seat and, in the back, all that Joey can think of is Maggie. *Tyler's Maggie*, he tells himself. In his head, he imagines walking through a crowded bar and in each seat at the counter are clones of himself hunched over their cocktails, depressed, hating everything, stabbing their limes and maraschino cherries with their straws, grumbling stupidly, thinking about Maggie, thinking about Maggie, thinking about Maggie, *Tyler's Maggie*. As he walks past them, he pats each one on the head and says, *Fuck you, fuck you, fuck you, fuck you-me, fuck you, Joey Carr, fuck you, Joey Carrs.*

Joey tells Chente to turn the tape up and, when he does, he hands Joey the tequila and Joey drinks.

KEARNY MESA, AFTERNOON

The next morning, Joey's phone rings and it's Rory and her voice is shaking and he knows something's wrong. "Joey, I've got something to tell you about Nicole," and he feels the air squeeze out of him. "Joey, I just . . . all I did was come over to see if she wanted to get coffee at Twiggs and I found her on the floor. The front door was open and *Wheel of Fortune* was starting."

What Rory heard when she walked through the door was the studio audience chanting "Wheel!" and then "Of!" but before they got to "Fortune!" Rory saw Nicole's bare legs sticking out from behind the kitchen counter.

Nicole died in the ambulance on the way to the hospital while Rory rode along in the front seat, calling Nicole's mom and brother over and over again. "Joey, I kept getting their voicemail. I didn't know what to say. I just asked them to call me back. They never did. I guess they heard from the hospital. The driver just . . . he, like, he sat next to me, going *so fast,* running all the lights on the way to the hospital. He never said anything to me. I looked at him and I couldn't believe he *ever* said anything. Like, to *anyone*. When we got to the ER and he finally turned to me and said, 'We're here,' his voice was so loud it was like being slapped in the face. I *felt* it. I felt the physical force of his *voice*. Like he grabbed my chin with one hand and slapped me full-on across the face with the other."

The paramedics shocked Nicole's heart back to life but she died again. They shocked her once more and then she was alive, and this time she hung on. After he heard from Rory, Joey drove as fast as he could to the hospital, then sat with Nicole in the room and held her hand. It was a child's hand, no grip, dirt under her nails. Nicole's mouth was ringed in black from the charcoal they gave her when her stomach was pumped. She looked small. She wasn't Nicole anymore, but when she opened her eyes, she was back. Joey could see the light that made her Nicole Alexandra Hale fading in her eyes; he would say something to her ("You thirsty?") and it would flicker back again; she'd try to talk ("Does my dad know?") and it would go dull.

Later, when Nicole's brother came, Joey walked through the sun-lit halls of the hospital and then out the sliding doors and down the smooth, even sidewalk, and then he was in his truck and then his head was on the steering wheel. It was him, but it wasn't him. It was him sitting in his seat staring out at the row of bright red hibiscus that lined the parking lot, and it wasn't him crying. It was him punching his steering wheel, and it wasn't him with bleeding knuckles. Joey sat in his car and he thought about her voice and the last words she said to him before he left: "I've had enough." She told him that as soon as they let her out, she was going to try it again. "You need to let this one go, Joey." Her breath smelled like a rotting animal. "Let it go," she said. Joey held Nicole's hand and he tried to convince her she had reasons to live, but she said he was just a kid who hadn't learned anything. "I don't want to keep doing this," she said. "It gets harder every year; just think how hard it will be when we're *old*. Oh my god, Joey. I can't *do* this anymore." Joey looked up to see her brother, eighteen and a man now, standing in the doorway, leaning against the frame.

A WEEK LATER

Chente and Joey sit at the bar counter at Tobacco Rhoda's and drink shots of tequila. "I remember how it was with my friend Morales," Chente says, his voice soft and low. "He tried to do it and I felt like he'd actually done it. It was just as bad."

"What was it?"

"The same. Pills and booze, and I don't think that works for *anybody*. A couple weeks later, I was in Calexico for my cousin Fudo's wedding and when I was gone, Morales tried it again and this time he did it—did it. Morales . . . he shot himself with his dad's gun. His dad was . . . he *is* . . . he still is . . . a cop. I didn't hear until later, after I got back, and I didn't get to see the funeral and I was . . . I was *pissed off* that he was already *gone* and I couldn't say . . . you know, *one last thing* to him. It wouldn't even matter what that thing was. It just felt . . . it was *unfair* that there was no way I'd ever be able to say *anything* to my friend again. My friend who was once such a big part of . . . I mean, I saw him *every single day* for years. We lived down the street from each other, so if it wasn't at school, I saw him *after* school. I saw him sitting on his porch playing guitar with his uncle Titi the welterweight boxer and I saw him at the Benito Arcade and I saw him playing soccer at the old middle school. My friend Jose Morales was *there*." He stabs the bar-top with the tip of his finger. "He was *there*. I didn't have to work to find him, and then he was so far gone he was off limits to me. *Forever*. That's why I'll never believe in god. No . . . no benevolent god would make a world where you lived just to *die*, where it ends badly for everyone no matter how good a person you are. It's an *insult* because you spend all this time becoming a better person. You learn and you grow and you do all these things to make yourself smarter. You pick up languages or you read books or you learn job skills; you get *good* at things and you store up all this information and history and experience, and after all that hard work . . . after *all* that hard work, this great thing you've become is just *tossed* into the ground and your life is over in an instant. It's over so fast you don't even get to *know*. I always joke around and say '*Que viva Satanas*' and write '666' on things and say I love the devil, but I don't believe in the devil, *either*. I just believe so *steadfastly* against the existence of god that I don't care what I say. I can say I love Satan. I can say I'll take a shit on Jesus's head. And I can say that because I don't believe in *any* of it. I don't think *anyone* believes. Why are so-called *believers* so upset when someone they love dies? Isn't that person in the best, happiest, magicalest place in the universe? Shouldn't they *rejoice* death? Shouldn't they be like, 'He got *lucky*. He found his way home and I'll be there someday too'? No, they feel just as bad about death as nonbelievers do. Death is awful and no one can deal with it no matter what they say and we drum up all . . . all sorts of *ideas* and *tricks* and, like, *myths* to make it seem less awful. When I . . . when I got back and found out about Morales, his mom Beti she told me, 'Doan worry, *mijo*. God had a *plan* for taking our José up to Heaven. God has big *plans* for José. God needs him for something *big*. It all happens for a *reason*. It was God's will.' God's will? If I ever doubted that I was an atheist that was the moment I reaffirmed my . . . my *dis*belief. If God's big plan for my friend José Morales was to 'take him up to heaven' and the way he took him was to make him *so profoundly sad* and *so desperate* he had to end his own *life* . . . if God's *plan* was taking him while he was at his darkest, most *devastated* hour and letting his *last fucking seconds*, his last fucking *memory*, his last *anything* be in total abject *horror*, then *fuck* god. No, *José Morales* took José Morales away. The shitty circumstances of José Morales' life took him away. Not god. God never did *anything*. There's no big spiritual reasons for . . . oh *shit* . . . shit, I'm sorry, *carnal*. I'm making this about me. I'm sorry. I think . . . yeah, you hit a nerve there," (laughing, but a sad laugh, tired) "I'm sorry. Hey, tell me about . . . tell me about what's happening right now with her. Have you seen her since the hospital?"

"She isn't answering her phone."

"I wouldn't, either."

"Why? I don't—"

"After that, I'd wanna lay low for a while and not have everybody I was around *thinking* about it all the time even if they weren't saying anything. You wouldn't be able to look people in the *eye*."

"I guess that makes sense."

"I don't think you should worry. You know me and Nicole never got along, but she's strong. She's a tough fucking girl."

"Yeah, I guess, but every time I call and she's not there I start thinking she's done it again. Rory hasn't heard from her, either, which makes it even worse. I drove past her house a few times. Once I stopped by. Knocked on the door. Waited. Jiggled the screen. Tried to see in. I don't know what to do."

"I'll tell you what you do, *carnal*." Chente nods at the bartender and she brings two more shots, full to the top.

"This one's on me, boys," says the bartender. "I overheard you talking. This one's on your Filipino fairy godmother. You feel better, alright?"

"Thanks, Lela," Chente nods. "Joey, you do *this*."

In the morning, Joey sits and reads his old City College textbooks. The *Your Golden State Studies* book. A list of California cities and missions named by Spanish priests, by region, south to north. The history of the mission at San Juan Bautista. The bandit Joaquin Murrieta hiding his gold in the tree by Camp Palomar; his head cut off and kept in a glass jar, pickled, on display. (Joey stares up at the ceiling and sees Murrieta's black hair swirling around his face, his eyes dead and white and his mouth gaped open.) He reads about Chinese immigrants in San Francisco and railroad camps and the killing of the Cauhilla Indian Juan Diego in front of his wife in 1883. He stares at an illustration of three native women, hair braided, kneeling at the top of Green Valley Falls, working holes into the stone to grind their acorns. But as soon as he stops to rest his eyes he sees Nicole.

Joey sits at home and then he sits at work and then he sits at Chente's, and Nicole hasn't called. He drives by her place again and it's dark inside. Knock. Shake the door handle. Knock again. Ring the buzzer over and over again. Wait on the stoop. Nothing. The steaming pavement after the rain as he walks back to his truck. Driving down University, and a sign twirler on the corner dancing to the music on his Discman and tossing his sign up above him, hands outstretched, catching it and dipping low to take the shock, rising back up again, playing the sign like an electric guitar, knees bent, leaning back, *wailing*. Light through the screen door at Chente's with *mariachi* music thumping through the wall and the smell of meat frying. Light through a row of brown beer bottles on Chente's window sill, one of them full of cigarette butts and ash.

In the park across the street from the old trolley deli, Joey listens to the sound of the sprinklers and pulls up fistfuls of grass until his wrists hurt and he stares at the clouds and he thinks about everything he can so he doesn't have to think about Nicole. He digs his switchblade into the soil and puts his mind on a (mindless) encyclopedic treadmill. He thinks about the landslides up in Malibu and why they happen. He thinks about Chente's bottlecap collection and tries to remember the name of the German beer Chente's been raving about since Christmas. He thinks about film crews and rattlesnakes (*where do they keep their poison?*) and *Pop Up Video* and god-awful skateboard art and muscle cars and Japan and boxing movies and CIA operatives and Tyler's lucky twenty-sided dice (*die? twenty-sided die?*) and plastic dog shit (*smells like nothing, like carpet*). He thinks about scratch-and-sniff stickers (strawberry, chocolate), Anza Borego, Palm Springs, Go-Bots, Thundercats, red glass, elf shoes with bells on the toes. He shuts his eyes and thinks about the tide pools at the Point, all the still life and cold, clear water. He thinks about the red clay tennis courts in North Park (so smooth, *impeccable*) and the red sunburnt skin of his uncle's balding head and the rainbow in the mist of the sprinklers across the grass from him. He keeps his thoughts tidy and full but then he slips up. He thinks about her. He thinks about her gone and then he thinks about her here again—alive but unwilling. She's slipped off the face of the Earth. Not in some reckless, torrential mess of a landslide but on her own volition. Her choice. Free will. But your choices aren't truly your own when people love you and you have to act in accordance. Or not. Sometimes you have to be selfish.

That night when the dinner shift is over, Joey and Tyler change out of their work clothes in the employee locker room. Tyler—happy and humming to himself and cracking jokes about Cosby sweaters and planes crashing (What did the rabbi do in his final six minutes? "He said, 'Ah, such is life,' and he broke *all* the windows! Get it?!") and Joey—listening, flat-lined, going through the motions.

"Joey, that was funny, right? You get it, don't you? He broke *all* the windows?"

"Yeah, I . . . no, I get it. It's funny."

"I dunno, *I* thought it was. Joey . . . you know . . . what we need?"

"Tyler, I don't know. I really—"

"I think you *knnnnnow* what we need."

Joey unbuttons his shirt and sets it in the locker. He pulls his undershirt off and drops it on the bench. As he looks up he sees himself in the mirror by the showers. Work pants and a belt. Shirtless. Rib bones and a humped spine. Face like a piece of white meat and eyes like black coins. The head turns and the coins stare at him. They're not coins. Holes. Black holes that go in for miles. Two boundless tubes you could thread a rope into, infinite. He looks away and the eyes are gone.

Tyler grins and makes a pyramid with his fingers and taps them together. "Joey, *I think you know,*" he sings. He shuffles his feet in a little dance. "You know. I know you know. You're gonna be calling me brilliant in about thirty seconds. Counting down. One, two, three, four, five, six—"

"I don't. Seriously." Joey pulls off his belt and lets his pants drop to the floor. "Seriously, *I don't,*" he mutters. He steps out of his pants and kicks them to the side.

"Okay, fine, even if you don't *know* you know, you *know* you know."

"Okay. Fine. What, *what do we need*?" Joey grabs his t-shirt out of the locker and pulls it over his head and rubs deodorant into his armpits and then slams the locker door.

"Vegas," Tyler grins, raising his eyebrows. "*Laaaas Vegas,*" he says with a nod. "You remember last time . . . aka the funnest weekend of my life."

"I have to work."

"Not every day you don't."

"*Pretty much*."

"Not every day."

"Tyler, I'm not in the *mood* for—"

"Vegas," Tyler says, crossing his arms in front of him and stomping his foot like a child. "Vegas," stomp, "Vegas," stomp, "Vegas, Vegas, Vegas," stomp. Tyler stops and narrows his eyes and waits for Joey's reaction. He does the shuffling dance again and puts his arms out and gives a big shaky grin.

And then it's too much for Joey and he's smiling, despite his best efforts not to. "Vegas. I think you're right. I think we need Vegas."

"No. You don't *think* . . . you *know*."

"I *know* we need Vegas." Now Joey can't stop smiling.

"Great! Vegas: Part Two, Journey into the Unknown. Me and you and a long weekend at the Circus Circus."

"Circus," Joey says.

"Circus Circus Circus Circus Circus."

"Circus Circus Circus."

"Circus," Tyler says with a note of finality, snapping his fingers. "We should get," whispering, looking around, smiling like a bad child, "*some crystal from Curt*."

"We could do that. Ask him. I'll go halfsies."

"Joey Carr and Tyler Monahan, up against the world yet again! The buddy cop movie to end all buddy cop movies! It's settled. Let's do this! When?"

"When should we go? This weekend. Friday."

"Good. I'll drive." Tyler shuts his locker carefully and turns the dial on the Masterlock (12, 13, 10).

"It's a plan. We could," a pause, "we could . . . I mean . . . maybe bring Maggie," pause, "maybe."

He says this as a question. He says it and it hangs in the air (three-and-a-half seconds). It hangs and then Tyler says, "Sure," but Joey still feels it hanging.

INTERSTATE 15 NORTH, 2 P.M.

Maggie in the rearview mirror, leaning against the car door, staring out the window. She's dyed her hair dark red since Joey last saw her and it blows around her face when she rolls down the window. Joey finds himself noticing new things about her that make his heart race. She's so small and soft back there and (arrogantly, and without regard to how strong she really is) Joey decides it's his duty to protect her and make her life as peaceful and easy as possible. *Maggie*. Desert going by in a bleached-out flash. Sand. Miles of barbed wire. As they pass the World's Tallest Thermometer at the Mad Greek diner in Baker the temperature reads 112. "Wow, *one-twelve*," Joey says and points at it through the window. Tyler nods and says nothing. Joey's voice barely there above the road noise, a sound washed out by sound. When he hears it come out of his mouth, it sounds like someone else. The song on the car stereo swings like a pendulum through its verses, quiet and dark and rhythmic, the singer singing, "Travel-ing swallow-ing Drama-mine!" It's Maggie's tape, her mixtape she made for the trip; side B, a collection of songs, side A, one band, this whole record, her favorite. Joey looks into the backseat. "One-twelve," he says again. Maggie and Jed sit up in their seats and look out the back window at the thermometer as it sinks into the landscape behind the car. Jed is Tyler's cousin he's only met twice. Jed Dickinson—a 16-year-old towhead from Laguna Beach, dressed in mall clothes, holding a kid's lunchbox full of weed and GHB. (Jed was sent to San Diego for the month to "visit family." The real reason is that Jed's father Marty is seeing someone new and he doesn't want his son to know. Jed's mother Nancy was killed in a very minor car accident in January and Jed doesn't talk much anymore. He smokes weed and he stares at the ground and thinks of his mother's voice and when he's home he plays endless video games and hides in his bedroom and listens to Slayer [he sits in his room and says "Slayer" to himself in a death metal voice, "Slaaaaayer, Slaaaaaaaaaaayer," deeper each time, but it doesn't sound tough and it makes him feel sad]. He's quit eating. He's looking for a way out. Passively, but looking nonetheless. In his [anonymous] LiveJournal he types, "July 3rd, 1999. I'm 16 today. If I'm still alive in two years, I'm joining the Navy. If I can't kill myself, I'll find someone to do it in a war. I just want to *scream* right now.") Jed and Maggie sit together, quiet. Their eyes silvery, narrowed against the sun. Jed's smoking a joint. He hands it to Maggie but she shakes her head no and he smiles sadly and looks back out the window. Maggie's wearing a white t-shirt with the Union Jack flag on the front. She has on skin-tight gray jeans with the knees busted out, a wrist full of rubber bracelets, and no shoes. Joey studies this until he can see her when he looks away.

2:27 p.m.

Motorhomes and semi-trucks block out the sun as they pass Tyler's car. Big-rigs carrying artichokes and grapes, hogs and cattle seeing the world for the first and last time. Maggie—staring out the window at a truckload of slaughterhouse cows. Tears are running down her face. No one sees this but Joey. She's there in the rear-view mirror and then she looks up and her eyes meet his and hers are wet green and red and hurt. He looks out his window and decides to quit eating meat once and for all. He stares and fights back the tears. An empty stretch of highway. Flat expanse of sand and rock. Mirage streams on the road that are nothing once they catch up to them.

"What's this band?" Joey asks, leaning into the backseat. An excuse to look at her. She tells him but she says it so quietly that he has to read her lips. "I've never heard anything like this." Maggie nods and smiles and Joey feels younger and taller. "This is really good."

2:45 p.m.

Desert. Baked-out trailers. Outlet malls. A cluster of gas stations like circled wagons. An abandoned diner with gray windows knocked through by rocks leaving black holes the size of fists—an old tire propped up against the front door, a sign above the diner that reads 'EAT'. A highway patrol motorcycle moves through traffic like a small shark.

2:46 p.m.

Joey uncaps the nail polish remover from his bag and huffs it until his teeth float in his gums and then he's lightheaded and the sound woozes in around him and his lunch starts to come up.

"Pull over! Tyler! Quick!"

"Huh?"

"Pull! Over!"

Tyler pulls onto the side of the road and Joey climbs out and vomits as the dust rises up around him. A splash of yellow on rock and sand with grainy curdles of egg and tortilla and the dust red and thick. He wipes his mouth as his eyes burn and defocus. A flattened beer can. Dust in his eyes. Pieces of broken glass pressed into the dirt like green and brown windows looking out from the earth.

Tyler gets out and urinates by the barbed wire fence and they share a can of beer on the side of the road until Joey feels better.

"Okay. Sorry. I think I'm ready now. Party foul."

"Here, take this. You'll feel better."

Tyler gives Joey a Vicodin and he drinks it down with the beer and they get back in the car and drive.

"Thanks. Ugh. That really hurt coming up."

Jed hands him a joint and he takes it and drags on it until his lungs are full of smoke. He holds it in as long as he can, and then he lets it out and turns up the stereo and he's instantly stoned. The desert. Everything cooled down now. His lips numb and he shivers and the music chimes slow and dark. It's the same band. The band Maggie loves. Her favorite and his favorite too. A shuffle of toms and shakers, a lazy chiming guitar, the singer singing mush-mouthed, lisping, tired, weary, "The custom concern for the people / Build up their mon-u-ments and steeples to weaaaaaar out our eyes / I get up just about *noon* / My *head* sends a message for me to reach for my shoes and then waaalk / Gotta go to work! / Gotta go to work! / Gotta have a jjjob."

Joey turns back to Maggie. The sun is setting. The tangerine light in her hair. Her skin death-white and her eyes hazel. She smiles at him but her eyes smile first and he feels it coming and he gets the chills. The music slow-plotting. Two guitars like twin braids of rope, one chiming, one a bottleneck slide, weaving around each other over the drums, and the singer singing, "Goes through the parking lot fields / Didn't see no signs that they would yield and then *fought* / This'll never end this'll never end this'll never . . . stop / Message read on the bathroom wall says, 'I don't feel at all like I thought' / And now we're losing all touch, losing all touch / Building a desert."

"This song," she nods, and her smile flows over him like dark, warm, muddy water.

LAS VEGAS

Las Vegas city limits—casinos on the horizon. The strip and then the hotel room. Snorting lines off the TV top. Drinking tequila and smoking speed, sitting on the bed laughing. Joey lying in the bathtub with one of the beds' yellow coverlets over him talking to Maggie for hours while she sits on the counter, swinging her crossed legs. Intense talks. Talks about everything. Family, death, marriage, birth, sickness, work, divorce, money. Serious, hard, sad, slow-building, then the funniest thing in the world, the kind of joke you'd never get in a sitcom or a movie.

Black sky outside with stars. Headlights blur in neon tube streaks seen from the overpass. The sun rising over the desert. Cars jiggle fast-forwarding in traffic on the freeway exit. Hotel doors open and shut. Bodies flood into casinos and then gush back out again, and two days are gone, a hot afternoon in the hotel room. Tyler—in the bathroom, rummaging through Maggie's makeup bag. Jed—sprawled out in the easy chair by the window mixing up GHB with

Evian and red food coloring. Maggie and Joey on opposite beds. Jed divides it up into Evian bottles. Joey holds it up to the light. It looks like blood. "It looks like *blood*," he tells Jed.

4:01 P.M.

The day slows to a crawl. All the sound in the city coming in through the windows. Mothers fuss with babies outside in the pool area. A sunburnt little boy shouts, "Look mom, look, look!" then cannonballs into the water with a great vertical splash. Joey hears voices in the lobby. ("Checkout tomorrow? No problem sir, I just need to see a major credit card," "Is American Express okay? Oh wait, you have my Visa, right?" "Uh huh." Across the lobby: "Ma'am, *ma'am*, over here, please," the concierge, tired, hating his life, proud and contemptuous.) Joey hears voices on the strip, in the casinos, in card rooms, diners, buffet lines ("Shrimp on pizza, *grrrrross*"), a coffeehouse ("Large mocha, um, shot of mint or peppermint or whatever you have." "Extra shot of espresso?" "Yeah, please. Thanks."), a chapel on the interstate, a mile away, three miles, six, ten, twenty. A scratchy voice over a drive-thru intercom says, "Welcome to McDonald's. May I help you?" Joey hears a lawnmower cutting grass in Reno and the back and forth slap of a father and son playing catch in Barstow. He hears two people having grunting pig-like sex in a bedroom and a wild squeal as the guy comes into the girl. He hears the ticking sound of a truck engine cooling in the Mad Greek parking lot and the sleepy murmur of the ocean back in California. He hears nothing. The dull roar. The TV. The air conditioner. He comes out of it sweating and sits up and laughs, scratching his face.

TWO DAYS LATER, BACK HOME

Joey on the phone talking to Rory: "The problem was Tyler wouldn't take his dose. He refused."

"Oh, bad, bad Tyler."

"He'd been awake since we got there and now he was drawing warpaint or whatever on his face with Maggie's makeup in the bathroom and snorting lines off the counter."

"Hahaha! Whoa, dude. I love Tyler."

"I stood there in the bathroom doorway and watched him and Tyler looked up and smiled but the smile . . . it was bad, Rores. It was all, like . . . *crooked* and his eyes were twitchy and they were, like, gross jaundice *yellow*. On each cheek he'd drawn a red lightning bolt with a blue one below it. It actually looked kinda cool.

"I always thought Tyler looked like *Aladdin Sane* Bowie."

"Yeah, he did, he does . . . I was . . . I was like, 'Tyler . . . Tyler, what are you *doing*?' and he said, 'Getting dressed to go out.' 'We're staying in.' 'I'm getting ready.' 'For what?' 'I don't know yet.' 'You alright?' 'Joey, here, one for me, one for you,' and he offered me a line and a rolled-up twenty, but it was like, no way, dude. Like, you're kinda *ruining* it for me, know what I mean?"

"Totally."

"I go back in the room and Maggie's lying in bed and Jed's smoking a joint and he offers me some and I'm like, 'Hell *yeah*,' and I take a hit. And then I hear the sound of the toilet flushing and Tyler comes out of the bathroom, his face covered in warpaint, a purple line down the center of his forehead, a blue dot on his chin. He's all sketchy and, like . . . *distracted* and all *jittery* and he's looking for something on top of the dresser. Maggie sits up in bed and she's like, 'Tyler, *whoa*. You look like you're in *Cats*.' 'It's warpaint,' he says, grumble grumble grumble, and he's pacing in front of the beds, all wound-up and shit. He has his glass pipe in one hand and he's tapping it against his hip. I'm like, 'Tyler, we'll go out later tonight. Okay? Change the channel and let's find a movie,' or something like that. And then, suddenly, there's this . . . this, like, huge ball of *fire*—"

"Dude. Whaaat?"

"—And Tyler has got Maggie's hairspray and a lighter in his hands and there's this burning torch blowing out in front of him and leaping back in again and the smoke alarm's going off!"

"No way. Hahahaha. Tyler's insane!"

"It wasn't very funny at the time. We're all freakin' out and Tyler's . . . he's standing by the TV holding the hairspray and the lighter, his eyes super big and he's . . . like, he's shrugging and grinning and frowning all at the same time, just all over the place, and he's like, 'No, no, it's, no, it's okay! *Hairspray torch,* it's okay!' and the smoke alarm's going off in the hallway and we're . . . we're fucking *scared,* as you might imagine. We're losing our shit. Jed starts hiding the drugs and I'm shoving things into the dresser and Maggie's just sitting there in bed staring at Tyler in disbelief."

"What hap—I mean, what was the *torch* all about?"

"He was trying to clean his pipe. Trying to burn out all the black residue. Which, of course, didn't work."

"What a loon. I love Tyler."

"Finally, Tyler tells us he's going to go out and, get this, knock on all the doors and tell everyone there's nothing to worry about, that it was aaaall a false alarm. Right? We, of course, talk him down from that and then he decides he's going to go out and buy *crack* and Maggie's like, 'Stop being a maniac,' and Tyler's tweaking out of his mind and pretty drunk and he's talking a mile a minute, 'No, it's okay, fine, it's fine, it's a false alarm' and then he gets going on pizza, 'I'm going to go get a pizza—a *pizza*—somewhere and bring it back and I'll buy some crack in the lobby from somebody's mother who's in town to watch the two men who have white tigers and do tricks with them and possibly, maybe, yeah, possibly magic tricks, illusions . . . funny things too,' and he waves his glass pipe at Maggie like a magic wand."

Rory laughs happily. "Oh *Tyler Monahan!* That sounds just like him. I can see him doing that."

"Maggie's like, 'Tyler, chill out. You're not going to buy *crack* in the lobby. You've never even *seen* crack. Stop acting crazy. Anyway, whatever, you *hate* pizza' which is true but he won't give it up. He keeps saying, 'Crack in the lobby, crack in the lobby,' over and over again and then he's distracted by a bag of spilled Doritos on the floor and squats down and picks up each chip, dropping them, one by one, back into the bag and he says, 'Some of these are stepped on,' really quietly and sad. Then he stands back up again. 'No, no, okay . . . no crack buying but a *pizza*. What toppings? Meat lovers, Hawaiian, mushrooms, bell peppers, extra cheese, black olives, vegetarian for Maggie, sun-dried tomatoes, red onions, Canadian bacon, Italian sausage?' and without waiting for an answer he grabs Maggie's sunglasses off the bureau-thing-or-whatever and he's out the door. Maggie and I both shout, 'Tyler!' at the same time but the door slams and he's gone and as soon as he's gone the alarm shuts off and I just, like, fell back in bed, *exhausted*."

Rory laughing over the phone. "*Duuuude*."

BACK IN LAS VEGAS, TWO DAYS EARLIER

When Tyler's gone, Jed mixes up another round of GHB. Joey turns the TV to a PBS nature documentary ("PBS is the only thing worth watching, you guys") and Jed lights a cigarette and gives it to Maggie and then lights one for Joey, and Joey sits on the edge of the bed and stares at the screen. He takes a drag. It's a show about beavers narrated by a famous tennis player from the 1980s. Beavers sleeping in their dams. Beavers in green, murky ponds, fish flitting around them in tinsely curtains. Beavers swimming up from hidden dens to the surface to take a breath, and Joey is high, and then he's falling asleep and then he's awake and laughing and he's nodding off again and he's back earlier in the day.

It was noon and they'd just left the strip and wandered into a casino to have a look around. Tyler, on speed, leading the way, stomping forward, singing the theme from *Annie,* ducking into bathrooms and passways to drink the tequila in his messenger bag. Maggie and Joey walking together, Jed trailing behind, stoned and mute and drifting. "The sun'll come *out* to-mor-row / Bet your bottom dollar that tomor*row* / There'll be *sun*!" Tyler—racing up ahead as they stood on a moving sidewalk passing through an African rainforest with piped-in jungle noise and a trickling stream and twin white tigers pacing behind the glass.

Joey looked at Maggie and shook his head and they laughed. “I feel like we should make a video of this to show him when he’s sane again.”

“No way, he’d love it.”

“I guess I’ve never seen him this bad.”

“Oh, Joey, you just wait. He’ll get worse.”

“Worse?”

“He’s on his way down.”

“Down?”

“To the very bottom.”

“Of what?”

“You’ll see.”

“He’s always so—”

“Composed?”

“Yeah.”

“This is the real Tyler Monahan. Campy and weird and totally insane. You should feel lucky. It’s like seeing a rare white rhino.”

“A tiger. White tiger.”

“Haha, yeah.”

“Right. Wow.”

“Joey, I’m glad you’re not being all kookoo-times like that.”

“He kinda takes the fun out of it.”

“Joey . . . I bet people who . . . y’know, people who see us think we’re together.”

“You think so?”

“I mean, Jed’s like *four years old* and so stoned he can’t even *see,* much less engage anyone in meaningful conversation. Tyler’s turned into, what, the campy psychedelic Big Bird or something. But me and you, we’re kind of dressed alike. We’re not acting all stupid and manic. We’re on the same page. We *fit*.”

“Yeah, we—”

“I think it’s pretty funny.”

“Funny. Yeah.”

Funny killed the mood.

The moving sidewalk let them off into the casino’s main room and they walked into the frantic wall of slot machine noise and cigarette smoke and flashing lights.

Joey comes to in the hotel room sitting on the edge of the bed in front of the TV and hears himself say, “Knowahmean?” The beaver documentary is over and the TV screen shows the skyline of downtown San Francisco—fog creeping over the bay, the Golden Gate Bridge.

“Totally,” says Jed, slowly, sitting sideways in a Lay-Z-Boy, legs draped over the arm of the chair, eyes glassy and lidded. “I was at the lodge at Squaw the first time I heard it. I was like, *Sausalito*? That's a *city*? I thought it was a delicious *cookie*."

"Uh huh," says Maggie on the other bed. "I wish we had those cookies right now."

The room is quiet again. Breeze blows the drapes with a billowing wave. Maggie lies in the bed, sheet pulled over her, her back to Joey, the curve from her shoulders to waist to hips silhouetted in the light of the window.

8 P.M.

When Tyler gets back to the room, everyone's up and ready to go out. Jed smoking a joint in the chair by the window and leafing through the Gideon Bible, reading passages out loud. Maggie going through Tyler's messenger bag looking for her missing eyeliner. Joey drinking a beer, showered and dressed up as cool as he can to impress Maggie.

Tyler opens the door, walks in the room. No one looks up.

Jed: (reading aloud, a low mumble) "'And we know that God causes everything to work together for the good of those who love God and are called according to his purpose for them.'"

Tyler, makeup smeared, tired, carrying two pizza boxes and a paper bag of breadsticks. "Pizza Hut delivery."

Maggie, Joey: (simultaneous) "Hey." "Jinx," mumbles Joey from behind his magazine (*Us Weekly*). He turns the page to see a famous model walking out of a Starbucks with her kids.

Jed: "Hey." Takes a drag off his joint, lets it out, coolly. Gives Tyler a wary look.

Tyler: (setting the pizza boxes down on the dresser, standing in front of Joey) "I'm—"

Joey: "It's okay."

Tyler: "You—"

Joey: "Don't worry." He sets the magazine down on end-table and sits up in bed, cross-legged. "It's cool."

Tyler: "Okay."

Joey: "Yeah."

Tyler: "Yeah." Tyler goes into the bathroom and comes out eight minutes later with the makeup washed off, his face scrubbed pink, carrying the baggie of speed and the glass pipe. "Yeah?" He offers it to Joey.

Joey: "No thanks."

Tyler: "Sure?"

Joey: "No, I don't—sure. Yeah, sure."

Joey flicks the lighter and runs the flame in slow circles along the bottom of the pipe's bowl. When the speed begins to liquefy and turn to smoke, he sucks on the glass stem and pulls the smoke into his lungs. Holding it in, he looks around the room as his face tightens up. On the clock radio next to the bed, a song plays and Tyler tries to sing along as he cuts a line on top the TV, "Doh-ohn't stop be-lieee-ving! Do do do dooo. Hold on to your *something* something." Joey lets the smoke out of his lungs and falls back on the bed still holding the pipe, and watches the ceiling fan spin circles above him.

1979

JUNE 30TH

It's been a while. This past year was one long train of twelve-hour days and when you're that close to the grindstone for that long, you lose track of yourself. Labor and action beats the ego out of you and maybe that's a good thing. You're occupied from waking to sleep and the lack of leisure means you have no time for introspection. The harder things are, the less you want to feel, and then you wake up one morning and you realize you've anesthetized yourself as a defense mechanism. It's medication and self-sabotage, all in one.

I'm twenty years old, but I feel like an old man. In school, each new thing was a revelation. When I was seventeen, I would come back to my dorm and take out my notebook and I couldn't *wait* to get it all down on paper and relive what I'd done, to re-experience the intensity of what I'd seen earlier. I felt everything so much more. Every sensation was groundbreaking. Now long blocks of time go by without me knowing the days were there to begin with. Weeks leaving no impression. My only consolation is the boy. Half-a-year old now and he gives me something to come home to.

I can see how people disappear (socially) once they have kids. Why *not* spend all your time with this wonderful thing you've made, this little creature that makes you feel less worried about your own stupid path—why not? Parties, work, friends, road trips, school, concerts, bars: The rest doesn't stack up. It's a case of greater than/less than and I can't find much of a pro argument for the opposition. I could sit with him all day and enjoy every laugh and smile, every little attempt at being a man, every grasp toward something bigger.

His mom and I hardly talk. I leave for work at six and (because I "believe" in what we're doing and because I want to be seen as "committed") I'm home by nine at the earliest. Weekends, too. The paper doesn't shut down until the issue is put to bed and those of us who give a damn stay until it's right. It's worse when you're an editor. The writers can walk away. We're the ones who do the heavy lifting. It's thankless, but there's something satisfying about the behind-the-scenes work. After a hard day on the job you get the same kind of tired as when you've been out running or playing baseball all day. The old high-school sports kid in me likes that. The mental transcends itself and becomes physical. You use your brain all day and your whole body hurts.

When I'm away from my desk, I feel guilty. And why? I know the paper isn't my paper. It's a job and it will be someone else's job after I'm gone with little or no affect (or record) of my time. Still, it's been worked into me that a lack of vigilance is bad character. What I've learned is that the best you can be is a workhorse. It's a noble thing. The strong, competent machine without sense of self.

Just the same: What's the measure of a man who knows he's a lever or a *gear* but won't act to change his position in life? Isn't the ideal course a steady rise in station? Ascendancy versus stasis?

I'm at a loss for truth, but I'm making money. I provide for my wife and the boy, and now that Channy's pregnant again, the solace of being capable is a good one. We live in La Jolla with a nice view of the sea. We eat out in fancy restaurants (when I'm home) and she and the boy have the clothes they want and our cars run and when they don't run, they're fixed by someone who knows their job. I hold on to that through the big news days, the nights when my eyes ache, the fights with Channy, the times when I miss Sorel's warm body. And the numbers of the calendar blur until I'm not sure they're numbers anymore.

It's summer now and I'm resolving to check in with myself and get this notebook going again. Some part of me knows that this is important, that identity is a crucial thing and making money is not enough. (I truly believe that as soon as you stop looking for yourself, you get old, but for this past year I've been a face in the mirror and a trusty set of hands and nothing but.) It feels as if I'm losing the part of me that once saw life as a game to beat. In the mirror, the face I see has aged. I went years without seeing a change. Haircuts came and went and summer tans faded away, but this weekend I saw myself passing in a shop window and my face was someone else's. It was harder, longer. I need to get up and—

JULY 1ST

Didn't finish that last one. It was noon and I was sitting on the back deck with my feet on the railing and the ocean was shimmering and the sun was on my face and my thoughts were coming in clear and strong and then Channy was behind me.

"Can you hold him while I fix his lunch?"

"Of course. Yeah, of course."

The boy is everything.

I got up and stuck the notebook in my work satchel and went inside and he was in his jump-up chair and I knelt down and he smiled the biggest open-mouth smile you've ever seen, and my heart was set right.

The boy looks at me with the purest love and he has an optimism that makes me want to fight for him until I can't anymore. His little bald head and the wisps of dark hair swept up around it, his blue eyes that are like some gemstone undiscovered.

I pulled the boy up out of his seat and walked around the house with him in my arms, and he held onto me and babbled his gah's and gee's and ah-goo's and a-yay-yay-yay's, and I could feel the goodness coming from him like the warmth of the sun. When I'm away from him, it's like I've stopped taking some vital medication. He's wholesome and I feel thinner inside when we're apart.

It scares me to think of the future he has ahead and that one day I won't be strong enough to protect him. The world is turning into something I don't want to be part of. I'm terrified for him.

When I look at the people around me, I see none of the excitement for life he has. What I see is bitterness and disappointment, *hardness*, people like hermit crabs that have died in their shells but continue to drift along the seabed. The only joy they have is being judgmental, *hating*, tearing things down. You can see the coldness in their eyes. They see their own faults (and are they really "faults"?) and they're crippled by them. So they lash out.

How does a man become a man without becoming a hard thing? How do you retain a sense of wonderment? Sure, you meet "childlike" people, but they're naive and no one trusts them with anything important. Is it possible to mature and have a realistic perspective, but still hold onto some sense of softness and joy? That's what I want for the boy above all else. But how? How does my boy survive manhood and still remain a boy? How does he stay clean-hearted while learning to survive? I don't want him to be disappointed or hard inside. I want him to see life as an adventure, but what example am I setting? Maybe it's too late for me and maybe the reason I'm here is to act as a buffer against the bad things around him, to be a *wall*. Does the parent cease to matter when the child begins to grow? Is it selfish to want something for yourself? Are you born with one set purpose, or can that purpose change as you change?

JULY 2ND

I've been thinking a lot about how my father never wrote to us. For that reason I've decided to write letters to the boy and keep them in this journal. One day, I'll give them to him when he's old enough and I'll say, "Here's how it was before you can remember."

Dear Son,

There's a lot I want to tell you and by the time you read this, I'll be a different person, and so will you. You and your mother and I are living in a nice two-bedroom house in La Jolla with an open view of the sea. We're not rich like I was when I grew up, but I have a good job and I've handled my money well and we're working our way up.

Son, I want to be perfectly honest with you because I love you and because you deserve the truth. Your mother and I have had a rough time lately. I'm not sure if we'll be together when you read this, but I hope we will and I hope we can all look back on this rocky part as something that happened in a past that has little or no affect on us. Something that "happened."

These days I'm working as an editor for one of the big daily papers here in San Diego. My job is a good job, but I run into a lot of bad people, and the bad people I meet are awful enough to make me think that humanity is a poison. I come home every night and I need to wash them from me. Seeing you does that. As soon as I pick you up and you grab hold of my shirt and start talking at me, I forget about all the awfulness of people.

From the moment I saw you I changed. As soon as you were born, I grew up and I figured myself out (as best I could). I've not made the best decisions in the past and maybe my heart wasn't always in the right place, but seeing you for the first time showed me that there are good, pure things in the world and that those things are worth changing your life over.

Every time I walk into a room and you smile at me, I can't help but smile back. There are no greater things than seeing joy in your eyes. That kind of happiness is antibiotic. It cleans you out, makes you walk straighter, taller. You have an outward-spreading benevolence that you can't possibly understand yet, but I thank you for that, Son. My uncle Roy once told me, "Some people are so kind and selfless and just *good* that it's like they bring the rain when you've got a drought inside you." That's you. You're the reason I'm here. You hold me in place and you ground me. You make me stay and fight and you make me forget myself and work for something greater.

Your father,
Merc

JULY 3RD

Just found out I'm working on the 4th and Channy's beside herself; says she feels like a prisoner in her own house. I told her she was being overemotional and said it was time to grow up and stop putting herself first.

She said, "If I'm putting myself first, it's because no one else does."

"Don't be so dramatic. That's not true at all and you know it."

"Yes, it is. I'm an *afterthought*. I'm a baby machine and a nanny." She stopped and shook her head and laughed and said, "I can't *believe* this is our life. I hate this. I hate our life. I never thought I'd say that. I *hate* our life."

"What did you expect?"

"I don't know. I didn't expect it to be amazing, but I thought it would be *better*."

JULY 4TH

I can see the fireworks from the window here at work. Karen and the new guy from A&E are sitting on the floor across from me under her desk laughing and sharing a beer. The newsroom has fallen apart. They're working but they're also drinking and the guys have their ties off and girls are in from sales with flushed faces and pieces of chocolate cake on red paper plates (eating it up close to their faces) and people are coming and going as they please.

"Hey, Merc, you old boat engine, lighten up and have some fun," shouts the new guy. He has long hair and a mustache and he looks like someone Jake would be friends with. When you're in news, you don't trust the A&E guys.

Karen's giggling—giggling and sipping the beer. "Yeah! C'mon, Merc! Have a *drink* with us! Don't be a lumpy grumpy pants!"

When Karen says "lumpy grumpy pants" the new guy gets hysterical and uses it as an excuse to lean on her when he laughs, and now he's got his hand on her knee, patting it, laughing, patting, slower now, holding her knee.

Karen's boyfriend, Charlie, is a great guy. Works over at KPBS. We go bowling together sometimes. He'd hate to see this. Even if nothing else happens but this. This would be enough. Goddamnit, Charlie.

"Suit yourself," says the new guy and they burst into laughter again.

There will be a paper on the streets with the date of July 5th, 1979, just like there will be a 6th and a 7th and an 8th. The new guy and Karen know this, but they don't understand what makes it so. They're just doing a job. I'm doing *my* job.

JULY 5TH

I slept at my desk last night. Didn't mean to but I was reading Jack Rosen's piece on the Baader-Meinhof and then there was daylight through the window and the cleaning woman was standing in front of me with her vacuum and mop bucket (a black silhouette against the light) and—

JULY 6TH

Didn't finish that one. The day began.

JULY 7TH

Channy says, "You only come home to shower." Channy says, "Are you having an affair?" Channy says, "Is there something you're not telling me?" Channy says, "Don't look at me like that. Tell me what you're *thinking*." Channy says, "We really need to—" and I throw my plate of spaghetti at the wall and she's up from the table with the boy in her arms and they're headed out the door and he looks back at me with these big scared eyes and reaches out to me and the door slams and they're gone. I hear her car start and then the headlamps light up the curtains.

JULY 8TH

At work, Leonard tells me I'm doing a great job and I tell him that means a lot and that it's good doing something you believe in, and he says, "Now, that being *said*," and my heart drops, "that being said, you look *tired*. Have you been sleeping?"

"Of course."

"You should skip out early. It's a slow news day. Go . . . go take the family to dinner at the new seafood place. Go to the movies, do something fun, *hell*," he lowers his voice, "get *laid*. You need . . . you need some *balance* in this line of work."

"I'm alright. It's just—"

"Listen. I've seen too many guys—talented, smart, capable guys—guys your own age, twenty-eight, twenty-nine, thirty—start up like rockets and burn out by thirty-five."

"Leo, I'm twenty."

"Yeah, haha, right, me too. I'm seventeen. I'm two and three quarters and I just shit my pants. You wanna see? Listen. Merc. You've been doing great work, *clean* work, but I want you to be around when you're my age. Don't be a . . . don't be a *Peterson*."

"I'm not Peterson."

"No, Peterson . . . listen . . . Martin Peterson was the best editor I had. Ten years ago, he was the strongest, smartest . . . he was a *fighter*, but he fought too hard. He didn't understand that sometimes, as much as you love something . . . as much as you *believe* in it . . . you need to find time away from it in order to be yourself again. What's that line from Abbey's 'outlive the bastards' speech . . . something like, 'It's . . . it's not enough to fight for the land. It is even more important to enjoy it.' Anyway, something like that. Peterson's a *wreck* now. You know. He's a rotting . . . a dead, rotting *bird* hanging onto the line by its feet," Leonard makes his hands into claws and holds them out at me. "Look, Merc, the indoctrinated make great soldiers, but a soldier only goes so far until he's blown to pieces or . . . or worse, ruined inside from what he's done. You need *balance*. I don't care what you do on your personal time. You can smoke *dope* for all I care," he laughs, "Half the people *here* do. I mean, what do you do?"

"What do you mean what do I do?"

"When you get home. How do you disconnect from this," he motions around the newsroom, "from this, from *deadlines* and *copy-editing* and the wire and Karen over there bitching about her stupid gook chink fuck boyfriend, and from *news*, from—" he looks down at the big underlined words on my notepad "—from the gas crisis and, what, NASA and SADR and from . . . from wearing—" he grabs his tie and holds it above his head "—from wearing this, you know, from *all* of this. How do you decompress? How do you level *out*?"

I shrug and tell him I'll keep it in mind and he says, "*Man*, you were sittin' there, staring at your notes, looking like you could use a friend."

"Hey Leo, what's the new seafood place?"

"Oh *man*! Bozic's on Clairemont Mesa. That little faggot from Arts . . . the new little faggot, Bippy or Bitsy or whatever his name is, did a piece on them last month and I've been going there ever since. Bozic's Ocean Floor. It's relaxing. Aquariums on the walls. Nice family owns it. Little James Bozic toddling around the place while his daddy cooks and his mama waits tables. One *helluvan* abalone sandwich. Get there early so you can sit in the front of the room by the big aquarium. There's this . . . man, this big fucking *lobster* in there the size of a *komodo dragon*. All the broadcast guys go there Friday nights. Best new place in town."

I tell him thanks and he smiles and goes back to his office and shuts the door behind him.

JULY 9TH

I took Channy to the seafood place and it turned into another fight. We sat across from each other with the candle between us and a bottle of white wine in an ice bucket (and behind her, tropical fish flitting around plastic sea plants and white stocks of coral, a grinning, moon-eyed eel bending itself in and out of the rocks). The boy was up in Julian with Channy's cousins on the farm for the night. We dressed up nice. It was a "date."

"So, nothing?" she said and I looked at her and she wasn't anyone I knew. The serene brow and noble, high forehead, the white blonde hair pulled back like a teenage gymnast, a Russian gymnast. Her big eyes, clear and sad, and her mouth, a grimace—tired, disappointed. "Don't you have *anything* to say? What are you *thinking* about? Just *tell* me."

Channy's pregnant but the child isn't mine.

That was tonight's big news.

"Whose, then? Who's the father?"

"That's not important. We need to—"

"What are you *talking* about? You're *crazy*. Of *course* it's important. Jesus, Channy. Jesus Christ."

"Don't shout."

"I'm not shouting, I'm—"

"Merc, we just need to—"

"*What,* Channy? *What* do we *neeeeed* to do? Tell me what we *neeeeeed.*"

"Don't be mean."

"Channy, am I being *mean*? Am I hurting your *feelings*?"

"What we need—"

"Yeah, you tell me."

"What we need to do is move on from this and raise them both as—"

And I let it pass all around me and out of my way until I heard nothing and saw no one but the stranger across from me.

1999

NORMAL HEIGHTS, 9 P.M.

"Just wait 'til she gets here, *cabron,*" Chente says. "Just wait." He and Joey walk into the bar, the black padded door closing behind them and blotting out the light and the noise of the street. "You've never seen someone drink tequila until you've seen Chavela. She drinks tequila like a *man*. *Better* than a man. She puts men to *shame*."

The bartender walks down the length of the counter, drying a plastic beer pitcher. He sets it on the rack behind him and nods hello. He has a mustache waxed up on the sides, hair slicked back and parted down the middle, and a pearl snap western shirt. "Gents?"

"Two Coronas for me and my *hermanito* here. Uh . . . stick of beef jerky, bag of that cheddar popco—no, *hot fries*. Joey, you want hot fries? Andy Capp's. Yeah. Please. Thanks."

"You guys want extra hot sauce for the Capp's? Lemon juice?"

"Yeah, lemon juice, hot sauce."

"Tapatillo or Cholula?"

"You guys have Chili de Amor, right?"

"Yeah, I think there's some in the back."

"Perfect."

"Right, be a sec." The bartender walks away.

9:15 P.M.

Eating hot fries from the bag with lemon juice and Chili de Amor, Chente tells

Joey more Chavela stories. 1) In high school, Chavela was the only non-*chola* cool enough to hang out with the *cholas*. Their girl-gang, *Seis Mal Milagros,* well known for its near-fatal beatdowns. Once, when Chente and Javier were walking through the neighborhood to get Slushies, a bunch of angry *cholas* ran out of a house and attacked them with sticks and broken pieces of branches that they picked up in the yard. Chente and Javier were no match. Ten seconds in, they were on the ground curled up in the fetal position, and then Chavela stepped out onto the porch like some Roman emperor and stopped the fight. "Ease *off* it, girls. Thas not Juan and Chato." It was a case of mistaken identity. 2) After one of her teachers caught her reading a copy of *American Psycho* in study hall and took it away, Chavela "declared war" on the school. She wrote a zine and a press release about it, sent both to all relevant media, and did an interview with the news. "Local high school girl declares war on school after teacher takes away controversial book." After the story broke, the book was given back and the war was over. 3) Chavela invented two of the school's biggest urban legends: a) That Coach Alan Vanderlyndy (baseball and P.E.) had his penis blown off in Vietnam. b) That the head cheerleader Mainsy Hawkins fucked the football team in the boys' locker room and contracted chlamydia, the stomach flu, and "a rare strain of Turkish gonorrhea," the three of which, by nature of their respective chemistry—a miracle of science—changed the color of her eyes to orange and that now she wore blue contacts to hide the truth.

10 P.M.

Chavela, a no-show, and the boasting of her greatness stops.

10:35 P.M.

Chavela hasn't shown and now Chente's drunk. He's gone from beer to tequila. Shots of Cuervo, then Sauza, now Patrón, moving up the shelf. The more he drinks, the less he cares about the money. Chente's fake ID says he's Ramón Juarez Almada, thirty-two, from Seal Beach, organ donor. Ramón looks like Chente, but it's an angry him—twelve years older, a wide, dark, thick face that says *bitter* when you look at it on the card. "Ramón fucking Juarez fucking Almada. Nothing I dreamed of as a kid came true. I'm going to rob your house and bash your face in with a glass salad bowl." The more tequila Chente drinks, the more he becomes Ramón. Two hours pass. No Chavela. More Ramón. The music louder, a DJ playing garage rock from the '60s. The bar filling up with people. A band setting up to play and passing out pamphlets with their "manifesto."

Joey and Chente move to the next room and sit on tall stools behind the pool tables.

"Joey, who are all these fucking people *anyway*?" Chente drags his eyes back and forth across the crowd, hunched over, feet on the top rung, arms folded across his knees, frowning. "Who are all these fucking *people*?" His eyes are red, tired. "This *fucking* hipster bar."

"Maybe she got the wrong day."

"I tol' her *tonight*. You can't get the wrong day from *tonight*. She's here one day." He shows Joey one finger then makes a fist and the fist becomes a claw. "One," fist, "day," claw, "that's it," a swipe of the hand, weary but violent.

"She could've got it wrong. People get—"

"You know what? *Fuck* what people get. Hey, Joey, *carnal,* less play some *pool*." He nods across the room at two men racking up a new game.

"I thought you hated pool."

"Fuck pool. Who cares. I *love* pool. Pool's my favorite, and I wanna beat *those* guys right there—*those fucking* gringos," he points with the bottom of his empty beer bottle, holding it by the neck, looking into the mouth of it, one eye shut. "Less' play some pool with those fucking *shorts-wearers.*" Chente stands up from the bar stool, staggers to the side, then holds himself straight again, cursing under his breath. "Those fucking *gringos*. Fucking . . . those fucking white people."

The men at the pool table are dressed in baggy shorts, white t-shirts, and baseball caps. The taller one's cap is the Padres, brown with mustard yellow letters. The shorter one, who has bad acne and a red goatee around his mouth, is wearing a Yankees cap, dark blue, almost black, with a bright white 'NY'. Both hats are new, but each man has had a similar hat since childhood. The Padres is hat #4. Yankees is #7, counting three signed caps at home: 1) David Wells, 1998, 2) Don Larsen, 1956 3) Andy Hawkins, 1989, all of which are in fine-to-perfect condition, besides the Larsen '56, extensive water damage on the left-hand corner of the bill. A flood in the basement, May 1990.

"*Órale,* Yankees and Padres, we wanna play teams with you *gringos*," says Chente, shuffling over.

"Naaaw, bro. Thanks, but we're cool," says Yankees, smiling. He tugs at the tip of his goatee, his eyes happy and relaxed. He has a gold wedding band and he turns it around his finger with his thumb. (Not nervous, just a habit.) "We're doin' this one ourselves. You guys can *totally* have the table next game, for sure. We're only playing one. We suck at pool, but I promise we'll be super quick."

"*No* we're playing pool with you right now, *cabrón.*" Chente takes a poolstick off the wall and rubs blue chalk on the tip.

"Bro, you guys *tohhhhhtally* got next game. I promise we'll be done *super*-mega quick. We already got the quarters in and—"

"Chente, no, it's cool. We can—"

"Joey, *carnal,*" Chente puts his hand up to stop him. "We're playing *this one*. *Ahora mismo, guey.*"

"We, like, y'know, it's *cool*," says Padres. "We just wanna do this one alone, so *adios*, okay?"

"*Adios?*" says Chente, stepping up in Padres' face. "You think you're *communicating* with me now, *Gringo Starr*? Are we essspeaking the esssame langueesh? Huh, *gringo*?" after *gringo* Chente spits on the floor at Padres' feet. "This may be California to you, but to me this is *Mexico.* You're standing on *my* ground right now, *maricón*."

Joey puts his hands up. "No, no, it's cool. What're you guys drinking? Beers? It's on me."

"We're not," says Padres. "Just soda. Sprite."

"Okay, then two Sprites. I'll just go and—"

"No, you won't go anywhere, Joey. Just—" Chente shakes his head and laughs. "Wait, *what did you say*, Padres? You said *Sprite*, you're drinking *Sprites*?"

"Sprite. Just Sprites."

"*Sprite* in a bar? Like 'Image is Nothing, Obey Your Thirst' Sprite?"

"Sprite."

"What kind of shorts-wearing pussies are you, *anyway*?" He spits on the floor again and Joey's stomach goes tight. Joey steps forward, then back again.

"Hey! Listen!" says Yankees, stepping in front of Padres.

Padres moves back against the wall.

"Hey, *yourself*, fucking *Sprite Drinker: Part Two, This Time It's Personal*, my friend Joey here wants to buy you drinks, and you and *Parte Uno* better be *polite* and *take* his drinks. *Sabes que*, Joey, no Sprites today. Four shots of *tequila* for us pool players. Patron. On *me*." He pulls his wallet out of his back pocket and fumbles with it and his credit card falls from his hand and drops to the floor. Joey stoops down and picks it up and tries to hand it back but Chente is staring at Padres and Yankees, shaking his head.

"Really, *listen*," says Yankees. "I mean, it's cool, but, y'know, we don't drink. Me and Brad, we don't drink. We just come here to shoot pool after our shift. And Sprite . . . Sprite is totally okay with—"

"*Sabes que*, I'll shoot pool up your mother's *ass*, Yankees."

"Come *on* now."

"Chente," Joey says, his voice shaking. "It's alright. They said they don't—"

"Yankees, you and *Brad* go shoot pool up your mother's asses, go fuck your mothers in the ass with a can of Sprite. I like *7 Up*. You hear that? 7 Up is better. 'Never had it; never *will*.' Never! Fuck Sprite. I wouldn't drink Sprite if it was for *free, cabrón*. 7 Up forever. Sprite up the ass, *por atras*," Chente grins a nasty Ramón Juarez Almada grin and thrusts his hips at Yankees. "Like this. *Por atrah-ah-ah-ah-s*."

"Look, okay." Yankees shuts his eyes and takes a deep breath and opens them again. "For your information—"

"For your *information*?" Chente says. "For your information, you're a bunch of *thirst* obeyers. Get the fuck out of here or I'll get all 7-Up-*crazy* on your ass, *putos.*"

Yankees swings at Chente but Chente steps to the side and now Yankees is off balance and Chente has him by the t-shirt and he's pushing him against the pool table, standing over him. Joey hears Chente's switchblade flick open and then it's at Yankees' neck. Chente holds the knife steady, staring into Yankees' twitching blue eyes. "Okay, Yankees. Alright, why don't you say *Sprite* just *one more time*."

"Bro, it's—don't—oh god—it's cool, we're c-c-cool—" Yankees stutters, his voice thick with Chente's hand on his throat. And now everyone in the pool room is gathering around the table, the bartender pushing through the crowd, yelling something Joey can't hear, and Chente holding Yankees against the table under the big Budweiser table light, the green felt glowing.

"Joey. Your *knife.*" It's an order.

Joey hands Chente the switchblade and he flicks it open but there's no noise this time. Joey hears his own heart; it's drowning out the room, urgent, a piston. Chente—holding Joey's knife in his spare hand, waving it behind him at the crowd. "Back up! Back *up*!"

The people move away from him as one wall of bodies and Chente points the knife at the bartender, who steps back against the crowd, raising his palms. "Okay. Alright, it's cool," the bartender says. "It's okay. You don't need to—"

"We were just leaving, *anyway,*" says Chente. He loosens his grip on Yankees without breaking eye contact. "Joey. *Hermano.* Take the cue balls. *All* of them."

Joey steps forward, his hands shaking. He shoves his hands in his pockets and they shake harder. "Cue balls?"

"Take them. They're *ours* now."

"Cue balls?"

"Quit saying *cue balls* and *take them*!"

Joey walks around the pool tables and gathers all three cue balls with everyone's eyes on him and then waits to hear what's next.

Chente backs away from Yankees and turns to face the crowd. "Part. Down. The *middle.*"

The people near the doorway step to the side and make a path.

Outside, Joey and Chente walk fast around the corner and then run down the darkened block. Joey trips on a cracked rise in the sidewalk and falls hard and then gets up, his hands and knees burning.

"C'mon! Go!" Chente, laughing, as they run. "Go! Go! Go! Go!"

Joey drops one of the cue balls and it bounces down the sidewalk behind him.

"Leave it! Leave it!"

They get to the car and open the doors and throw themselves in. Joey's jeans are ripped at the knee; blood soaking the denim. Chente revs the engine and hits the gas and the car peals out and away from the curb.

They make a left onto University and run the first red light and then the second. Chente turns right, squealing around the corner, and then another right into an alley and hits the brakes. They jerk forward in their seats. The car is stopped and Joey's out of breath and sweating. (The car—Chente's new one, a two-door '71 Chevy Nova he's named Mariah Carey—primer gray but fast and dependable, a good engine under the hood.)

"You see that, Joey?! 'Part down the middle!' I was *Moses* back there! Let's see them play pool *now*. Get the tequila," he says, laughing. "From the glove box." He's laughing, but it's an order, like back in the bar.

Joey pops open the glove compartment and a flat pint of Cuervo slides out with Chente's registration papers and a white plastic spoon.

"Okay, just a sec."

Joey unscrews the lid, his hands still shaking and the pulse in his head working with his heart. The alley lights and darkness all around them. The lights and darkness. Darkness and lights. The alley. "What are we drinking to?"

"Joe DiMaggio and Tony Gwynn back there. Tony Gwynn Stefani."

"What?"

"Baseball players. *Yankees. Padres.* You don't know anything do you? Just drink, *carnal*."

Joey sips his first shot and then gulps the next until his hands stop shaking and then he drinks again and his nerves are calm. He hands the bottle to Chente and Chente takes a drink and starts the car.

The streets are thick with fog as they speed down University, running stoplights and passing the bottle back and forth, and then Joey's drunk and he's okay and he's laughing so hard that he can't open his eyes. "Red light!" yells Chente as they run each light. Joey rolls the window down and leans out and throws a cue ball at the newspaper box on the sidewalk and hits it square on. "Direct hit!" He throws the second cue ball at a van driving at them in the opposite lane and it honks its horn and swerves and they run another light."Red light!" He pulls himself back into the car and Chente hands him the bottle.

"*Padres and Yankees*!" Chente says, laughing and shaking his head. The headlights cut through the fog in front of the car and the windshield wipers beat back and forth. "I bet that guy shit his pants. '*Uh, well, we, well, uh, we drink Sprite, me and Brad*.' I bet that one's name was Todd. White people are always called Brad or Todd, aren't they? I'm glad your name's Joey. It's almost José. Your new name is José Carro, *carnal.* Joey Carr is *dead.* Let's see them play pool now. Let's see them play pool *now.*"

The fog socks in around the car and they move through it past Normal Heights into North Park then Hillcrest, Mission Hills.

They race down the Washington Street hill and the whole harbor and bay sprawls out below them, dark with red and blue lights, buoys, a construction barge, boats out on the black water. They hit the bottom of the hill and the car bounces and they lift up in their seats and hit their heads on the car roof and Joey yells, "Ow!"

Chente runs the intersection.

Now they're in Little Italy, driving slow. Cops everywhere. Bars. The waterfront tavern. Pasta places with '-inni' and '-io' surnames. Well-dressed people stand outside clubs smoking and talking. Girls with long legs and bare backs shivering in short black dresses, holding their purses in front of them, hunched forward. Guys with sports coats and ponytails or shaved heads gleaming. An open-air cafe filled with people eating and drinking magnum bottles of red wine next to outdoor heaters with glowing orange tops.

"Let's see them play pool now," Chente says to himself.

"I could go for pizza right now," Joey says.

"No way. *Chorizo.* We'll get *chorizo burritos* later. *Sin huevo,* like men. *Chorizo para Chente y su compa José Carro . . . José Coche.*"

The tequila's gone, the bottle empty on the seat between them. They drive down Kettner by the waterfront. All the storefronts boarded up and closed down. Black plastic trashcans in front of warehouses. An old favorite bar out of business. A place where Chente and Javier got drunk and tried to beat up a famous singer in town playing a secret show. Dark windows, one of them taped up where it broke. A stray dog walking past, sniffing a spot on the sidewalk. Lifting his leg. A 'Closed' sign and a 'For Sale By Owner' sign. Joey watching the old bar pass, the glass dusty, the neon sign smashed and dismantled and lying up against the front door, wires strung out its back end like some kind of mechanical jellyfish.

At the Casbah, they sit on stools with their backs up against the bar and drink tequila and Dos Equis until last call. The band on stage plays a listless set to three girls and a man in a wheelchair who sleeps through most of it. The club is full but everyone's out back on the patio, smoking, talking loudly.

When the lights go up and the people begin to file out, Chente leans in to Joey.

Joey sees his shape. His outline. Light around his black-brown featureless face.

"*Ay carnalito, José Cochino,* less go to Ti*juana.* Iss time to go fuck some horse. Some . . . *whores.* Some *whores.*"

Joey nods and does his best to follow Chente.

Outside the club, the fog rolls down Kettner toward the airport. Chente floats down the street and Joey trails behind. Chente stops. Joey stops. A plane roars over them as it prepares to land at the bottom of the hill, its belly silver, blinking lights on the wing. The wind whips through their hair and the sound is crushing. "Biiiiig Johhhhn!" shouts Chente, pointing up at it.

Ahead of them on the sidewalk, an older guy Joey had seen throwing up in the bathroom is standing along a row of hedges, pissing, eyes closed, teetering back and forth on his heals, mouth gaped open, vomit down the front of his white shirt. And now Chente walking past him, shoving him with one hand without looking, the guy falling silently into the hedges. The guy doesn't get up and he doesn't move; Chente stumbling forward, unknowing. As he walks past, Joey looks at the guy, facedown, passed out.

2:05 A.M.

In the car, the radio blasting a wild swell of *mariachi* music. The car smells like beer.

2:08 A.M.

Chente talking about Mariah Carey (the singer and the car) and Joey nodding along but half-conscious. "The fat Mariah! I like the fat Mariah!" yelling over the road sound, the windows down "I don't care what anybody thinks, the fat Mariah is the best! Those big legs and that . . . that *ass*. If she was my girlfriend, I'd make her eat turkey and steaks all day! Ice cream! Lasagna! Get fatter, Mariah! Do it for rock 'n' roll! I love you!"

2:10 A.M.

Joey vomiting out the window as Chente drives.

2:15 A.M.

Joey passed out in his seat.

2:34 A.M.

Joey awake and Chente driving in silence, black and lights all around, a quiet Mexican folk song playing on the car stereo (scratchy, old, haunted, bluesy). They will remember nothing of the drive. What comes next comes in fractured time: 1) In the day-use lot on the U.S. side of the border, Chente arguing with the brown blob silhouette of the parking attendant, saying, "and a fucking disgrace to Mexicans *everywhere*." 2) A taxi in Tijuana, and Joey's eating a *churro* and drinking a Mexican Coke from an old-fashioned glass bottle and the lights of the city wild like Las Vegas and the driver and Chente singing together, "*Laaa paloma blancaaa*!" and then Joey asleep and he sees a black bull sleeping in the shade of a tree and then the bull is just bones and a great horned skull and then the river flows over his land again and the land is now a sea and the clouds race across the sea and go around the curve of the Earth and then he's out of the taxi and Joey's awake. Stars wiggle and smear above and the moon is bouncing in the sky like a sing-along ball and then it's concrete, cold, bits of sand and gravel, his knees stinging, and he's on his back on the sidewalk. The world spins. The ground tips left and right, heaves forward, pitches back. Lights again. Darkness. Lights. A struggle. A voice shouting, "Geet the fuck outta *my texi*! Geet outta Mehico!"

Chente standing above Joey, pulling him to his feet, and Joey's up and he takes a wide stance to balance himself but the ground moves in a rippling wave like someone shaking out a blanket and he falls again. Chente—blood streaming from his nose, screaming in Spanish at the taxi driver. The taxi driver—on the other side of his cab, shouting back in English.

"*Espero que tu se mueras*!" Chente spits blood on the ground.

"Doan *ever* come bek to Mehico!" The driver climbs into his cab and starts to drive away, then slams on the brakes, and opens the door again.

"What now?! What, *maricón*?!"

The driver gets out of his cab and throws the empty Coke bottle at Chente and the bottle hits Chente's chest with a thunk, and he catches it in both hands and throws it back as the taxi drives away.

The bottle hits the street behind the cab and sprays out across the asphalt.

Joey's vision spins. He sits up and then falls onto his side and pulls himself up again and sits with his back to the fence alongside the road. The border wall. He turns and looks through an open space in the fence. The cool metal is nice on his face. The U.S. side. Dark brush and the hill below, desert. And now a break in traffic. Quiet. The night breeze. The rattling of loose metal somewhere. Clanging. The empty street next to the border fence, floodlit, yellow. A family of three cuts across the street from the housing block, running low, backpacks and full black trash bags in hand. The young father and mother carry a long aluminum ladder together like a surfboard. The ladder goes up next to Joey and Chente. Chente doesn't look. He stares into the street, swaying. The father throws a trash bag over and then another. He checks the ladder to see if it's steady. "*Listo*," the father whispers. "*Leti. Ahora.*" And they begin to go over. The mother first. She gives her backpack to her husband and looks him in the eye. She's afraid. Frowns. Eyes well up. Starts to cry. "*No,*" the father says, "*No, mjia, no, querida. Vamos. Cuidado.*" She turns and climbs to the top of the ladder while the man holds it steady, looking up at her.

She stands on the final step, arms out for balance, and jumps over the top of the fence. The man throws himself to the metal wall of the fence, desperate. "*Leti!*" He looks through it, palms to the metal siding, frantic. "*Leti?!*" he whispers through the fence. "*Leti*!" But she's fine. Through the slat, the man and Joey see the woman run into the bushes. The man throws another trash bag over, then his wife's pink backpack. "*Listo, listo.*" His son goes over. Jumps and falls onto the cushion of the trash bags. Gets up. Grabs his mother's backpack by the strap.

The boy looks back at his father's face through the fence then runs off into the brush.

The man throws his son's stuffed giraffe over, then another backpack, and then he climbs the ladder.

He stands at the top and looks back at the housing block and then down at Joey, uncertain, then expressionless. He jumps. Hits the ground. Cries out. Something's wrong. Cries out again. Muffled. Rolls to the side, holding his knee. Gets up, limps off into the bushes, dragging his bags.

The ladder is left behind.

And they've crossed.

Chente stands in the light of the passing cars. He staggers and steps to one side but stays put, staring squint-eyed at the spot where the taxi sped up, turned, and disappeared.

BOOK TWO

A BOOK OF LISTS

"He had seen the dead march on Karpathos."

—Ed Distler, *The Light in the Window*

1999

BOWLING ALLEY, MIDNIGHT

At the start of the big Christmas week rainstorm, Tyler and Joey meet Maggie and her friends from school at Clairemont Bowl for "Cosmic Bowling." Outside the rain comes down in sheets that drift across the parking lot.

Joey and Tyler sit in Tyler's Mazda waiting for it to pass. For a while, they play Maggie's Hank Williams tape and talk about movies and animals, but when the rain drowns it out, they turn the music off and listen to it come down.

"Tyler, I hate to say this, but my time spent as a weather prophet in . . . in Nepal tells me this rain isn't going to let up."

Tyler laughs. "Yeah, I guess not."

"We need to make a run for it and . . . I think you should be aware of the risks. We could be killed. You know that, right? We'll *probably* be killed. It's been good knowing you, bud."

Tyler nods gravely then breaks into a big, shaky grin. "We can do this."

"Do it for rock 'n' roll."

"Okay. For rock 'n' roll."

"The rain's strong but we're stronger. I'll drink this whole rainstorm if I have to. I'll get a straw and suck all the clouds into my stomach like Superman. Oars? You got the . . . the oars?"

"Oars . . . got the oars. Aye, aye, captain."

"Life jackets on?"

"Life jackets, aye, aye."

"Okay. Go. Go!"

Joey opens his car door and the sound of the rain is deafening.

"Whoa!" shouts Tyler as they climb out of the car into a solid downpour.

"Nooo!" Joey yells, laughing as he pulls the back of his jean jacket up over his head. They slam their doors and run across the parking lot to the green-lit entrance.

Inside, Tyler and Joey stand in line to rent their shoes, dripping on the carpet, thrilled, alive.

"Soaked!" Tyler says happily.

"Soaked," Joey confirms.

Over Tyler's shoulder, Joey sees Maggie sneaking up to surprise them, walking soft and low.

"Soaked," Joey says again, low and distracted. He pretends to wring out his shirt and Tyler laughs.

Standing behind Tyler, Maggie puts a finger to her lips and gives Joey a smiling *Shhh* and he can't help but grin.

"What—" Tyler says and starts to turn and Maggie screams and leaps onto his back, wrapping her arms and legs around him. Tyler spins around with Maggie hanging on. She shrieks and laughs as they turn in big, loose circles, her twin braids flying, and then tumble to the carpet. One of her shoes comes off and Joey sees her sock. Dark red with bright blue stripes.

Tyler stands up, offers his hand, and pulls Maggie to her feet. She looks down and steps into her shoe and laughs. "Hey, Joey," she says, happy to see him but composed. With Tyler, it's different. She wraps her arm around Tyler's waist and pulls him close. "You guys are totally *wet*! What're you *doing* tonight?"

"We're hanging out with *you*," says Tyler. "Cosmic Bowling. We're getting all Cosmic-y."

"Well, you better start drinking, because I'm *drunk*!" she says, flushed, smiling, her eyes full of light. "Don't tell anyone, but Byron's got" whispering "a flask of *whiskey*. We stole it from Vons! Shhh."

Joey hears a bowling ball race across polished wood, followed by another one, while yet another hits the pins, and another is dropped and rolled.

"We'll meet you back there," says Tyler, nodding to where her friends are gathered around their lane. One of them is dancing ridiculously, holding his bowling ball under his t-shirt like he's pregnant. He makes a surprised face and lets the ball drop and puts a palm to his mouth.

The bowling alley's bar is decorated with silver tinsel behind the pinball machines. A line of Christmas lights stapled along the length of the counter blink darkly. Tyler and Joey belly up to the bar and Tyler picks at the lights aimlessly. He unscrews one of the tiny bulbs and the whole string goes out.

"Tyler!"

"I know." Tyler gives Joey a shaky smile and screws the bulb back in and the lights are on again.

"These always look like they're gonna be too hot to touch, but they aren't." Joey pinches one (a dusky magenta) between his fingers. "They never are. The color is hot. But they aren't even *warm*."

An older woman in jeans, a red t-shirt, and a short white apron comes out from the kitchen, carrying a plastic tub of lemon wedges. She sets it on the counter next to the maraschino cherries and green olives, and straightens up the stack of napkins and the bin of cocktail swords and paper umbrellas. The woman has graying blonde hair in pigtails like a little girl, her shirt cut low to show withered pink cleavage. Joey has seen her at the bowling alley since he was a kid, but she never remembers him. She *ughs* painfully as she bends to the side to get something from under the counter. A Santa hat. She puts it on and smiles. Good teeth. "Some IDs for me, kids?"

Joey shows her his and she looks at it and hands it back and gets his beer. "Here ya go, hon. Happy hour's five more minutes. Three bucks. You Merc

Carr's kid? Merc from Julian?"

"Nope."

"Same last name. Old Merc," she says, shaking her head. "*Mercury Merc.* Where's *he* gone?"

Joey shakes his head and shrugs.

"Well, a drink to old friends not present," she says nodding at Joey's beer. "Sometimes people stop coming in and you never see 'em again."

Joey pays with a five and tips one of the dollars she gives back and puts the other in the front pocket of his jean jacket. "Thanks, Jacey."

"How you know my name, kid?" She looks at him crooked, a sly smile.

"A guess," he smiles.

"You sure you ain't Merc's boy? *Cowboy Merc, the Julian Jerk* my brother Keith used to call him. Man, we were *kids*."

"No, ma'am."

She looks at Tyler's fake ID. "Nuh-uh, sweetie. I don't know who Peter what Fillan . . . ahuh . . . imoreimore?—is but it ain't you. Soda?"

"Coke"

"RC?"

"Sure. Thanks."

She pours it from the spout gun and drops a cherry in the glass and hands it to him. "This one's on me. Merry Christmas, kiddo."

Tyler and Joey sit at a booth on the level above the lanes and watch Maggie and her friends bowl.

It's Maggie's turn. She takes off her coat and steps back before shuffling forward and pitching it at the pins. The ball rolls wide to the right, then swings back left and knocks all the pins down. A thundering strike. Her friends jump up and yell and she gets high-fives and one of the guys from the group bear-hugs her, swinging her around in a circle. On Maggie's second roll, the ball drops into the gutter and her friends cheer as if she's scored another strike and she tries to do the moonwalk.

"Maybe you should've called me Peter back at the bar," Tyler says, bored, his soda sitting in front of him, untouched. "Or Petey . . . that might . . . might imply *history* between the real you and the fictional me. Petey? P. Dog? Dog P.?"

Joey hears him but his answer's a grunt. *Mhhmn.*

"You okay?" asks Tyler, reaching across the table to take Joey's beer. He sips it and narrows his eyes at him.

"Huh?"

"You alright?" he passes the bottle back.

Joey rubs his face and opens his eyes and shuts them and opens them again. "Yeah, yeah, I'm okay . . . I don't know . . . *spacing*."

"So, Chente . . . off to *New York*. Crazy."

"It's a relief. I mean, to be honest. The stuff we got up to . . . you know. I'm not surprised he left. And anyway, whenever we hung out we drank *so much*. No matter *what* we did. We never hung out without getting drunk. I know I've said this before, but I think I want to take a break from drinking—drinking to get *wasted*. For a while, at least. Right now I feel great. *One beer*. A nice . . . pale ale like this." Joey lifts the bottle and toasts it at Tyler. "I love this. This's all I need."

"You think he'll stay?"

Joey sets the bottle down and slides Tyler's soda across the table and takes a sip. "In New York or with Chavela?"

"Both."

"She's in school, Columbia or NYU—I always get those two confused—and she's there four years minimum. I don't know, he's pretty serious about her . . . she's *great*, she's really amazing . . . and, theoretically, he still has that record deal waiting for whenever he gets a new band together."

"How's Nicole?"

"Better. *Way* better. Thankfully."

"Still, I can't believe he moved to *New York*."

"Huh?"

"Chente."

"Oh."

"You'd never move to New York, would you?"

Before Joey can respond, Maggie slides into the seat next to Tyler.

"*Heyyy boyyys,*" she says, batting her eyelashes, pretending to flirt.

"Hey," Tyler and Joey say at the same time.

Maggie takes Tyler's glass and fishes down into it with her fingers and digs out the cherry and pops it into her mouth.

"Contaminated," Tyler says looking down at his drink.

"You like it. Hey, you guys bowling or what?"

"I dunno," says Tyler. "Probably."

"Probably," Joey echoes. He looks down at his beer and shuts one eye and stares into its brown glass mouth. The mouth of a well and the amber light shining through it, the dark puddle inside. He takes a drink and in his head he sees a snowy road at night and he sees a car crash into another car over and over again, backing up with reversed film, crashing. Crashing then backing up again. The first car spinning out, the second car into the ditch. Then crashing again, backing up, crashing. Now the snow lit up orange with fire as the second car burns.

"So what's up with this *rain*?" Maggie says, taking the cherry stem out of her mouth, showing it to them, tied in a knot. "They saying this's another El

Niño? I'm getting a boat and putting it in my mom's driveway if it is. I'll camp out in it. I don't care."

"It's crazy." Joey's eyes wince as the words come out of his mouth.

Just then, a tall gangly flash cuts across the periphery and grabs Maggie and pulls her out of her seat and Joey's arm jerks and knocks over his beer and it spills across the table.

Maggie and the boy fall to the floor, wrestling and laughing, and then he jumps to his feet and helps her up. His big, thick-framed glasses have fallen off. He picks them up, rubs them on his raggedy green t-shirt, and puts them back on. "Better," he says, pushing a strand of oily black hair out of his eyes. He turns to Joey, bows extravagantly, and sticks out his hand. "Joey Carr, right? I'm Ben Frank, defender of the universe."

1979

JULY 15TH

It's been hot and clear and sunny since I came down here. I wake up late every day to the sound of traffic on the street, and then they bring my breakfast and I spend the rest of the day on the roof in my deck chair.

My apartment in Tijuana is small and clean. It's a one-room adobe shack on the roof of a six-story tenement building in the *Coahuila* district; the rooftop is large, the size of a tennis court, but I'm the only thing up here.

Every day, the woman from the taquería knocks on my window and I get up and let her in and she lays out my breakfast on the table by the bed. Today it was *machaca*—shredded beef, onions, and green peppers fried with scrambled egg. A bowl of that, a bowl of refried beans, a mason jar of strange black coffee flavored sweet, a dozen steamed tortillas wrapped in foil, and an orange. (The orange is dessert. She sets it on my table last, next to the coffee, and sometimes—like today—she smiles sad, like it's an insult giving me something so humble.) After I'm done with everything, I take the orange and my jar of coffee and I go outside my door and sit on my deck chair in the sun. The oranges are like nothing you've ever tasted. So sweet, and so bright in color, the pulp clear like orange glass.

My day is spent in the chair, reading and letting the sun work into my skin. I eat the orange slowly and I make the coffee last until dinner.

The roof is enclosed by a wall, like the battlement of a castle. From up here, I can hear the city down below, a quiet, dull roar that sounds like the sea. It bothered me at first, but now I'm not sure I could do without it.

In the evening, the woman from the shop comes back with a tray and sets up my dinner on the small, round table next to the chair. Last night it was *carnitas*, a fatty, dark, fried pork. It came as pre-made tacos. Six of them in foil-wrapped corn tortillas with diced onions and cilantro and half a lime. The night before last, it was a soup with spicy, oily broth and tomatoes and peppers cooked down, earthy and red and dark. (It felt like you were drinking clay and muddy water in the best possible way.)

At sundown, the woman comes back to take my dishes and, when she does, she brings me an earthenware jug of water. The water has an aftertaste of soil and iron and it's invigorating after a day sweating in the sun. Another thing to savor.

By nightfall, if I've left a message with Robi (the errand boy) and set a time, a girl my age (a Haitian called Reyna) comes up and we go into my apartment and we lie in bed with the door and the windows open and the breeze coming through and touching our skin. When I do this, I close my eyes and I think about Sorel when she was still Egyptian. Channy I can't see if I try. The problem with Channy (and I know this now) is a problem with myself. I never went out of my way to know her. We were together for a very short time in the beginning and then she was pregnant and I was away, and when I came back we were together, but I was working and then the boy was born and then any time together was time with the boy. I knew her in the beginning, but by the time I came back, she was someone else.

The boy I miss. I can't think about him. When I do, I push it away. *Time will make you forget how you feel about him,* I tell myself every day. I don't believe it but I'm trying to.

JULY 16TH

Shaving in the mirror today, I realized I've picked up a lot of Channy's mannerisms. I guess that's how it works. You grow to become the person you're with.

How do you grow back to yourself?

JULY 17TH

I've been paying Robi to fetch books from the English section of the library. Right now it's *Zarathustra*, which I read as a boy but wasn't ready for. This stood out earlier today: "Did their hearts perhaps grow faint because solitude swallowed me like a whale?"

Dear Son,

A while back, I vowed to write you letters during the time of your life when you would have no memory of. When does memory start? For most, it starts in your first few years, but it's sparse and by the time you're an adult, your memories of childhood are patchy at best. I was lucky to be born with what they call a photographic memory, so maybe you will, too. Regardless, the sad fact is that most people have a memory or two they can bring up from each year of childhood at best. Of all that living . . . and a two-minute scrap of vacation here, five minutes of birthday party there, an image of the sea from a place they don't know, and then nothing, blackness. What a shame. All that early joy you won't remember, all those good and gentle days when no one wanted anything of you but to be happy and safe.

The early part—the part you're in now—will be gone forever. I know there's a difference between thinking something over and over-thinking it, but I can't help but dwell on what you'll lose and it's shaking me up a little. I'm not doing well, Son. I hope this is a temporary thing and that when I meet you next you will see a stable, secure, well-adjusted man. I don't want you to know your father like this, but I'd be remiss if I didn't tell you the whole truth. One of the worst things you can do to someone you love is lie to them. No matter how horrible or hurtful the truth is, don't hold it back.

Son, I need to tell you that your mother and I are not together anymore. I'm not sure whose fault it is, or if it was anyone's fault to begin with. It's hard to make things work, no matter how much you love someone. We've all got too much going on in our heads. We sabotage ourselves

JULY 18TH

I didn't/couldn't finish.

JULY 24TH

A bee flew into my room yesterday and I stumbled all over the place trying to kill it. When I finally had it trapped inside an upturned mason jar, I didn't have the nerve to do it. I tore a blank title page from a book on Cabeza de Vaca and slipped it under the mouth of the jar and carried it outside and let the bee fly off.

Robi's going away to work on a ranch in Sinaloa, so no more books. I paid in advance for the girls. Three months' cash, just like my rent (which feels awful, now that I really think of it).

I have $800 left and, for some reason, I want it gone. I'm not sure why, but knowing that it's under my mattress makes me nauseous.

This morning, I woke up with the flu or something like it.

It never rains here but it's raining today. I stayed in for the first time since I've been here.

"I paid in advance for the girls." Reading that back makes me feel sick. What am I doing?

I used to think I was decent, honest. The more I'm alone with myself, the more I know that it's not true.

I wonder if my father would have been disappointed in me. If I knew anything about him, I'd be able to answer that.

If the boy was like I am . . . I can't even think about that.

I don't want the boy to grow up to be me. Channy's better than I am. She'll raise him to be what I'm not.

It's better that I don't go back.

JULY 27TH

Still sick. The fever dreams last night were awful. Tiny, bristling hairs growing out from between my teeth, and as I pulled them out, more grew in their place. After that: driving down the hill from my old apartment into downtown, the brakes cutting out, faster, faster, no control. Then I began to hit bodies. They rolled up over the hood and hit the window with a terrible crunch, and fell off to the side. I drove through a crowd. It was terrible. After that: Jake sitting at a table with a napkin tucked into his shirt, eating Sorel's severed left hand on a plate with Worcestershire sauce and mashed potatoes, holding it down with his fork and cutting into it with his knife. Sawing, fighting against the tough flesh and bone and gristle. I keep seeing that one. I can't get it out of my head.

JULY 28TH

Today Magda, the woman from the shop, brought a plate of *chili rellenos* with a side of *habanero* peppers, diced ginger, and minced garlic. She told me to eat the peppers and ginger and garlic first and drink them down with a lot of water to drive out the sickness.

She also left with me with a red candle in a glass jar and told me to light it every night at dusk and stare into it thinking of the face of Christ. Deep breaths. Fifteen minutes. I'll try anything.

Tonight I heard firecrackers and music and some kind of parade passing by and I wanted to be a part of it.

A few minutes later, it was gone. It didn't fade away. It just cut off. Noise and voices and music and celebration, then nothing but the street sound below. I'm not sure why, or how.

Yesterday, there was a shooting down on the street. I heard the shots and I got up from my chair and looked down from the battlements and saw a man in the middle of the street, and the cars stopped all around him at odd angles and a pool of blood circling his body.

It's getting hotter and there's a nervous energy I can feel from down there. People are frazzled and bad things are happening.

I haven't gone down to the street once since I've been here and the thought of it terrifies me.

JULY 29TH

The face of Christ. Deep breaths. Fifteen minutes.

I felt nothing.

I tried it for an hour. Still nothing.

I wish I could believe like Channy did . . . or does. Still does. She still believes even if I'm not there to witness it.

The world didn't end because I left. It went right on going.

This will get better. Time will make it better.

AUGUST 2ND

Is optimism a reflection of an unconscious faith in divinity? Do atheists without worry believe without knowing?

AUGUST 5TH

I think I'd like to work in a pet store and have my boy as my co-worker. I could do that forever. The other fantasy: the boy and I as cowboys, riding the range together, just him and me, father and son. That's how my life would've played out had I stayed on Roy's farm in Weston. Of course, if that were the case, there would be no boy. The idea of that I can't fathom. The boy is here. He was always here because I can't imagine him not. Where was he waiting before he was born? *God*, if I could hear him *talk* right now. If I could touch his hair. See him for a second. Even if he didn't see me. I can't do this without him.

AUGUST 8TH

Last night a different girl came. This one was Ecuadoran. I asked her to leave but she said, "Later."

"Later what?"

"I'll leave later."

She was dark as night and dressed all in red, and around her neck a string of bones.

"What kind of bones?"

"Human."

"Human bones?"

"Yes, my ancestors. *Their fingers.* Fingerbones."

As she moved above me and I pushed up into her, I held each bone between my thumb and forefinger and kissed each one and each time she cried out. In the throes of it I thought of Channy, and as I came into the Ecuadoran's body, I could see Channy in the way I saw her when I first loved her. Channy as the soulmate I knew, and then didn't know.

When I woke up this morning, I was relieved, and then I realized I had nothing to be relieved about and that was one of the worst feelings I've ever had.

What is a soul if there's no god? What is a soulmate if the soul is nothing? I wish I could believe like Channy does. It's not that I don't want to believe; it would be so much easier. What a *weight off* knowing for sure that heaven is real.

Today feels like the end of something. What end, and what thing? It's hot and humid and all morning I thought of my brother in Vietnam, walking the jungles, looking this way and that, his rifle pointing into the black-green. Was it the war that changed Jake or was he like that to begin with? Uncomfortable in his own skin, waiting for an excuse to step outside of his role as the son that would succeed . . . .

What was my role in the family? My parents had a lot of faith in Jake, in the things he would go on to do. What did they think about me? What did they say to each other when no one was around?

AUGUST 13TH

This morning, I watched a hawk kill a small bird in the air without dropping it. Today, I realized I have no sense of humor anymore. I don't want to laugh and I don't want things to be funny. I'm not sure what that means but it was a mistake coming down here and I know that now. Just the same, where else would I go? If I went somewhere else, I would have to be someone else.

AUGUST 14TH

Last night, the Ecuadoran came back and I asked her if the bones of her necklace were really human, and she laughed until she had tears in her eyes and said, "No, no, no, I am sorry, I thought you knew . . . it was joke. I was making joke. They are . . . they are, you know, *wood* bones. It is a . . . what word. . . a decoration? No, a . . . *cómo se dice* . . . a necklace for costume, you know? I come directly from party, costume party? I was voodoo . . . voodoo . . . ."

"Voodoo priestess?"

"Yeah, yeah." She laughed. "Priest—est."

We fucked for hours.

AUGUST 17TH

Is the me who wanted Sorel the real me or is the me who loved Channy me? Could I be both? Could I be with both, if each knew about the other? I always thought I loved Channy as a person and Sorel just physically, but I think it was the other way around. I got to know Sorel but I still don't know Channy. Channy I was attracted to the moment I saw her. Sorel grew on me and, the more I think about it, the more I think I might have loved her after all. That's so strange to admit. Was I in love with Sorel and in lust with Channy and not the other way around?

AUGUST 18TH

Channy loved candy canes; she always had a few stashed even when it wasn't Christmas. Sorel had a Band-Aid on her knee almost every time I saw her, even when we fucked and I had her on her knees, it never came off. Channy loved taking taxis. Sorel was best in bed after her dance class. Channy cried the last time we had sex. Sorel hated the beach. Channy said "never mind" when she didn't feel like repeating herself. Sorel loved any movie where an ape was the co-star. Channy ate all of her movie food during the previews. Sorel's hiccups went away when you gave her orange juice. Channy sent out one short story a week to the journals no matter how busy she was. Sorel was a mouthbreather. Channy was allergic to pineapple. Sorel loved to draw hieroglyphics in the margins of magazines. Channy loved Felipe's Pizza because they gave the boy a wad of pizza dough to play with before the meal. Sorel hated the '50s music I listened to in my old apartment. Channy eyes were always dazed and glassy after a kiss. Sorel said too much eye contact was "evil." Channy made the best grilled cheeses you ever had. Sorel liked to have sex with her sneakers on. Channy wanted to take sailing lessons. Sorel could never open a jar and I felt strong doing it for her. The back of Channy's neck always smelled like pine sap. Sorel said "Wed-nes-day" just to piss me off. Channy always dressed like she was cold. Sorel liked a finger in her ass when you went down on her. Channy had no friends. Sorel loved anything glow-in-the-dark plastic. Channy cried when she saw kittens. Sorel could never remember her social security number. Channy only listened to one record, Elton John's *A Single Man*. Sorel had armpit hair in her new "natural woman" phase and it looked good on her. Channy made great Denver omelets. Sorel always burned the popcorn and liked it that way. Channy said, "Jesus, Jesus, Jesus," when she came. Sorel wanted to have kids. Channy thought Walter Mondale was "cute like a little fat baby." Sorel liked doing the flower game, 'He loves me, he loves me not.' Channy wanted to invent something that could shrink things like cars and buildings down to toy size. Sorel hated nuns and called them "dumb-fuck nuns." Channy made her own birthday cards for people. Sorel always said, "I wish I had a death ray on the front of my car that I could shoot bad drivers with." Channy loved Bobby Kennedy and cried sometimes when she talked about him. Sorel could list off all the presidents in alphabetical order and always giggled when she said, "Garfield." Channy loved Tolstoy, Vonnegut, and C.S. Lewis. Sorel bought jewelry all the time but never wore it. Channy's face looked crumpled-up before her first cup of coffee. Sorel brushed her teeth six times a day. Channy's IQ was 10 points higher than mine. Sorel covered her freckles in makeup until one of her co-workers told her not to. Channy left the house a lot without saying where she was going and came back without saying hello. Sorel loved to make chocolate chip cookies (but most of the time she just ate the dough). Channy loved the smell of fresh house paint. Sorel believed in ghosts and swore she saw three Civil War soldiers walking through the woods back in Alabama. Channy loved Coke but never drank it. Sorel hated the words "watches," "apricot," and "planted." Channy wouldn't drink milk unless it was chocolate.

2000

NORTH PARK, EARLY EVENING

Joey sitting alone in his new apartment, smoking weed in an easy chair, staring at the wall, thinking not in words but pictures, sensations, mood-infused, painful, bright-colored, excited. *Christmas comes and goes and, by January, you've forgotten who got you what. And all those things you saved up for and bought your friends? Not even a memory. New Year's slips by—the clock ticks 11:59 and the excitement of the countdown and confetti snapping out into the air and drizzling back down. Champagne corks pop across the room and you laugh and cheer while the bottle foams over. People hugging. Kissing. Shaking hands. And so-and-so dancing in novelty sunglasses with lenses made to look like the numbers of the new date. So-and-so's girlfriend throwing up outside while so-and-so's sister holds her hair and sings softly to her. And who was it raiding the closet and giving everyone funny hats to wear . . . and now . . . a fedora? Top hat? "Yeah. This year." "This year's gonna be the one. My god, this last year was fucking shit, wasn't it, wasn't it shit straight through, like shit wall-to-wall?" And everyone singing the song they sing each New Year, and no one knows the words—old acquaintance? All acquaintance? Two thousand years of history rolled over. The new millennium. It was nothing.*

February starts off cold and blustery, but it warms up a week into the month. After Valentine's Day, you quit the retirement center and take a job as a paid intern in an office building that the fiancé of a distant relative works at. On St. Patrick's Day, you move out of your aunt and uncle's house and get a one-bedroom apartment in North Park. The next morning, Tyler, Maggie, Nicole, and Rory help you move in.

You move all day and then before sunset it's finished. You carry the last box into the bedroom and there's Maggie sitting on the floor, looking through a photo album, turning the pages.

"Joey, who's this?" She takes a photo from its plastic slip and holds it up for you to see. Wallet-sized. You and Allysia Joseph smiling in formalwear in front of a sky-blue backdrop with the name of her school in gold lettering.

"Allysia Joseph. My first girlfriend. That was the spring formal, hers."

"Joseph?"

"Yeah."

"Good thing she's not a guy and you're not a girl and you didn't get married and become Joey Joseph."

You laugh and it feels good to laugh with her. "Good thing."

"She's pretty." She sets the photo aside and turns the pages of the album, looking at the rest of the photos, touching some of them through the plastic. She's quiet and patient and serious. It's what you like best in a girl.

"It was a long time ago." Was it? You kneel on the carpet and take the photo and stare at Allysia—fifteen years old, pale skin and bare shoulders, flat chested, her green formal dress, cranberry-hair parted down the middle and pinned to the sides with yellow plastic barrettes. This was a conscious choice. She loved My So-Called Life and knew she looked like Claire Danes. Some people are happier as someone else.

You and Allysia sitting on the boardwalk at night under the streetlight and pretending you were drunker than you were so you could get away with trying to kiss her. "I think I'm drunk, Allysia. I think I might be." "I think I am, too. I'm pretty sure." And silence and her looking up at you in the moonlight and streetlamp light and how beautiful her eyes were, big, dark. "I want to kiss you but I'm afraid I'll miss." "That's alright. You should try. I won't be mad." And kissing her and it was your first kiss (not hers), the thing you'd wanted for so long. And that next morning at home in your bedroom with the radio on, dancing around your room like a crazy person. I'm in love. My first kiss. My first kiss! Allysia's terrible baggy jeans, her flannel shirts with the cuffs over her hands. Her brother Maury with his gentle, cow-eyed stare. Down's Syndrome. It broke your heart. "Sistuh! Sistuh, bring me hugs!" Sweet, kind, little Maury. You loved him like he was your brother, too. "Maury the champion," you called him. Gone four years now. Four years in the Sherman Cemetery. You cried so hard when you heard the news. It all happened so fast. And Allysia and her tough sister Melody off across the country, running away from their stepdad who touched them when they were toddlers and ruined them forever. You swore you'd kill him, but you didn't.

The smell of her room in Linda Vista, incense, old carpet, lotion. The horrible sour cheese and dog poop smell of her sneakers the day you picked her up from school in the rain in your first car. The ripe tomato smell of sweat that was gross but turned you on just the same. The salt-chlorine smell of her on your fingers the first time she let you put your hand down her pants. You were so ner-

vous. You always asked first, Is it okay if I do this, Is it okay if I take this off, Is it okay if I touch you here?

Allysia's mother cooking dinner in their kitchen, greasy vegetable soup, the best you ever had, a steaming, clattering pot, her little sister sitting at the kitchen table doing homework, small and long-haired, singing along with a car advertisement on the TV—"Mossy Nissan, Mossy Nissan, Mossy Nissan moves you."

Allysia sitting on the edge of her tiny bed, fully dressed again, tying the laces of her shoes after you'd fooled around for hours, hours of kissing and at the end just down to her panties and socks and nothing else, her bra off finally after weeks of dreaming of it and her white body next to yours, and the sadness and shock to be back in clothes and knowing you had to leave. Two virgins. The singer on the radio singing, "Ohhh my liiife, it's changin' ev-ery day / In every poss-i-ble way," and you were aching at all the change. You told yourself that you were no longer a boy, but you were wrong. You were in love, and when you're in love, you say wrong things and you believe them.

You see her clunky pink phone and its coiled white cord and the answering machine next to the bed covered in cartoon cat stickers and you see her drawings of angels on the walls, her schoolbooks in a stack by the door—some of them with covers made from grocery bags. Drawings of crosses and bandit-masked raccoons in colored pencil. One of them with your name and hers in Crayola marker—curled together with green ivy. On her wall, the famous painting of Jesus you see everywhere—kind, sad, blonde-brown hair and a beard, white robe, brown background, a faint white light behind him, eyes heavenward. You went to church with her out on Kearny Mesa Road. Her youth group. How did you forget that? She believed so sweetly that you almost believed, too. You called yourself a Christian for three weeks and you wore a cross. You were so in love, but she's a ghost to you now—someone you saw on TV and knew as a character. A face in the newspaper.

"I think she goes to art school in New Hampshire. Or Vermont. Yeah, Vermont. Vermont. I barely remember her."

"Oh, I don't believe that. She's cute. She looks like a little field mouse. You guys look happy."

"We were. I mean, for a while we were. You know how it is."

"I've never seen you look that happy. You're always so 'Grrr, grrr' dead serious about everything and walking around like you're this—" she stops herself and her cheeks flush red.

She's blushing over something she was going to say about you.

She's thought about you and what you are and what you mean to her.

Shut up. Listen to yourself.

"Alright, we should probably leave. We need to beat traffic at the border.

We're burning daylight."

"We're burning daylight. We're burning daylight?" She says it like she's turning it over to see it from behind. "Yeah. Let's do it." Maggie slides the picture into one of the empty photo sleeves and shuts the album.

In Tijuana, you eat tacos and drink margaritas as the sound of Spanish guitars drifts out from the back of the restaurant along with the oily butter smell of frying tortillas. It's a warm night and you're the only ones here.

Maggie sits next to Tyler. You sit between Rory and Nicole. As it gets later, Tyler and Maggie scoot their chairs closer until they're shoulder-to-shoulder. She makes excuses to touch him. He puts his head on her shoulder to show how tired he is and she says things that you can't hear.

"You guys'll never believe who Rory's dating," says Nicole, her eyes bright and mean like a bird.

"Nicky!" Rory acts like she's mad, but she's not. She pulls her hair back into a ponytail, lets it fall loose around her face, and waits for Nicole to break the news.

Nicole says the guy's name. A name you don't know. He's a "super, super famous pro-skateboarder. He calls himself Little Jay," she says and Rory shakes her head and sits low in her seat.

Tyler laughs. "Really? He's mega famous. Like in-movies famous."

"The one and only. And whenever he leaves the room he's all, 'Little Jay's out,' and does this weird hand motion thing. Like this," Nicole holds the pointer finger of her left hand in the fist of her right and pulls both hands away from each other and shows their palms, fingers spread out dramatically. "Like that. Like a magic trick that doesn't do anything. He thinks he's so effing cool but he's such a dork. At least he doesn't add jazz hands in there but I wouldn't be surprised if he—"

"Nicky, c'mon," says Rory, playing embarrassed. "He's not dorky. He's sweet."

Tyler tries it. "Little Ty's ouuut," he says happily and Maggie snuggles up to him.

*More drinks arrive. Beers, lime slices set gently in the mouths of the bottles. Strawberry margaritas in frosted glasses with salt along the rim. The restaurant fills up and a three-piece mariachi band comes in from the street to play folk songs for people at their tables. "*Y agaraste por tu cuenta la parranda / Paloma negra paloma negra dónde, dónde andarás? / Ya no jueges con mi honra parrandera / Si tus caricias han de ser mías, de nadie mas.*"*

Plates are cleared. Red candles lit. Desserts served—fried ice cream (Maggie's favorite) and caramel flan. Tyler has his arm around Maggie now and she's talking to him, smiling. She looks down at the candle in front of her and flicks her finger through the flame. Their faces glow.

When you drop Maggie off, Tyler gets out at her house and they walk to the front door, holding hands under the porchlight.

AFTERNOON, INTESTATE 5

Joey driving his truck, lost in a new neighborhood near the border, staring out the window. *Take a new way home from work. You can afford to get lost for a while; your apartment's empty and no one's waiting there for you. Leave the freeway that wraps around the malls and head up into the hills by the old Spanish mission, the jungle of trees beside the road, the palms and eucalyptus and walls of ferns. Catch a glimpse of the sea so faded by sunlight that it's nearly aluminum. Then trees again. The winding road. Sun splashing through your windshield. And the bay below you, the shore in coves like puzzle pieces. Then the mission, the white walls and arches and bell-tower. Your head plays back a song they taught you when your elementary school class visited the mission for Old Town Week. Singing and walking with your backpack on in the group lead by a college volunteer, walking across the grass lawns below the mission, singing, "Long ago we baked adobe bricks / Sunshine drying did the trick / Pounded apples, grinded corn/partied on fiesta's morn." (And on the bus ride back to Pacific Beach, "Tall" Tim Sanders turned it into "sucked adobe dicks" and "farted on fiesta's morn" and it made you sad.)*

Drive down the hill and across town and around the golf course until all the houses are turquoise and pink and green in Mexican neighborhoods. Iron-wrought gates and fences choked with honeysuckle vine. Lawns of yellow-green crabgrass. Churches on every block—Christ Harmony Valley Adventist, Mt. Hope Calvary, New Fellowship Zion, Centro Cristiano Maranatha, Iglesia del Nazareno, Puerta Al Cielo, La Luz del Mundo. Then the tamale cart. A black family outside a car lot with ropes of colorful flags flapping in the breeze, their daughter your age and beautiful. The seafood restaurant with a pirate's name. Chicken shack diners. A gray-blue afternoon now. Windy. Darkening.

You think about the rowboat, but you push it away.

Drive past the preschool with its Spanish tile fountain, past junkyards with high fences and warehouses, around closed down factories at the harbor and over the railroad tracks. K-chunk.

The rowboat.

No.

Tomorrow you work. The next day is yours. Sunday is yours, too, and then you work five more.

Finally lost. Where did Limón Street go? Or did you come down Montemorelos to get here?

The rowboat.

You and Nicole found the rowboat at the foot of Santa Clara by the Sailing Center. It was on the bayshore at low tide with two oars, a coil of gray rope, and a jug of water inside. There was a wallet but the wallet was empty, a salt-stained fold of black snakeskin, worn down to the leather in the middle. You poured the water out into the water and stuck the wallet in your pocket and then you tied the rope to the cleat on the nose of the rowboat and cuffed up your jeans and you and Nicole walked the rowboat through the shallows and lead it back to the foot of your street. You loved the rowboat. It was yours. "I have a boat," you told yourself.

This was near the end. You traced the course of events after she left. It was the week she and David Horowitz first started . . . the week they first started.

You decided it would be romantic to take the rowboat out onto the water. You would row in the back and Nicole would sit in the front and do her homework. You'd get to a good spot out past the noise of the bayshore and tie up to a buoy and rest. You could bring some sodas and make some sandwiches.

You left the rowboat on the sand and walked back to your aunt and uncle's and she got her backpack and you changed into swim trunks and a t-shirt. You made a peanut butter and banana sandwich for her and a tomato sandwich for you. You sliced up an orange and put it in a Ziplock bag. From the fridge, two sodas, a Dr. Pepper for you, a Mountain Dew for Nicole.

At first it was easy. You sat in the back and she sat in the front, in the bow. The sun sparkling on the water in patches so bright you couldn't see. Jellyfish below the boat. (You leaning over the side, gripping the rail and staring at them billowing through the water, rising and falling. Nicole lighting a cigarette and ashing into the water). It was easy and it was perfect. The sounds of gulls and the smell of the bay, the oars through the water and the wake from boats hitting the bow with a hollow clunk. But then the wind came up and you couldn't row straight. The oars would turn in your hands and come out of the water. Instead of forward, you were pushed backward and to the side. You tried to row to the shore but the boat went in circles. And then she was yelling. Calling you so many names. Pulling out all the old fights. The first time you ever got drunk—Johnny Taylor's party on New Year's and she had to watch over you while you puked in your sleep and she hated you for it and never let you forget it. The time you forgot to pick her up from work and it rained. The time you didn't call every day when you went up to Lake Tahoe for Christmas. And then you were useless. You couldn't row and you couldn't argue and you weren't a man. And then you were in the front, looking down at your hands and she was rowing to shore. She was angry and when she was angry she was sure of herself. She rowed straight to the shore and you left the rowboat there.

Keep driving.

BAY AREA, NIGHT

The first day of summer. A party in the scrub-brush hills overlooking the bay. It's a mild, clear night. Quiet, spacey folk records play on the turntable. People sit on couches or stand in the kitchen holding their drinks. Kids playing grownup in a three-million-dollar house. No one smokes inside.

Joey and Ben Frank sit outside on the curb drinking wine from a gallon jug of Carlo Rossi. The wine is cheap and it's too sweet, but it goes down fast and they're getting drunk.

"Ben Frank, this shitty *Dawson's Creek* rich kid party can go fuck itself," Joey says, hoisting the jug and taking a swallow. "Fuck itself until it gets pregnant and gives birth to a better party." He spits a stream of wine out on the asphalt in front of him and it looks like blood. Some of it dribbles down his chin. He wipes it off with the neck of his green t-shirt.

Ben Frank laughs. "You sound *old*."

"I *feel* old. You ever get, like . . . like, where everything in the world makes you angry? It's like one fucking house fly that keeps landing on the same spot on your arm and it lands so many times it feels like your skin is being rubbed raw? Chinese water torture or whatever. You know what I mean?"

"No."

"That's . . . maybe I am getting old. Ugh. Maybe I'm just tired. I had a long day. Work *sucked* today. It suhhhhhhhhhhhcked."

"Quit your job. You should go on the road with me."

"I'm too broke."

"I doubt you're as broke as you think."

"You have money in your account, right?"

"Yeah, some."

"Enough to pay rent?"

"Yeah, enough for that."

"Utilities? Water, trash, electricity?"

"I don't really . . . they're included in the . . . they're part of the rent."

"You're better off than most people."

"I guess."

"Trust me. You are." Ben Frank—dirty, tired, just in from Chicago by way of Florida by way of Texas. He wears horn-rimmed glasses and an old suit with a giant paperback book shoved in the side pocket (Ed Distler's *Ghosts and The Amazon*). His leather dress-shoes are giant, like clown shoes. One has laces, untied. One is wrapped with duct tape. Across the duct tape is the word PIZZA written in black marker. Ben Frank pulls his knees up under his chin, wraps his arms around his legs, and tells Joey how he spent the spring. Greyhound buses, cross-country on a faked Ameripass. San Diego to Atlanta. Shoplifting his dinner in Salt Lake City, paranoid about Mormons. Hitchhiking through Arizona. Coming down off pills and dazzled by the lights of Boulder. Evading arrest for shoplifting in Sioux City. Sleeping under an overpass and nearly killed by a flashflood. Hiding out with Henny Lee Bluefeather, a beautiful Native American girl (blind since birth) at her brother's cattle ranch on the edge of town. (Stories concerning Henny Lee: 1) Listening to raindrops while sitting inside an old fridge in a vacant field. Her idea. 2) Reading Ed Distler's *A Book of Lists*, "The tank was hit by the shell and they felt nothing. You don't wake up dead like Private Carvelle told Morris. You don't wake up at all. Sixteen years later, a field of purple flowers shuddering in the breeze, and in the soil the shattered bones of Carvelle's face." 3) Climbing the water tower and firing her dad's Colt .45 into the great deep-red dusk. A eulogy to her father Tom on the anniversary of his death.) "Joey, the worst part was the cops. I'm on the road all time but I've never *seen* this many cops. Iowa cops are the worst. Sitting in their fucking highway patrol cars, spitting dip into a Gatorade bottle, just *waiting* for you. What kind of person *voluntarily* becomes a cop. Why would you be like, 'I want to be *evil* when I grow up.' Why?" He tells Joey about superhuman kids across the country who shoplift all day and dig for food in the dumpster and hop trains and drink wine by the bucket and give themselves tattoos with each other's names. He tells him about the photocopied magazines they make with the stories of their triumphs, their battles with society, their great heartbroken tragedies. It's the Old West all over again, he says. The New Old West. The frontier, now that the frontier is a stripmall.

"Rory told me you died for five minutes on an operating table. She was like, 'Oh my god, Joey, you have to get Ben Frank to tell you his near-death story if you see him tonight!'"

"Rory?"

"McKellen. Gonna-be-a-lawyer-Rory. Goes to UCSD."

"Huh. I don't think I know any Rories. But yeah, I did."

"Died?"

"Twice," he says with a nod and shows him two fingers. (The nail of his middle finger is painted baby blue, but chipped.) He pulls a cigarette out of his pack and sticks it in his mouth. "You want one?"

"Thanks."

"Here. No problem. Twice in two weeks. Whiskey and Vicodin. *Dumb*."

"And each time they brought you back."

"Yup." He lights the cigarette and takes a drag. "Takes more than that to kill me off. I'm like Bruce Willis, *Die Hard, Part 7: Internal Secret Office Memo to All Terroristic Douchebags and Crooked Cops: 'F' and 'Y' to the Goddamn 'I', Ben Frank Cannot be Killed. Stop Trying Now, It's Getting Ridiculous. Thank You. Yippee Ki-Yay,* et cetera, ad nauseum, aut viam inveniam aut faciam."

"How'd you feel? I mean, afterwards."

"Fine. Better than fine. For a second, I was like, Does this mean I'm a zombie because that would be *awesome*," they laugh, "and then I walked out of the hospital—actually, I *ran* out, in my gown, orderlies chasing me, and I ducked into the first alley, and caught my breath and my heart was pounding and I felt freer than I'd ever felt. I actually stole clothes off a clothesline. Like in movies. I walked back to the squat dressed like some hip-hop dude in baggy jeans and a Bulls jersey. There was no belt, of course, so I had to hold my pants up with one hand. Straight-up crip-walking *thug*. That was the first time. The first time I died, I mean. The second was uneventful, boring."

Joey laughs and shakes his head. "You know you're my hero, right?"

"I'm everybody's hero. Ben Frank . . . it's like . . . it's like a brand name at this point." He lies back on the grass and stares up at the stars. "Someday there will be Ben Frank endorsed cereal boxes, signature model skate shoes . . . Ben Frank brand candy bars, energy drinks with my grinning caveman face on it."

"Ben Frank plastic trash bags," Joey says, "shovels, race cars, McDonald's Happy Meal toys, theme bars."

"Shovels is a good one," he says, sitting up and scratching the back of his head. "How 'bout Ben Frank brand coffins, microwaves, bicycles, umbrellas, cookies, doors, cats, dogs, fake teeth, fishing rods."

"Poisons, law degrees, planets."

"Revolutionary War cannons."

"Phantom gas clouds."

"Snowplows, philosophical tangents, rare chameleons, tidal waves, STDs, toxins, religions, Friar Tuck robes, varying degrees of shame, pepperoni, feudal street gangs, death rituals, designer impostor fragrances, underwater cities," he laughs. "What are we even *talking* about? Whenever we hang out we get so *absurd*. I love you, Joey."

"We're talking about . . . what are we talking about . . . about Ben Frank brand moon landings (both real and faked), senators' teeth, Missouris, Dalai Lamas, Bowie knives, Alamos, coleslaw, shredded cheese, new ideas."

"'Stupid moves, nightmares, or dreams come true,'" Ben Frank says, quoting a song.

"'Mucho work, minus play,'" Joey continues, singing now.

"'Tension mounts in a twisted face.'"

"Ben Frank visions, a radio hit with combination dance move, leap years, Louisiana Purchases, WWIIs, Submarina locations, Jimmy Carters, Al Gores, Indiana Joneses, Britney Spearseseses, Napoleons, John Travoltas, River Phoenixes, Marilyn Monroes, smoke signals, atrocities, shark teeth . . . and . . . that's it, that's all you get. That's the limit of your celebrity. Sorry."

Joey laughs and passes Ben Frank the wine jug and looks back at the house—Tyler and Maggie framed in the light of the front window, arguing soundlessly, his hands out to his sides, her arms crossed in defiance. She's shaking her head. His mouth is open and now he's punctuating what he's saying by shaking his finger at her. Through the kitchen window Joey sees the party's host, Fat Fred Hernandez, talking to a group of smiling girls, as wide as all four of them. He says something and shrugs comically and smooths down his big, black beard. They all laugh and one of them touches his shoulder.

"Fat Fred Hernandez is the worst person on Earth," Joey says bitterly.

Ben Frank laughs. "He's a good guy when you get to know him. Look, Joey, San Diego's a dead end. California's done. We missed the boat by, like, thirty years. Look at all this," he waves his hand across the skyline. "There's nothing here for people like us. This party just illustrates my point. Have you read Ed Distler?"

"Not really . . . I mean, no. I'm not a big reader, I guess. I always . . . I always just read the same book over and over again, the same . . . like the same five books."

"You really need to. His best one." He pulls the book from his pocket and shakes it at Joey. "*Ghosts and The Amazon*. I'd loan you mine, but you have a job. You're rich. Use that shit for something worthwhile. Go to Borders tomorrow. Buy every copy on the shelf."

"Alright."

"I'm serious. You need to put some fire into your life."

"I have fire."

"You could use some more. Look, Joey . . . Joey . . . us, me and you . . . everybody here . . . all our friends . . . we could have adventures but we don't. We sit around and . . . what? We drink and do stupid drugs and talk about bands. Boring. If we're lucky, we go to a show but we don't watch the band. We stand outside and drink and talk about bands. Drink and talk about bands, drink and talk about bands. It's awful. That's not living. We should be hopping *trains* together, me and you. Find some horses and ride 'em off into the desert and see what *happens*. We should build a junk boat and sail it down the Mississippi. Get the hell outta Dodge. Adventure, Joey. Adventure."

"I guess."

"No, not 'I guess.' I'm *right*. You need to move to Chicago. I'm going out there at the end of summer for school."

"No way. It's too cold."

"'It's too cold' . . . listen to you. You sound like somebody's stupid shitty dad. Look, me and a couple kids from here (Aaron Cunningham and Matthew Crispin and maybe Byron) are moving into this abandoned storefront in Chicago that's been turned into . . . it's like a palace from antiquity. I'll email you photos. Kids've built pathways and lofts and catwalks and secret rooms all over the place. It used to be a grocery store. It's a squat like the old office in La Jolla—you've been there."

"I don't think I have."

"Anyway, but it's . . . like, professional or whatever. I'm only paying forty bucks a month rent. Forty bucks! I won't have to work. The place is called El Supermercado."

"Have you *ever* worked?" Joey tries to say it funny but it comes out mean.

"No, and proud of it. You could quit your job. I know you don't want to work in an *office*."

"I like my job."

"No, you don't. You're too young to have such an old life. You need to quit as soon as you can. How much do you make an hour?"

"Thirteen . . . with full benefits."

"So at eight hours a day, that's about a hundred bucks a day, right?"

"I dunno."

"God, you're *rich*. Five hundred a week, give or take, before taxes. Would you let someone pay you five hundred bucks to go to *jail* for forty hours a week?"

"It's better than food service."

"No, it isn't. It's worse. Food service, offices . . . Joey, we don't have to live like that. We can cut expenses, find smaller rents if we have to rent at all, get rid of our cars and ride bikes everywhere, live with friends, pool our resources, grow our own food. We can do it different. Just think about it at least. Tell me you'll think about it."

"I will."

"Listen to you, 'Uhhh, Ah weeell.' I don't believe you."

"No, I will."

"Promise me or I'll come back in the dead of night and climb through your shitty stupid window and cut off your head and take it back to Chicago with me in a burlap sack and use it to turn people to stone."

"Okay. I promise."

"Now we're talkin'. Joey, you need to be better than you are."

"Doesn't everybody?"

"Yes, totally, of course. Me too. Especially me. Everybody. Everybody, Joey."

Ben Frank hands him the wine jug and he holds it up to the cityscape below, the red blinking lights of boats on the bay, headlights and brakelights on the freeway, all glowing through the bottle's hull like a Christmas tree. He unscrews the cap and takes a drink.

By midnight, Ben Frank has gone off to see a house show in Golden Hill and Maggie and Tyler are fighting again. Joey sits on the sofa watching people drink; he watches them go from excited to slack-faced and extinguished.

The couch sags as Fat Fred Hernandez sits down next to him.

Fat Fred lights a joint, takes a drag, and hands it to him. "Hit it, *ese*.

This shit is *kiiiiller*."

"Thanks." Joey takes a hit and coughs and then takes another and passes it back.

"Have some more."

"No, that's okay."

"Joey, you see what me and Lani just did?"

Lani is Laniele Nguyen, Fat Fred's girlfriend, a poli sci major, concert cellist, a rising star of young classical music.

"No."

"We made out with that girl Maggie. All three of us together. She and Maggie got drunk together on the couch and Lani's on E and they just started making out a little and I was like, 'Dude, fuckin' sweeeeet!' I sat down and joined in. I even felt her tits! Both hers and Lani's. At the same time. One in each hand! Maggie got up and left after that and Lani got mad. I thought I was gonna fuck 'em both. I was like, '*Hell yeah*, getting my dick wet in *two* pussies tonight,' but no. That was it. Bummer."

"Oh."

"You okay, Carr?"

"I'm—"

"You look a little pale, *ese*," he says. "You alright? You havin' a good time? I got some" (whispering) "coke in my room. You want me to get you something? Beer? Wine? Vodka? Food? There's *hella* food left. I'll heat up some *empanadas*. You're not vegan, are you? There's some jalapeño poppers left. When you come to my house, you want for nothing. I can mix you up a killer Fat-Fred-brand blackberry margarita. Let me make us a couple. Just chill and I'll be right back."

"No, I'm . . . I need to go, like . . . outside." And Joey gets up and walks, the world curving in around him, a tunnel, the ceiling dipping low above his head like tree branches, and then outside, fresh air, night air.

When Joey started middle school, he had panic attacks every few months for three years. Now when he feels one coming, he goes outside. It works. Most of the time.

Across the street from the party, he finds a couple sullen, ratty kids sitting on the hood of a car with New Mexico plates sharing a bottle of off-brand tequila. Ben Frank's friends he met earlier. Train kids. Travelers. He nods to them. They nod back. He sits down and they drink.

As the party dies down, Joey stumbles through the house looking for the bathroom. The place is endless. He keeps coming back to the same rooms: back to the bedroom with the 'Off Limits' sign on the door, back to the room with Lani's cello.

And now, in the bathroom with the lights off, he's on his knees throwing up into the toilet and then he's crying with his face over the bowl and puke is clogged up in his nose and then there's light at the crack in the door.

The door is opening.

He looks up, and wipes his nose.

Maggie.

Maggie's silhouette in the frame of light from the hall.

"Maggie?"

And then he's standing up and she's hugging him and he's crying and his shoulders are shaking and he's telling her he just wants to die and she's calling him 'baby' and she's smoothing the back of his hair.

The next part happens fast. She kisses his neck. Just barely. Just a touch for the smallest second in the dark while all his hope is crashing and his heart is in a rage and everything is useless and stupid, and then, suddenly, it isn't.

BAY PARK, MORNING

It's gray and sprinkling when Tyler's mom picks them up in the morning at Fat Fred's. She and Tyler sit in the front. Joey and Maggie in the back with their hangovers like leeches eating them. Joey puts on his sunglasses. Maggie digs around in her bag for hers and then sticks them over her face.

They drive down the winding hill and turn at the 7-Eleven, then cut back north on Morena, Mission Bay below, dark clouds overhead, gray waters.

"Tyler! What's wrong with them?!" Tyler's mom says so loud it cracks Joey's skull.

"They're hungover. They got waaasted last night," says Tyler, sarcastic.

Tyler's mom laughs loudly and says, "Tsk tsk, you guys! Tsk tsk!"

"Tyler," groans Maggie.

"What? You *did,*" he says, smiling at her from between the front seats.

They pass industrial lots, a line of bicyclists with matching yellow jerseys, the indoor shooting range, a sailor bar with an old man out front smoking in the rain.

The raindrops hit the windshield now in a wild, drumming spray and Tyler's mom clicks on the wipers. She turns up the radio. A speech from one of the candidates: "My father was the last president of a great generation. A generation of Americans who stormed beaches, liberated concentration camps, and delivered us from evil. Some never came home. Those who did put their medals in drawers, went to work, and built on a heroic scale . . . highways and universities—"

"Tyler you better vote in November," she says.

"*Mom.*"

"—suburbs and factories, great cities and grand alliances—"

"You better vote. It's your right. Who are you voting for? You better vote. Tyler, you better vote."

"Mom. Please."

"—the strong foundations of an American century. Now the question comes to the sons and daughters of this achievement—"

The hangover howls and Joey's dried up inside and everything throbs and hurts but there she is, she's sitting next to him, and he remembers everything.

"—What is asked of us?"

1979

AUGUST 20TH

When the Ecuadoran came, I made her stay the night and gave her the rest of my money. She shook her head and I laughed handing it to her. "Here! All of it! All of it!" She dropped the money and ran out of my room and slammed the door behind her.

AUGUST 21ST

Tonight, the Ecuadoran came back, and when we finished she cried. I gave her my money and she took and it left. If she comes back, I want to ask her to marry me. She's strong, capable. Her mind is good and she has a great sense of humor. I need a new start.

AUGUST 22ND

The Ecuadoran didn't come tonight and I sat up for hours freaking out about it. They sent a mean, slit-eyed girl with dyed blonde hair who was incredibly drunk and I asked her to leave. When she argued with me, I told her I had a gun under my pillow and threatened to shoot her and she left. I'm so confused. If I had a gun, I'd shoot my brains out and be done with it. I'm done. Ready. Ready to be free of this.

AUGUST 23RD

No one came today. Not the Ecuadoran. Not Magda with the food. Why eat? I've eaten every day of my life. Who cares.

AUGUST 24TH

Still no one. I could go down to the street. I could. I was hungry all day and then it stopped. Now I couldn't eat if I tried. I won't try. I won't.

AUGUST 25TH

What happened? No one came today. I drank the last of the water and ate a stale shard of tortilla I found between the bed and wall. It was as hard as a bone. One of my back teeth is loose. It wiggles. Wiggles left and right but I can't pull it out. Maybe I should tie one end of a string to the tooth and the other to the door and then slam the door. Does that work? I don't have string. Stupid.

AUGUST 26TH

Again, no one. Drank rainwater, sat in bed and laughed all day. The world ended and there's no one left down there. The sound of the traffic, I once joked, was the sound of the sea, has been the sound of the sea all along. Jump off the roof, fall into the sea.

AUGUST 27TH

The tooth came out last night. I was pushing at it with my tongue and it came out. I don't know what to do with it. I got to thinking about how I would put my baby teeth under my pillow and my mother would trade them out for a quarter and I cried so hard I couldn't stop. Mom. Jesus Christ. Where are you? Why can't you do anything for me?

AUGUST 28TH

Slept all morning. Morning. Channy Morning Greene? The sun rising. The sun is the center of a red flower. What flower? A sunflower. I'm an empty barrel. I pulled my shirt up this morning and I couldn't see my stomach. It was gone. My ribs jutting out and I had to lean forward to see my belly button.

I could go downstairs. I could. I could put my shoes on and change my shirt and walk out the door. I could get out of bed. I could.

I'm waiting for my mom to come save me. She'll know I'm here and she'll know what to do. My dad's dead. He's dead: What a strange thing to be, dead. My dad's a pile of bones, and he doesn't even look the same. He's been dead for almost as long as I've been alive. Jacob's alive. As far as I know. What about Sorel? Alive, I guess. Channy? Alive. The boy? Of course he's alive. I'm alive, too.

AUGUST 29TH

Yesterday Señor Dueñas, the owner of the building, came up to the roof. Magda from the *taquería* was with him and she laid out dinner for he and I and we ate together. The first course was shrimp *ceviche* and fish soup. (Ten minutes into the meal, I went back behind my studio and threw up.) The second course was grilled lobster tails with a sweet red sauce and a honeyed Bundt cake Magda called *rosca de miel*. Dueñas brought a bottle of *mezcal* and two glasses and we sat in the deck chairs and he talked until late.

Dueñas told me about his father and how he came up from Oaxaca and made his money on horses at *Agua Caliente* and went into real estate and film financing when the track was closed. He told me about the Revolution and about his family, how they traced their line back before the Spaniards (and how they kept it a secret when doing business). What his family was most proud of was their small *mezcal* factory back home. "A hobby, really. We built the factory because we had the money, and then when we had no money, the factory closed down and my father was brokenhearted and never touched a drop again." Dueñas said, "When my father drank *mescal*, it was not like this. He would pour some on the ground first—a little bit, just a drop. My father said this was an offering to *Mayahuel*, the fertility goddess of the maguey plant that this wonderful drink"—he held up his glass—"is made from. And he ate *oranges* when he drank it. That I do not understand. For me, a glass, nothing else, no lime, no fried larvae, no chilies, no salt. I am a purist, but a purist is no fun," (laughing.) "My father, he was an adventurer in all aspects. A purist like me . . . not so much." Dueñas poured the *mezcal*—I had a glass, he had six—and spoke slowly and clearly. His stories were stories of family, how this uncle's marriage meant this, this son worked and then achieved this, this cousin was nothing because of this. The more he drank, the darker and later it became, the more stories he told of his wife: how, without her, his drive to succeed would be "nothing but capitalism." He said, "You must understand the ambition I had was not mine. My name is Jesús. Jesús Carlos Zubieta Dueñas. An important name, a name handed down from my great-great grandfather, who was burned alive for cheating the men of his village out of money . . . burned alive, if you can imagine . . . *roasted* like a screaming pig, tied back to back with his business partner, a man said to know weather before weather would come. Another crook. I come from a long line of men who shaped the world around them for the good of themselves. The good of self. *Personal gain*. Some of them were criminals. Some, like my father and his brother, were powerful men for a very short time. Their wives, they were there to provide heirs, and to watch the home. When I met Jesika, she consumed my world. I made a lot of bad choices because I wanted nothing but to know her and absorb the . . . the," he waved his hand in the air, "the I-don't-know-what . . . the *vitality*, the *life force* that came from her. It was magnetic, youthful . . . voluptuous, exciting. Jesika, she was full of this . . . this *energy* that would infect you. If she was happy, you could not help but be swept up in the feeling. Her joy, it was *narcotic*. When you felt it, it was pure and clean and it was *satisfying*. It made you hungry and it made you laugh and do brave, wild, *terrible* things. I wasted away for years in her joy. We lived in poverty. I worked a dozen jobs and not one of them honest. I robbed people. I stole. I killed. I admit this. I killed men in the name of work. I am not proud of this, but everyone here knows how I spent my youth. I remember each one. Felipe Salinas de Zedillo. Ernesto Luís Echeverria. Lazaro Raúl Avila Calles. Three men for . . . various reasons. With Jesika, I lived, like you, here in that same apartment, but unlike you (respectfully) we did so without money. We lived in that room—thirty years ago—and we lived on beans and rice and tortillas and the occasional chicken brought by my mother. We were no one, but we were everyone to each other. To the rest of the world, to this neighborhood, to Tijuana, to Mexico, we were as good as invisible. Did we care? No. The world around us, it did not exist because we were a world for ourselves. Jesika, she got me reading. Rulfo, *Les Paradis Artificiels,* Nervo, de Balbuena, Juan Ruíz de Alarcon, Castellanos, Rudolfo Usigli, Villaurrutia, *Areopagitica* and *Tretrachordon,* Nezahualcoyoti, *Songs of Innocence and of Experience* (Blake was a favorite of hers and mine), Gardiner's work on Cromwell, *Worship of Silence and Sorrow* (which was a flawed text but a beautiful idea), Mariano Azuela . . . Jesika, she said, 'Pico,' my nickname, 'Pico, a man who does not read (and read *well*) is not a full or worthy man. Any man can carry a gun or go to a job with a briefcase or a wrench or a hoe in his hand, but a man who knows the music and truth of William Blake or García Lorca or Nervo is a man who knows *completion.* We lay together in that bed . . . in there . . . your room . . . and we drank *mezcal* and we read to each other and we made love. The books came from her mother's library in Hermosillo and the *mezcal* was her father's—a great man, another Oaxacan (by birth alone), a man who would later become a god to me but a man who killed and killed and *killed* and left his mark in the graveyards across Sonora. Me, sometimes I worked. Not much. Here and there. Enough to pay the rent in our room—your room—and for a little food. Like now, there was no electricity, no phone, no nothing. Nothing to . . . complicate the arrangement. We had two chairs—like these, different ones, long since firewood or sawdust—and we had our shrine to Mary in one corner with a dozen candles and we had the table—the same as yours—and a pile of books that came and went like the seasonal birds. Stendhal, the writings of Julius Caesar (his *Commentarii de Bello Gallico*), *The Two Gentlemen of Verona,* Proudhon and the radicals, Sappho, Pindar, Aeschylus, you know, Xenophon, von Eichendorff, Skameta, even Marx (who she loved and I hated, and *still* hate). I had three shirts—white with buttons like this—a pair of hard shoes I shined myself, and two pairs of pants, one nice, one for working. She had one dress . . . but *what* a dress. It was like wearing a *color* instead of clothes, the cotton was so thin and to me she was like the mother of all Earth in that dress (her grandmother was full-blooded Tarahumara). The dress . . . thin, the color of red clay. Jesika in that dress was a force, silent when silence was necessary, loud as the Earth shaking when the Earth must be shook," he laughed. "When she washed that dress here in a bucket and hung it out to dry on the line, she wore nothing and I sat in my chair and I watched her and listened to the bedsheets flapping on the line and the world was good, us under the sun and stars, *Jesika y Jesús*. These stars. Orion! There! His belt. Look. This . . . we were like this for a few years until it was time to change. For her, because of her, I became a man, after years as a boy. I went into business with her father and soon our lives were different. Different, but better. I worked for her father but I worked for *her*. Not as an employee but for the good of her, to give her a life worth *remarkable* things, worth the end that comes for all and comes no matter how much you build up around you. I worked so that when she would leave this world, she would leave this world *satisfied*. When her father died, I took over part of his business, the rest split amongst his brothers and cousins and sons, but I made it a *clean* business. I made it a business where no one was hurt unless . . . sometimes unless it was deserved . . . but a business with good intention and noble heart. All this for her."

For a while we sat back in our chairs and didn't say much. Dueñas was very drunk then and a few times I was sure he'd fallen asleep. Finally, he said, "What about you?" He raised his arm and waved his fingers. "You wear a ring on your finger but you are here alone . . . and you have been here a very long time . . . I know this, you are a curiosity, we have been . . . been keeping *tabs* . . . and then, then with the recent . . . occurrences . . . *well*." He leaned forward in his chair with a sound of comfortable pain and found the jug at his feet and filled his glass.

"My wife . . . Channy . . . she's back in the States with my boy." I brought my glass to my lips but I decided against it and didn't drink. "She's back in San Diego."

"Your wife, you are not together?"

I set the glass down and shook my head. "We're not."

"I am sorry. What was she like?"

I tried to bring Channy into my mind but there was nothing. "I don't know. I never got to know her."

2000
THE COURTYARD OUTSIDE THE UNIVERSITY'S ALL-AGES MUSIC CLUB, SUNDOWN

"We took Polaroids of the whole thing."

"While it was happening?"

"While it was happening."

Maggie and Joey sit across from each other at a black, iron patio table. Joey sees them in bed. Maggie losing her virginity. A pile of photos. Maggie swats at a fly and leans back with her bare feet up on the chair next to her (her shoes are under her chair). She's wearing a ragged blue and yellow dress that's cut off and frayed above the knees. Joey's changed clothes since work, but he still has his work clothes in the bag and he knows they're in there and it makes him feel claustrophobic and guilty. He puts his sunglasses on and stares at her knees, white and soft and small and perfect. He gets guilty about that too and takes the glasses off and puts them in his bag.

"We went to Target for supplies." She tells him about the black sheets she bought for the occasion, how it hurt and how she cried a little when it was done. "It made me wonder what everyone was making such a big *fuss* about." She tells Joey the guy's thing was huge ("like a large banana at the grocery store") and how she was afraid it wouldn't fit and how hard it was to get the condom on and how they broke three of them before they got it right. "You're supposed to roll it on but we were pulling it on, like a sock, and that doesn't work. When I finally rolled it onto him it was fine." She tells Joey it was the guy's first time too and how they're going to wait a while and then she'll be on the pill and they won't have to use protection anymore. The actual event, she says, was quick and awkward. "It was like, okay, wait, that was it? It's done? Was I supposed to feel something?" She tells Joey about the guy she lost it to—a friend of a friend from their social group. Nice enough guy. Genius musician. Smart, serious. A guy Joey knows from parties. She tells him how the guy isn't her boyfriend ("officially," she says) and how he says he loves her ten times a day and calls her and cries and how he's jealous and tries to be more to her than she wants. "At least for right now," she points out. For what she wants right now.

Joey's jealous. He feels small and weak.

"Are things still happening with you and Tyler?"

"Sometimes."

"Sometimes?"

"Not as much. We haven't slept together—if that's what you're asking."

"No, I didn't mean that, but yeah."

"I don't think we will. I don't think I could, y'know, *sleep* with more than one guy at once, but Tyler comes over and when he comes over we usually end up doing stuff. Just because . . . I mean we've been doing stuff for so long that it's just what happens. I wouldn't know how to *not* do stuff with Tyler. The day I . . . after, y'know, after it *happened,* Tyler came by and one thing lead to . . . it just happens. It *happens.* I'm not even sure if I want it to happen, but it happens."

Joey sits back in his chair and listens to the creaking of the trees above them. He smells the eucalyptus leaves and the smoke from a stick of strawberry incense burning somewhere and he feels his blood moving, his heart beating steady.

Maggie—serious, quiet, looking across the courtyard. A group of kids with backpacks standing around a small blonde girl holding a kitten. Maggie stares at them and squints. "Joey, you know what the worst part of this whole thing is? My friends. They think I'm a slut. They're always talking about me behind my back now and it *sucks*. It's a shitty way to treat somebody you're supposed to be friends with." She stares up into the patch of dimming blue above them. "I hear about it all the time." The tree branches move in the breeze and divide the sky and light. "I hear about it, y'know, *secondhand*. So-and-so was saying this or that about me. So-and-so overheard so-and-so talking about what I did on some night at some point."

"You're famous." He says this to make a joke. "You're a celebrity."

"If I were, it would make more sense. This way, it's just sad."

The singer of the band inside the club checks his microphone, "Check, check, one, two, ch-eck. Okay, that's fine for me."

The sound engineer: "Sure?"

The singer: "Yep. I'm good."

The sound engineer: "Cool. Let's do backup vocals, okay?"

Maggie: "I think I could deal with it better if it was just every once in a while. I mean, everybody talks shit at some point in their lives, no matter how above it you think you are. But they talk about every little thing. They talk about me if I get *drunk*. They talk about my *clothes*. The stuff I *say*. Who I say it to. It's not like I'm doing anything *freakish*. Everybody else does that stuff. Except them. It's normal for *everybody else*. God. Goddamnit." She looks away and Joey can tell she's pushing back tears.

"Maybe they're bored. People do ridiculous shit when they're bored. I know *I* do. I dyed the palm of my left hand orange with fake tanner once just to see what would happen?"

"What happened?"

"It turned orange."

She laughs, and then she stops. "I guess . . . I guess I always imagined my friends would be more grown-up by now, y'know? And less *prudish*. This stuff is just so *inconsequential*. There are so many more *horrible, awful* things to concern yourself with other than who someone's seeing at the moment or what dress they wear to a party or what word choice they used that might not be . . . might not be rigidly, morally perfect, or if they flirted with some kid they'll never even *see* again. I keep thinking, Man, it must be nice to be *perfect*. I wish my friends would man up and let stuff roll off their shoulders a little more and stop judging everybody all the time. *Fuck*, man. That shitty moral high ground . . . ugh. I'm kind of . . . I guess I'm sort of disappointed with how they're turning out. I thought being eighteen would be an endless party. I wanted this time of my life to be . . . like, violent. Is that a weird way of saying it? Violent? Like, rowdy and wild and full of life? I wanted it to be like *Velvet Goldmine* or something. Really sexy and trashy and wild and all the rules thrown out the window. I guess I'm overthinking this. Does that make me a hypocrite? Like, me saying that I want my friends to be wilder and more careless and less concerned with insignificant drama but here I am getting all judgmental on them? Am I a total hypocrite, or just lame?"

"No, no, not at all, neither. Okay, Maggie, check it out, this is super embarrassing to admit, but a while back I found an ad in a magazine that was like, 'You think you're too tired to go out? Wait until you're eighty! If your life was a movie, would you want to watch it?' It was super cheesy now that I look back on it, but I wrote it down on my school binder my first year of college and I'd look at it all the time just to check myself and make sure I was being . . . I don't know, being, being . . . being worth paying *attention* to. You know what I mean? I didn't . . . I *still* don't want people to say, 'Oh, what's that kid Joey Carr all about?' and have somebody go, 'Oh, he watches a lot of TV, works this boring-ass job, plays Sega, sits around a lot.' I don't want to be one of those dead-inside wastes of space who're just, like, *online* all the time or watching cheesedickish sitcoms and biding their time until . . . like, until something real happens. I want to do things I'll *remember*. Does that make any sense?"

"Definitely. *Totally*. Fuck *yeah*, it makes sense."

"But whenever I look at my life, when I really *think* about it and *analyze* it and when I'm really *honest* with myself, it seems like the kind of movie that would bore me to death. I'm not doing anything real or authentic or . . . or being at *all* adventurous. All this judgmental shit about me not doing it like everybody else is just bullshit and, yeah, like you said, me being a hypocrite. What I see when I look at my life is a lot of, y'know, *sitting around,* a lot of *talking* or just *hanging out* by myself doing nothing. Or working. In that stupid fucking *place* I work, *emailing* people all day about something I don't even *care* about, something that's not totally *vital* to my happiness and survival. That's a terrible movie. It's not even a good *TV show*. It's like one of those comic strips in the paper no one really likes but they all still read every day; one of those shitty comics where the character does the same exact thing every strip with little or no variance to mark the difference between days. Just getting . . . getting *through* the workday, the big conflicts being . . . being, like, some stupid-ass shit about fixing a copy machine or dealing with a mean boss or a quote-unquote crazy girlfriend or a mailman . . . I mean, a paperboy . . . that always throws the paper on the roof. Life as an unfunny *joke*. Unless I'm hanging out with somebody exciting and over-the-top, like Ben Frank or Chente or my friend Ted Boone, my life goes on and I don't even noticing that it's passing. And then a month'll go by and I won't remember what I did, and that scares me. One day it'll just be, like, 'Holy shit, it's *August?* Where did July and June and *May* go? Where has the fucking *year* gone?' And pretty soon your life is over and you don't have anything to show for it. What did you do? You went to school, you worked, maybe you fell in love, or maybe you tried to believe you did, and then you got old and you fucking *died*. Know what I mean? Think back . . . how much of, say, 1997 or 1998 can you remember? 1996? How many memories from those years can you pin down and be like, Yes, that happened that year, that *happened*. 'If your life was a movie, would you want to watch it?' Fuck *no*, I wouldn't. Not at all. It's funny the cheesy fucking shit you see that inspires you. And when it's an advertisement. I mean, an *ad*? Is that where we're getting our truth? I feel ripped off."

"I wouldn't watch my movie either," she says, looking up at the sky, her head tilted against the back of the chair. "Sometimes, I wish I had a PR person following me around and telling me when people were looking. It's tiring if you think about yourself on stage all the time, but if someone could be, like, 'Okay, Maggie, now, do something good. People are paying attention. The microscope is on you. Show us what you got,' that would be okay, right? 'On cue, start living.'"

"Yeah. Totally. I want that too. The Joey Carr Public Image Department."

"Somebody that could be like, 'Maggie, you look tired today. Stay in, alright? Take it easy. Sleep in. Get some rest, eat some chocolate and Chik Nuggets and rice, and try again tomorrow.' Somebody watching out for you all the time. 'Go on the BRAT diet for a while. Build yourself back up.' That sort of thing."

"The BRAT diet?"

"That's what my mom always put us on when we were sick. Bananas, rice, applesauce, toast."

"That would be nice . . . the PR thing. I'd pay good money for that."

"Me too. If I had money."

"I'll pay for both of ours."

"Deal."

"I'll get the contracts ready tomorrow."

"Whoa, fuck, man," she says, laughing, "this is totally *not* stuff I'd ever want *anyone* to hear me say. Jeez. What a buncha nerds we are. How lame did we just get back there? Can we strike everything we just said from the record?"

"Deal." He says 'deal' and he laughs when he says it, but inside he's proud. *You're a 'we'*, he tells himself.

10 P.M.

The band in the club starts its set and Maggie and Joey stay in their chairs and watch through the wall-length windows. Inside, it's dark and the kids in the middle of the room are thrashing around and knocking into each other and condensation is forming on the windows and dripping down.

The first song is over quickly and then the next song opens with a squeal of feedback and drums and loud guitars and then it goes to a slower section and the singer who was hanging from the low rafters by one arm drops back onto the stage, and he's singing loudly over the quiet part while his bandmates stand around him, hunched over their instruments, nodding their heads with the rhythm of what they're playing. And then the song explodes loudly again and the singer throws himself around the stage, smashing into the drum set, bouncing back to the front of the stage, graceful, one arm in the air, sing-screaming earnestly into the faces of the kids in the front row who stand packed up against the stage, eyes closed, nodding their heads to the music. The small blonde girl who had the kitten outside holds a camera above her head and takes a picture without looking and the room lights up with the flash.

HOME, 2 A.M.

When Joey gets home, an answering machine message is waiting for him. "Joey, it's Ben Frank, captain of industry, king of the Planet of the Apes, leader of the Autobots. This is for you from the Distler book I was talking about, (clears his throat, laughs, clears his throat again), reads: "Yuri Yevgenyevich Lvov heard the knock on the front door. The knock he had been waiting for since morning. He got up from the bed and checked the pistol for shells. Two left until Aeneas and Karolos arrive with the cargo from the *Lucia*. Yuri limped to the door and slid the board free and opened it quickly. He pointed the pistol out into the night, braced at his hip like an Old West gunfighter. He felt confident. Sure of himself. Who's out there? Who? No one. Hello? Anyone out there? Aeneas? Karolos? Boy? He stepped out onto the porch. Beyond that the hills and the sea and the night—black and then white flashes of electricity in the clouds, lightning, soundless. No. Not lightning. The Germans shelling again. Of course. He stood on the porch and listened. Yes. The distant thud of artillery. Why now? The boy was out there looking for Ioannis—somewhere in the woods by the ruins of the village—but he would not be coming home tonight. Tonight Yuri would sleep. He was convinced of that, happy. The plans would wait another day. Yuri closed his eyes and breathed in deep and he smelled the sea and the rain coming. Pleasant. Not a bad place to be stuck. He shut the door and slid the board back in place. Then a knock at the back door. Steady knocking. Okay. Yes. One moment. Yuri set the pistol on the table and turned and walked to the back door, favoring his left leg. Of course. Yes. The boy was playing his knocking joke again. A joke. It wasn't funny before but now it is. Okay. Haha. But before Yuri could reach the back door, the knocking stopped and he heard knocking on the front door again and he turned and walked to it. A joke? Of course. But now he heard knocking on both the front and the back doors and he was stuck in the middle, indecisive. Which door should I answer? The front or the back? How do I know which is more important without seeing behind the door first? Just then a curious thing happened in a long line of curious things since Yuri Yevgenyevich had been shot down three nights ago: He heard someone begin to knock on the wall to the *right* of him. On the wall by the bed. The wall which was no wall but the side of the mountain, solid stone, a piece of the earth, immovable. Yuri picked up the gun and checked the shells (again) and held it in his right hand, unsteady, shaking. What is this? This is not the boy or the cargo shipment. What is this? What is happening? He was sure it was either Satan or Christ and that if given the chance he would shoot either. But then he wasn't sure anymore. He was sure of nothing. A new thing was happening than had happened before. Why is this happening to me? Why is it happening when I'm here alone? Yuri dropped the gun at his feet. More knocking. Someone—two sets of hands, four in all—knocking, drumming on the opposite wall along with the front and back door and the wall which was not a wall. My God. And soon it was as if every inch of wall outside the boy's mountain cabin was being knocked upon, a dozen fists, two dozen, and now they were banging on the walls, hammering, and Yuri Yevgenyevich knelt down in the middle of the room as his urine ran hot into his boots and he put his hands over his ears and he screamed the first thing he could think to scream, the name of his mother. He screamed to drown out the sound of the knocking but he could still hear them and new hands were joining in, hundreds now, thousands; fists, fists, fists! He could feel knocking through the floorboards and he could hear it on the rooftop and the walls were shaking and a thousand fists beat below him now and the floor rumbled and the dust rose up around his feet and Yuri knew that soon the cabin would rattle to pieces and then he would finally see who was doing all this knocking. He took the pistol from its place on the floor and put the barrel in his mouth and, without hesitation, pulled the trigger. Click. A dead shell, old, wet. He tried again. Another dud. Of course. The pistol had been with him when he crashed into the sea. Enough. Enough fear. I can be afraid and nothing will change, I will be afraid until the danger confronts me. Or I can confront the danger myself. Yuri Yevgenyevich (pants soaked, shrapnel festering in his left leg, fractured ribs on his right side, hungry, tired) stood up and walked to the door. He pulled back the board and opened the door and spread his arms wide. 'Here I am!'"

HOME, 10:11 A.M.

At home the next morning, Joey cooks a pan of bacon, humming one of the band's songs from last night and singing the words he can remember.

When the food's done, it lies in its puddle of grease and it looks like something dead. Joey stares at it in the pan for five minutes then shakes it off and dumps it in the trash. Singing again, he makes miso soup then drinks it from a coffee mug with the name of the company he works for on the side.

He paces the living room and rearranges his furniture. He stands at his front window and stares out at the concrete staircase that blocks his view of the parking lot. Ten minutes pass. He pulls himself away from the window and listens to his answering machine messages and listens to the ones from Maggie once more. "Hey Joey, this is Maggie. Tyler said you were going to the Ché on Friday to see Physics. I just wanted to see if you needed a ride from us." "Hey Joey, this is Maggie. I just wanted to let you know you left your jacket at my mom's. I'll be home all day Monday if you want to pick it up. Okay. Bye." Joey listens to Ben Frank's message once more and sings a song that Nicole made up about being afraid of the sharks they saw when they went snorkeling in the Cove in front of the Marine Room: "The leopard sharks are my friends / They're not bad / They're nice to me when I'm sad." He sings a cereal commercial to himself from his childhood: "Smurf Berry Crunch is fun to eat / A very Smurfy breakfast treat / Made by Smurfs so happily / Something something some-thally."

He stares into the refrigerator even though he's looked already. Top shelf—Dr. Pepper six-pack with one can missing, expensive peanut butter in a glass jar, eggs in a half-dozen carton. Middle shelf—various cheeses in plastic, gray lunchmeat like sick skin, leftover burrito wrapped in oily yellow paper, half log of salami in white and green paper, various bottles of beer—brown bottles, green bottles, clear bottles of yellow Mexican beer, a lone forty of Olde English left over from a party two weeks ago (on the label someone has written "Mine" in black marker). Bottom shelf above the vegetable crisper—a hard green lime with a brown patch on one side, carton of milk, carton of blackberry kefir from People's, produce bag of Roma tomatoes, plastic container of cherry tomatoes, bag of red grapes, bag of watery baby carrots. Vegetable crisper—empty. Door—full of condiments, Miracle Whip, two mayos, Heinz ketchup, plastic lemon, a ranch dressing—unopened, caesar dressing, a jar of green olives with orange pimentos, dill pickles, sweet pickles, three bottles of store brand Dijon mustard, French's yellow mustard, Chinese hot mustard, Grey Poupon (says to himself in a bad English accent, "Pardon me, would you have any Grey Poupon?" "But of course!")

Twenty minutes pass. Joey makes himself a tomato sandwich and eats it standing up at the island counter that separates the kitchen from the living room. 1) Tomatoes, Roma, musky and fresh, cut in quarter inch slices. 2) Just enough mayo, a careful spread on each piece of bread. 3) The bread, a nice heavy San Francisco sourdough, cut in half diagonally. Before eating it, he leaves the sandwich on the counter for five minutes to let the mayo and tomato (specifically, the water of the fruit and the seeds) seep together.

He finds his ratty, old copy of *Harriet the Spy* in a stack of textbooks on the floor and thumbs through it and reads a section where she's talking about a skinny friend, "When I look at him I could eat two thousand tomato sandwiches." Joey laughs and reaffirms his hero worship for the title character, then puts the book back with the rest, 1) *Your Golden State Studies: Pre-history to Statehood and Beyond,* 2) *Political Science: A College Introduction,* 3) *Chicano Studies New Morris-Henry Edition Comprehensive,* 4) *Math Tips for the Algebra Anxious,* 5) *Asi Es, no? Third Year, Tercero Año,* a collected summation of his final semester before dropping out.

It's Sunday—a hot one, quiet outside, nothing but the sound of the freeway and the occasional cheer or dull knock of ball to bat from the softball field behind the complex. But most of all it's endless Maggie. Maggie from all angles. The problem is that he knows what Maggie's doing right now—she's with him, with her boyfriend—and he can't shake it. He knows where she is because when you start a new relationship, you spend every moment with that person. Their body is new. The things they say are exciting. The things they love are the things you love. This is the idea he can't get around: On Sundays you choose to spend your time with the person you most want to be with. Who is he with? He's alone. *What does* that *mean?* he asks himself.

Outside, a breeze blows and the palm fronds rasp against each other. It's a Santa Ana wind, hot and dry from the desert to the east. The kind of wind that spreads brush fires in the hills. By sundown it's on the radio. "California wildfires once again." "East County in peril." "Horses at risk." "Evacuation." "The man on his roof with a garden hose has been airlifted out with both of his cats!"

The later (and hotter) it gets, the more frustrated he becomes, until he's pacing the room and cussing to himself under his breath. He starts to call her but he hangs up. He grabs the receiver again and puts it back down. Sweating down his back, he drinks a beer. Two more. Three. He drinks six while sitting in various chairs and he's drunk and his mouth is dry and his thoughts are unclear and that helps nothing. He drinks from the half-empty bottle of Malibu that he's had forever. Three gulps and another two and it's sweet and warm and awful and the world woozes in around him, fades to gray, and then opens up like a movie screen. He hears the clicking of the projector and he sees them sitting on the edge of her bed. Or maybe it's his bed, the guy's bed. The bed he's had since he was six. Hand-built by his dad from a Mervyn's kit. *Star Wars* sheets. No, *Return of the Jedi* sheets. Faded. Teddy bear Ewoks holding their spears next to Luke and Han and Leia, Vader and the Emperor looming behind, Chewbacca and C-3PO and R2-D2 in miniature below them, the unfinished Death Star hanging in space above everything. And Joey sees the guy lifting her dress over her head and she's letting him. She's holding her arms up. He sees him kissing her neck and she has her hand on his back. And then they're lying in bed afterward, her head on his chest or his on hers—yes, his on hers, he's sensitive, she's not—and him talking in a low, deep voice about the things they'll do together the next day, where they'll eat breakfast (IHOP), what shared friends they'll go see (Ben Frank?), the movies they'll rent at night (*Goonies* and *Stand by Me*) and what candy they'll buy to eat while they watch it (watermelon Sour Patch Kids, Red Vines, peanut M&Ms). Joey sees them doing it again and this time she knows he's getting better at it and that maybe she could love him if it keeps feeling like it does now. Maybe it could work. Maybe it could. It could! No, it *will*. It *is*. And he's on top of her with the sheet pulled over his lower back and he's breathing hard and pushing against her. She's flushed, eyes to slits, mouth open, a half smile, a gasp, and now he's smacking into her and then her eyes are shut tight and she's nearly there. She's there and she's digging her fingers into his back. Her hips are jerking in place and then she's done and he pulls out and yanks off the rubber and tosses it behind him. He grabs hold of himself and looks down at her, and then does it right onto her and then drops back next to her. He kicks the sheet to the bottom of the bed and puts his hand on her ribcage and she whispers something to him. He laughs and she touches his hair. They're out of breath. She shuts her eyes and smiles and the picture fades to black.

And then, eyes closed, kneeling on his bedroom floor in the darkness, hand gripped in his lap, Joey comes onto the carpet in front of him before he realizes he's forgot to feel it happen, before he realizes it was *him* she was with. In Joey's mind, he made the guy into him and now he's drunk and he's alone in his room, Maggie off with the guy, the falseness, the coldness of the fantasy, it all hits at once and Joey stands and pulls his boxers back up and he's in the middle of his room, the middle of his apartment complex, neighborhood, city, state, country, continent, and as the camera pulls away and shows the blue and brown world in the blackness of space he's not even a speck.

Here I am.

1979

AUGUST 31ST

The next day, I left my rooftop for the first time. Out on the street I hailed a cab and took it to the *Plaza de Toros Monumental* (on Dueñas' recommendation). As the car neared the arena, the bullring rose on the horizon like some relic of old Rome, the ocean stretching gray-blue below its coliseum walls, a great nothing of blue sky above.

I found my seat halfway up the steps and sat down. Below me, in miniature, the first matador turned a half circle in front of the bull, stepping across the yellow sand with his cape on his arm and the blade of his sword catching the sun. The man was agile and quick and the bull staggered, head bowed, knees unsteady, spears dangling from its side and its flank slick with blood and blood pouring from its mouth (his mouth) onto the sand. He was half-dead and when the matador drove the sword in for the kill and the bull fell to his knees, there was no surprise or excitement or joy. After that, another man ran out and cut off one of the bull's ears with a rough, sawing jerk of his knife and wrist, and ran back to the sidelines and I knew I had made a mistake.

I watched three bulls killed and lost my stomach for it and left my seat and walked up the tiered slope of steps to the top of the arena.

At the highest point, I looked out over the wall to the sea and let the sound of the crowd and the brass band drift off on the breeze.

With no one to hear me, I spoke out loud. "What do I do *now*?" That was all I wanted to know. Just that. An answer to that question would be enough. Just give me that. I'll know it's a sign if it comes right now.

The sea like mercury, silent, the vastness complete, an endless plane of bright gray water and then sky and sun and rippled clouds overhead. The air salty and clean and cooler than it was in the center of the city.

I listened.

Nothing.

Someone once wrote that if you live with monsters, you'll become monstrous. What if you live alone? Do you become solitude? Who is Channy Morning Greene? She's not even a Greene now. She has my last name, but what does that mean? What did she need from me, and what did I offer?

Summer's ending. You can feel it marching away and you can see the change in the air, the sky pale, the sun there but distant. When I was a boy, I had this feeling of shrinking at the beginning of fall. Back to school. The loss of freedom. Shoes. Change. Growth and new faces. It was a sad feeling but it was okay. Still, there was a pressing down, a sense of days growing shorter and the nights longer, of your life with a few less hours to it.

You grow up tall and you move more quickly to the end of your run. As a boy, it made me sit inside and stare out the window for hours without moving. The trees. The leaves falling off the branches in a yellow flurry with the wind. The people in coats and sweaters and scarves. Umbrellas. Gray and rain. The trees bare and the patches of sky empty and light. Then Thanksgiving, the smell of apples going soft, a hot kitchen and steaming windows, a kettle, cider, molasses, the early dark, pancakes, chicken and dumplings, a table covered in papers, hardback books, the sound of jazz on a radio, Christmas, snow.

SEPTEMBER 3RD

When the Ecuadoran came last night, I told her to go but she stayed and when we were done I knew it was time to leave Mexico. I'm in a taxicab stuck in traffic as I write this. Tijuana swarming around us and shops with open fronts, music and noise and bulb lights and neons. My last sight of Mexico—the evening heat and the dark blue dusk. It's humid and I have the window down and the driver is yelling and honking at someone (at who? The car in front of us? The line of cars?)

He looks back at me. "Sorry, *señor*, the border no very far. Ten minute if the traffic it move. You wan' some music?"

"Sure, that would be fine."

"Okay, *señor*. I find something you like."

The driver turns on the radio and music comes on loud, a scratchy Mexico polka, accordions and trumpets and tubas and the singer shouting above it all, the sound of celebration, vigorous life.

"Hey, what kind of music is this?"

"*Mariachi*, *señor*. Is good, huh?"

"What's the band?"

"*Pobres de Jalisco*."

"I like it. Turn it up."

"Okay, *señor*. "

A pack of elementary school kids is moving around the cab in white and blue uniforms and backpacks. Some of them slap their hands on the hood of the cab as they walk or look in and make faces at us. The driver honks his horn and they keep coming—holding hands, shouting, marching, laughing, singing in groups. One of them knocks on the window and then presses his art project up against the glass. A painting of mountains with a plane flying over and a smiling sun. His name at the bottom. Marcos. Then he pulls it away and joins the pack. They come until they fill the street, and then they're gone.

The brakelights of the truck in front of us switch off and it moves forward—slowly, then faster—and now we're driving. The light is violet. The light is burnt orange.

"Sorry, *señor*, no much time more. Sit back. Relax."

The driver turns up the radio as we move forward through a street fair, the lights of the bazaar flickering all around us like church candles.

2000

SEA WORLD DRIVE, MIDNIGHT

In the morning, Joey goes to work with a hangover. He sleepwalks through the next nine hours and ends up at a cocktail bar with his co-workers. Happy hour cocktails (vodka cranberry, cosmopolitans) turn into shots (Jack Daniels) and then the four of them are loud and someone's singing, "Hey now, you're an all-star / Get your game on / Get *paid*," (and one of them, the funny one with the bulgy eyes, changing "paid" to "laid") and even that Joey can ignore because they're buying and everybody loves everybody and the world is a big, red flashing heart.

Now Joey's driving back to his apartment with Yesenia Lopez, a short, loud hipster girl who works in the sales department. On the car radio it's a talk show ("The problem is no one believes he'll make good on even the most *minor* of his promises,") but what Joey hears is the singer from two nights ago and the band's still in the club and Maggie and Joey are still listening outside and the singer's singing, "In a smaaall ghost town there's a little arcaaade / Where the poltergeists play their vid-e-o gaaames! / 'Game over,' they said / 'Game over,' they said / 'Run and get your quarters in!'" Joey's driving Yesenia's car and Yesenia's giggling in the passenger seat next to him, small and hunched over, smoking a tiny joint she can barely hold, her spring-curls bouncing around her face. She passes it to him and he takes a hit and it burns his fingers and he drops it onto the floorboards. Downshift to third. Pass a minivan full of movement inside with a school name and the year on the back window in colorful soap paint; driving fast, hands beating on the glass, waving at Joey and Yesenia, cheerleader uniforms, a pom pom flashing, a lot of hair, a football star with his shoulder pads on, celebration. Grind through the gears. Look down and see the joint like a red firefly near the accelerator. Stomp on it with the brake foot. Kill it. "Hey, J.C., I wasn't *done* with—" Taillights on the I-8. Left turn signal flashing green. Brakelights hot and blurring in smears of red. Yesenia takes off her granny glasses and puts on Joey's Ray-Bans and looks at herself in the rear-view and makes a pout face and laughs. The globs of white from the oncoming traffic blooming and then showing big then bursting past them. "In a small ghost town, there's a little arcade where the poltergeists play their video games." *In a small ghost town, Yesenia talks about low-fat burgers in the seat next to you, your sunglasses like a big stupid blindfold around her face.*

At the apartment, Joey and Yesenia sit in Joey's living room on the carpet with their shoes off and smoke grass and drink beer. The room fills with smoke. Yesenia doesn't notice. To Joey it's green, a special smoke made from burning piles of dead flies. He laughs at this but Yesenia doesn't notice.

"*God*, I just can't take this *job* sometimes," she says, letting out a cloud of dead fly smoke as she talks. "I mean, Marcella is such a *bitch* to me. Like, I know I'm out of place on the sales team—*the boys' club*—but she treats me like I'm lucky to be *around*. She makes me feel like such a *monster*. You know what I mean? You ever feel all *yucky* and *monstery* when you're there?" She puts her hand on his knee when she says this.

"No. Not really." Which is a lie. A small one, but a lie nonetheless. Joey sprawls out on his back and tries to listen to what she's saying but he got too drunk at the bar and now he's too stoned. *In the arcades of the small poltergeist office town, I feel lucky to be working like a video game ghost. Sometimes I feel like the ghost of a monster. Sometimes I feel like a monsterless child.*

"J.C., I mean, if you weren't around, I would be so *out* of that place. I could go get a writing job somewhere. A fashion magazine, culture, New York, D.C., Frisco, pay more rent . . . but this *place* . . . I can't *believe* it sometimes. All a bunch of arrogant fucking surfers and frat boys. I've told you before, J.C., it's bro culture in this fucking town. You can quote me on that. Man, I . . . I fucking *hate* surfers. Fuck beach people. They wouldn't know art if it dropped like a dumpster from the sky and smashed them *flat.* Someday I'm going to get out of San Diego and move somewhere artsy and hip and write a *huuuuuge* bestseller about the *vapidness* of bro culture and the *New York Times* will review it and I'll be in *Vice* and I'll be on all the talk shows talking about it and then everybody will want to date me. I mean, I'm dateable, I think I'm dateable. What I need is fucking *Oprah*. Naw, that bitch needs *me*. I'm dateable, right?" She hands him the joint and he doesn't want it but he takes it anyway.

Suck in. Cough. Eyes burn. Dodge the question with another cough. Stall. Cough again and laugh and hand her the joint.

"Joey, I've been having a *drought* lately. I don't think I've been out with a decent guy in a *year*. Twenty-eight is *totally not old*. It's not old, right? Oh, wait! Check it out!" She unsnaps her pink leather purse and pulls out a clear orange pill bottle with a white cap. She shakes the bottle and gives Joey a sly look. "Check it. Oxy*fucking*codone. My oral surgeon put me on them after I had a couple gnarly root canals but he gave me *two refills*. Who needs two refills of Oxycodone? Not for a couple *root canals* you don't. Maybe he made a mistake but I was like, 'O! M! *G*! *Best. Doctor. Everrrrrrrrr.*' This stuff is *great*."

"What does it do?" His voice comes out flat like the anonymous witness on *America's Most Wanted*.

She puts a pill between her lips, puckers it out at him like a tiny white tongue, then drinks it down with a beer. "They just make you all numb and tingly. *Especially* if you're stoned. It's nice. Trust me. You'll *tohhhhtally* love it. I'd be a *mess* without this stuff. Like my *abuela* without her glass of white wine. One after work every day. One before bed and my *dreams,* oh, *man*, I could write a fucking *book* about my dreams on this stuff. I should start *painting*. I could paint some crazy-ass shit about my dreams. Sometimes . . . sometimes I even take one *during* work on the really, really nasty days . . . keep that on the DL. Not like you would—tell anybody, I mean. Oh Joey, I'm so glad we're *doing* this!"

The more weed Joey smokes, the more of Yesenia's pills he takes, the less he thinks. More, more, equals . . . less. The music on the stereo drags slower like its batteries are dying. Joey smiles at Yesenia for no reason and laughs before he knows he's laughing—and at what? At nothing. He's an island without the danger of a sea, an island alone and happy because no one knows he's there. Better than an island, a mountaintop. Enclosed inside castle walls with all his own food growing in gardens around him, alone forever, safe, laughing in the sun. A mountaintop you can't fall off. (The guy on the record spinning next to them says, "I'm a maaay-ahn ahhn on the mayow-tun / Come ahhhn UP / I'm the plahhhwman in the vaaalley with a face fulla MUD.")

Joey on his mountain, laughing.

"Huh?" she asks, cut off during a story about scarves.

"I was just . . . laughing."

"At what?"

"At *what*?"

"I asked *you*."

"Asked me what?"

"J.C., what were you *laughing* about?"

"Oh."

"Well, what? Helloooo, you in there? Change the record. I hate the Stones. Put on something new. Hey! You wanna do a line? Curt got me some *killer* MDMA."

"Okay."

"Hold on."

"For what?"

"You're fucked *up*," she says proudly, poking his chest with a finger. "You're *totally* fucked up. You know it and *I* know it and you can't say you're *not!* I'm so glad I found out you're fun."

Yesenia cuts a line on her Locust compact and she and Joey snort it.

Joey feels nothing. And then he does.

"J.C." (whispering) "let's do some *more*."

"More?"

"Let me take the reigns . . . you're . . . you're obviously in a good place, stay there. Hold on a sec. This . . . this stuff's good for you. It's like . . . it's like vitamins. There. Okay, right. Perfect. Here. Take it. Like . . . ," (laughing, leaning closer to him, touching his shoulder) "like this."

Joey and Yesenia on their backs next to each other, staring up through the smoke of her cigarette and he listens while she talks about the college classes she's taking online. Greek and comparative religions, interior design and Roman architecture. The classics. ("Fuck the classics," she says.) She talks and he listens. She talks and he stops listening. She talks and he listens to the music. She begins to make plans for them, trips to the mountains, drugs she'll get him, famous people they'll meet—famous because they'll be famous, too. She tells him that she'll be a famous sex and dating columnist, touring the world, all over the magazine covers and that he'll figure out his life and be famous for something too. Just what? It doesn't matter, she says. "Everyone will know us as the coolest people in the world. They'll care what we do. And we'll do it together. J.C. and Y.L., me and you living in LA and just soaking that shit *up*." The music flutters and trills on the breeze. It sighs down to a low, chiming valley, drones as a breath. The singer is a Japanese girl and her baby-voice fills up the room while Yesenia talks about film festivals and apple season and skiing. And then the girl is singing about being lazy when it's raining out and staying in bed and smoking cigarettes all day and living like cats—and Joey's asleep, dreaming for a humid, strange second—a flash of gray highway, desert on all sides, the desert in black and white, lightning on the horizon. Then awake. The lights above him bright and spinning. One light becomes twelve, a ring of lights, turning. Yesenia's voice. "—and have you ever been to *Rome*? You *totally* need to go to Rome. I *adore* Rome." And asleep. The candidate jogging in running shorts with a team of reporters behind him, the camera zooms in and shows the audience what he's got in his chest instead of a heart. It's a mason jar full of blood and it's sloshing as he runs. But no, it's more than that—a tiny shark in the jar and that shark is God. Detroit tenement apartments—cops in riot gear flood the building. Up the staircase. Beating on the door with a metal ram. Bursting into the room. The black guy falls off the bed half-naked and makes a run for the bathroom. The girl yanks the sheet up to her chest, screaming. The guy turns back and looks at her and the cops shoot him in the chest and he slides down the wall, eyes open, a smear of blood on the wall. But he was innocent. We all know it! The *cops* are the bad guys! The whole system is crashing! Awake. Yesenia moves closer and then she's on her side curled up to him with her little stubby hand on his chest, drumming her fingers, and her thigh rubbing his knees. He can smell her perfume and her booze breath and she's telling him a story about Washington State wine country and the Columbia River Gorge and then she's leaning over him and he's looking up at her face through the black forest of hair. "Hey, J.C.," she smiles and bites her bottom lip and tucks a strand of her hair behind her ear and it drops back down again and she laughs (breathy) and leans down to him. She comes in for the kiss and her eyes close and her lips part and he smells her dark red lipstick and he thinks of ashes and earth and decay.

And then he sees Maggie in all the places they've been. He sees her on the hotel bed in Las Vegas, the gauzy afternoon light all around her. He sees her in Tyler's car, smiling when he looks back to tell her something. He sees her in a jean skirt and a faded gray *Les Miserables* t-shirt standing in her mother's yard, and he sees her room, her cotton Dust Bowl dresses on hangers, the rhinestone cat collar she wore all winter. He hears her big, wild, unashamed laugh (the best laugh) and he sees her sitting across from him on her mother's couch next to her little sister Jolie and her cousin Molly and the other one whose name he can never remember, and Maggie's talking happily about the cop drama she loves, her sister playing *Tetris* on a Gameboy while the nameless cousin looks at the TV and Molly's half-asleep, and then awake, yawning. He sees Maggie in the wholeness he knows of her. This isn't the Maggie that Tyler knows or the Maggie her boyfriend knows. It's the Maggie Joey knows. The real Maggie. The real Maggie, or the one he's made her into?

Yesenia says something Joey doesn't hear. He sits up. *You need to stop this or you'll never be able to face her again. You'll regret this even if it's great.*

He turns his head away and rolls to the side.

"Whoa, Jesus, I'm wasted," he says, sitting up. *You've lost control.* He stands. "Let's get, like . . . some fresh air. My head it's just . . . zooooom, y'know? You need some fresh air? Cigarette? Let's go have a cigarette outside. Let's smoke." He stands with the world swelling around him and he sees Yesenia get painfully to her feet. She's barely five foot without her tall shoes. He looks down at her and she looks down at the floor, the lenses of her glasses gone white.

"Joey, I should go. I need to go." She doesn't make eye contact. "I really need to—" Shaking her head, eyes cast down. Her bare feet and the red nails with a white heart on each. Pulling on her green leather shoes. Standing up tall again.

"No, but—" he starts to say. *But what?*

She's blushing. "I should go, Joey." Looking down again. "I should. I really should, like, really *go*."

"No, you don't have—"

"I have to get in early and put the web feed together." She digs through her purse and finds the bottle of Oxycodone. "Here, have the bottle. I have refills."

"Okay, but—"

"I need to . . . I've gotta go. See you tomorrow."

And then she's out the door.

Joey hears her car start.

And now the space between the window blinds lighting up as she backs out of the parking space, then going dark again and she's gone.

HOME, 8 A.M.

Joey learned this one fast. If you want a day off to fight a hangover, you call in sick before your boss gets to work. Catch the voicemail so he can't argue with you. "Hey Rob, this is Joey . . . Carr. I woke up sick this morning. I think I had some bad sushi last night at King Samurai's. You know, the new place in Mission Valley? I think . . . I think I'm going to stay in today if that's alright. Alright, hope everything's . . . alright. See ya Monday. Thanks. Bye."

An hour later. Voicemail: "Hey Carr, it's Rob. Thanks for calling, bro. Yeah, *totally*, dude, *stay in*. Get better! Food poisoning is the *wwwworst*. I'll try to stay away from—what was that place? Samurai's Something? Thanks for the word of warning, bro-ham-bone. Alright, hope you're feeling better. 'K, laaaates."

Joey's apartment complex is full of noise—banging sounds, a crash, someone moving furniture above him, dragging a dresser or a couch, a couple arguing in Korean (*"Cheoncheonhi malhae jusipsio. Ihaega ankamnida! Nugu? Nugu?!"*), a game show on TV ("Survey *says*!"), and then the calls start and don't stop all afternoon.

Voicemail: "Joey! This is Tyler! Call me!"

Voicemail: "Heyyyy, J.C. (pause) it's Yesenia (pause). I saw you weren't at your cube today. I hope (long pause), never mind. Hey, maybe I'll see you Monday. Marcella is being a total cunt today, FYI. Alright, byyye."

Voicemail: "It's Ben Frank. Fun is happening tonight. Call me ASAP or I'll feed you to a lion and feed the lion to a whale. I promise."

Voicemail: "Joey! It's Tyler again. I called you at work. *Where are you*? We're meeting a bunch of people at Hillcrest Landmark. You should come. They're doing a private midnight screening where it's just us and our friends . . . our friends that work there and they show a film and you can drink in the theater and it's free and it sounds really fun. I don't have all the details. It's the Ben Frank kids. You should come. I'll send you an email too."

Voicemail: "Joey, your uncle and I are worried about you. We haven't heard from you in forever. You sound weird on the answering machine, Joey. You should change your message. It sounds . . . you sound weird. Joey, your sister decided not to come. She thinks she might be out in the winter. Thought you'd want to know. Come by, Joey, okay? We're worried. Call us. Okay?"

Voicemail: "Joey Carr, this is Ben Frank, king of the dogs. Call me back on Nate's phone. (858) 272-1578. Fun is going down tonight and you better be there. Call me on Nate's or you're dead to me forever. Don't make me put you in a paper bag and light the bag on fire and set . . . set it on someone's porch and ring the doorbell because . . . because that means you're shit. Don't be shit, Joey."

Voicemail: "Joey, this is Nicky. Let's get Italian tonight! Old Spaghetti Factory! Yay! My treat! Spumoni ice cream for evvverrryone!"

Voicemail: "Hey, it's Rory. You should go to Old Spaghetti Factory with me and Nicole. I think we're going to the Ché afterwards, if that sounds good. Some band with members of Tristeza."

Voicemail: "It's Ben Frank. I hate you. If you don't hang out tonight I'm going to dig out your eyeballs with a spoon and eat them and then I'll see what you see and I'll tell everyone how boring your life really is. Tonight. Hanging out. Call me on Nate's."

Voicemail: "Joey! Call me! This is Tyler. Let's go to that midnight screening. Maggie and I will be at your place at ten. You better be ready. Where are you? *Ten*. Ten o'clock."

Joey throws back the covers and steps onto the carpet and looks for his shoes.

HILLCREST, 1:30 A.M.

The streets are wet and dark and foggy and Joey spins circles. His ankles move and his sneakers step below him—spinning—his arms out for balance, one finger through the ring of the wine jug—spinning—as the stoplights and storefront neons on Robinson Street blur into one streak of night and color and movement. Joey—losing his balance and falling forward, tossing the empty wine jug into the hedges, a hook shot, and then he's on his hands and knees, dizzy, the world tipping and heaving as he tries to stand.

Joey pulls himself up and the world tips again as he walks to Tyler's car, which hops in front of him with the street and the whole neighborhood, smashing, bouncing as if on hydraulics, slowing now into the pace of a seesaw. Tyler and Maggie. Tyler and Maggie on the hood of the car. Sitting. Tyler and Maggie sitting on the hood of the car watching Joey stumble toward them and Ben Frank spinning his own circles in the middle of the street.

"Joey! Tell Tyler he's mean!" shouts Maggie, sloppy-drunk and playful, her arm wrapped in Tyler's. "Tell him!"

Out in the street, Ben Frank falls and rolls onto his back. "Bring me my boots and my cape!" he shouts. "Bring me my guns and my . . . hats." He crawls to the sidewalk and spoons himself around an orange rubber traffic cone in the gutter.

"Why's Tyler mean?" Joey, still off-balance, sits on the edge of the hood next to Maggie, breathless, smiling. He pats the pockets of his jean jacket for cigarettes. "Jesus, I need to quit." He looks across at Maggie, her breath in the air, a puff and trail of steam—Tyler next to her, frowning, staring straight ahead.

"Ask him."

"Okay, I'll ask."

"Please and thank you."

"You're welcome. Tyler, why are you mean?"

"To *Maggie*," she says.

"Mean to Maggie."

"I'm not. It's nothing. I'm not mean."

"Tyler's being a mean, grumpy, old man. Tyler, tell Joey how mean you are on a scale from one to ten. Tell him all the mean things you do."

Tyler rolls his eyes.

"Don't ignore me. Tell him. Tell Joey Carr why you're mean."

Joey laughs. "Come on, Tyler. Tell me why you're mean."

"I'm nice." Tyler sits on the hood with his arms folded, slouching, his dark blue cardigan buttoned to the top. Maggie in her brown rancher's coat over her trademark camisole. The red and white lights of the Rite-Aid behind them. The Starbucks on the corner closed up for the night.

"Tyler, you're mean to me and I'm moving to deepest, darkest Peru. You know where deepest, darkest Peru is, Tyler? It's where I'm moving because you're so mean."

Tyler shakes his head and yawns and holds his fist up to his mouth until the yawn is done. "What are we *waiting* for?"

Across the street is a gay bar, house music pumping from inside. An older man standing outside in jean shorts and biker boots, a black leather vest, shirtless, hairy, paunchy, a cop visor cap. He's smoking a cigarette, nodding his head to the beat, watching them.

A Mexican girl, drunk, on rollerskates, clatters past the man and shouts, "Hiiii Dennis!" She's wearing an old ratty prom dress cut off above her knees and she has cat glasses and short pigtails. "How's it *going*, Dennis?!"

"Same as always, Sweety! Say hi to Mom for me!"

"Headed there right now!"

"Bye, Sweety!"

The girl skates across the street and turns right, stumbling at first on the curb ramp then clacking past them, disappearing down 6th into the fog; a long red ribbon tied around her waist, fluttering behind her like a sign towed by a plane. And then she's gone. Swallowed up by the fog.

"That girl was *incredible*," says Maggie. "Why isn't she hanging out with *us* tonight? Who's this *Mom* person?"

Tyler mumbles something negative.

Joey laughs. "Do you think her name's really Sweety? Because that's the cutest thing in the world."

"Tyler," says Maggie, shaking his arm, "Tyler, go get Sweety and bring her back here and tell her I want to make out with her. I love her little tiny *skates*." When she says 'skates', she bumps Tyler with her hip. "If we were friends, I'd name her 'Skates.' She'd be my friend *Skates*. Joey, isn't that cute?"

"It's cute. I don't know what's cuter, Sweety or Skates. They're both pretty cute."

"Skates," says Maggie. "Skates is the cutest."

"Skates it is."

"Tyler, stop being mean and go get Skates and bring her back here."

Tyler frowns. "No, Maggie, come on."

"Tyler, Skates is my new best friend. I love her."

"Stop being crazy."

"Tyler, go get Skates. Get her! Tyler, get Skates!"

"Maggie, stop. Shhh, Maggie, shhh."

"Skates! Skates, Tyler!"

"Maggie, no. *Stop*. I'm *tired*. Joey, tell Ben Frank to come on. I have school."

"Skaaaates!"

Ben Frank is up again, standing in the middle of the intersection, spinning through the fog with the traffic cone gripped by the nose. Spinning, he shouts, "I'm gonna fuck North Carolina," spinning, "North Dakota, South Dakota!" spinning, out of breath now, "South Carolina! I'm gonna fuck Maryland," spinning, losing his voice, "with a . . . Spanish . . . galleon," spinning, fighting to get the words out, "made out of pizza," spinning, "strapped to my," spinning, "jackhammering," spinning, "crotch!"

"You tell 'em, kiddo!" shouts the man outside the bar.

Maggie laughs. "Joey, is Ben Frank's name really Kiddo?"

"His name's Sweety."

"Skates, Joey. It's Skates."

"Oh right."

"Don't forget."

Ben Frank comes to a stop and lets go of the traffic cone. He falls to his hands and knees and the cone sails across the street and hits the door of a white Aerostar parked in front of the Mazda. The alarm goes off with a horrible, alternating, lurching sound.

Ben Frank stands up, staggering to the side, left, right, down onto his knees, up again. "I am the kiddo that tells 'em! I am the last hope for the monarchy!" From his belt he pulls a snapped-off car antenna and whips it through the air. "Ben Frank!" he shouts, slashing at the fog, "Ben Frank, Ben Frank!" He swings the antenna sword side to side, slicing it through the fog. "Ben Frank, Ben Frank, Ben Frank!"

Maggie laughs and shouts, "Ben Frank, Ben Frank, Ben Frank!" She takes a beer can from her army bag and cracks it open and throws it at him.

It sprays in a foaming arc as it flies then hits his back and falls to the ground, emptying in gushes of foam on the concrete. Ben Frank stops and picks up the can and pours the rest of the beer on his head, shrieking, "Ben Frrraaaannk! King of the men!"

The man outside the bar flicks his cigarette in the street and shouts, "Honey, you made my night!" and goes back inside. (The music louder as the bouncer opens the door for him then shuts it. Quiet again. Muffled beats, dun dun dun dun-dun-dun. Tonight, the man will do ecstasy but he won't feel anything. A dud. A sugar pill. He'll go home alone, eat leftover chicken strips from

Hamburger Mary's, and watch the 1997 film version of Ed Distler's *A Book of Lists* and fall asleep halfway through, bored.)

Joey climbs in the backseat and slams the door behind him.

Maggie gets in the other side and scoots up next to him and slaps a drum-roll on his knee with her hands.

Ben Frank steps out of the fog and drops down into the seat next to her, giving one last out-of-breath "Ben. *Frank*. I make nights."

Joey pulls beers from the six-pack of cans on the floor and passes them down the line and then opens one for himself.

"Nobody's sitting up here with me?" Tyler says this so softly that Maggie and Ben Frank don't hear. Joey does. And he pretends not to. Maggie's sitting next to him. Up against him. He can smell her hair and he can feel warmth from her thigh next to his.

She cracks open her beer and shouts, "Drive like the wind, old woman!"

Tyler starts the car and puts on his signal and the seat-belt warning dings.

Ben Frank shuts his door, beer dripping from his hair. He scoots up to Maggie and Maggie moves closer to Joey. Ben Frank puts his seatbelt on and the warning goes off and he begins to sing, "*I'm* Henry the *eighth*, I am! / Henry the eighth, I am, I am!"

And Maggie joins in, "I got married to the widow next door!"

Now Joey, "She's been married seven . . . *times* before / And every-one was a—"

Ben Frank and Maggie and Joey: "Hen-a-ry! Hen-a-ry!"

Tyler turns up the radio and drowns them out with Jammin' Z-90.

"How *rude*," Maggie whispers in Joey's ear and her breath is wet and hot and he gets the chills. "Right?" she says. "Right?"

"Uh," Joey stammers. "He's—"

She tries again. "I'm Henry the eighth, I am!"

Ben Frank joins her, "Henry the eighth, I am, I am!"

Tyler drives in the slow lane, his headlights shining on the wall of fog.

"This is the thickest fog I've ever seen," says Maggie, smiling happily and staring out the window. "What if it was always this foggy? How peaceful would *that* be? You'd just . . . *float* through life like a little . . . bitty . . . *boat*."

"I, Ben Hur Rodney Dangerfield Archeopteryx Dr. Becker Frank, do openly declare I farted this fog and it came out as mustard gas and killed half of Europe."

"Which half?" says Tyler from the front seat, disinterested.

Joey cracks open another beer and it foams onto his jeans. "Oh no."

"The one that *deserved* it," Ben Frank says. "Can I get a what-what?"

"Here's to that," Joey says and he and Ben Frank touch their beer cans together.

"Fiddlesticks," says Maggie looking out the back window.

And now a police cruiser emerging from the fog, pulling alongside them.

"*Fuck, man*," whispers Maggie.

"*Ben Frank*," whispers Ben Frank trying not to laugh.

"Sit up straight. Hum. Hold your breath," Joey says. "Act natural."

They hold their breath and hum nonsense tunes and try not to laugh.

The cop car hangs in space, slow and predatory, matching their speed, before moving forward, disappearing into the fog.

When it's gone, they let out a big gasping laugh and Maggie gives its taillights the double middle fingers.

Ben Frank clears his throat dramatically. "I, BEN HEGEMONY ANDRE THE GIANT FIDDLESTICKS FRANK, HEREBY RELEASE THIS STATEMENT TO THE PRESS: FUCK YOU TO ALL COPS EVERYWHERE, PAST, PRESENT, FUTURE; FUCK ALL COPS TO BE BORN FROM HERE TO ETERNITY; FUCK ALL COPS FROM ANTIQUITY TO CENTURY 21 INSURANCE COMPANY; FUCK ALL COPS FOREVER 21 A GOOGLEPLEX," (laughs, coughing) "AMEN, SOUND THE GUNS CHRISTMAS DAY HEROES IN A HALFSHELL MACGUYVER SPAGHETTI BIRTHDAY CHICKEN BURRITO MADNESS BLACK PLAGUE MOTHER*FUCKER*!"

Joey laughs. "I hate that I'm afraid of cops even when I'm not *doing* anything."

"Like drinking in a car?" says Maggie.

"Not guilty," Joey says, his right hand on his heart, eyes closed, smiling angelically.

"*Never* guilty," says Ben Frank, doing the same.

Joey laughs and looks into the front seat at Tyler staring straight ahead, his face cold and his jaw set. Tyler shifts gears. They catch and grind. Joey looks out the window again. Fog. Darkness. The canyon.

2:14 A.M.

At Maggie's they spill out onto the curb, laughing and knocking each other over as Tyler drives off without saying goodbye.

They sit on the lawn outside the house. Ben Frank—hunched forward with his knees to his chest and his arms wrapped around them. He pulls a family-size bag of Ruffles out of his pack. "Ruffles?" he says, offering it around.

"You are a fantastic man," Joey says, reaching in, taking a handful.

"Hold your applause." He opens his bag again and takes out a jar of Queso cheese dip and unscrews the lid. "Hillcrest Ralph's dumpster. I found a *case*."

Joey dips a Ruffle in and pulls it out dripping cheese. "I could *live* off this stuff."

"I *do*," says Ben Frank.

"Alright, chip-eaters," says Maggie. "Here's the story. We can go *inside*, but we've gotta be quiet until we get to my room because my room will *kill* us."

Joey laughs. "Nice."

"I mean, my *mom* will kill us."

Ben Frank laughs and picks a Ruffle out of the bag and puts it in his mouth, crunching down. "I want your room to kill us. Life is never good enough to justify death until rooms kill you for being too loud. Goddamn, fuck the world. Fuck it all at once. I'm done. Lead me to your murderous room."

"Your murderous roooooom," echoes Joey, staring up at the sky.

Ben Frank pulls a paperback book out of his pack (Thomas Wolfe, *Look Homeward, Angel*) and stretches out on his back in the grass using it as a pillow.

Above them the full moon shows from behind the clouds, bright and yellow and pockmarked.

"It's *big* tonight," says Joey.

"Alright," Maggie says, squinting up at the moon. "Let's go. Let's go in."

Joey laughs. "I always forget that you're afraid of the moon."

"Come on, Joey Carr."

"It's cute. It's fine."

Ben Frank sits up. "How did I get so *wet*? Is there anything I can wear to sleep in?"

Maggie taps a finger on his chest. "Dresses. You can sleep in *dresses*."

2:24 A.M.

In Maggie's room, Ben Frank and Joey sit on the edge of the bed while Maggie digs in her closet, throwing handfuls of clothing behind her.

A sneaker sails past Ben Frank and he jumps back to catch it and falls off the bed with a crash.

He pulls himself back up, holding the shoe above his head. "Quarterback Ben Frank scores the touchdown and wins the Superbowl yet again."

"Do quarterbacks *score* touchdowns?" Joey asks.

"I don't know. All I know about football is the words 'quarterback' and 'touchdown'. Oh, and 'Superbowl'. And I know that some people just . . . they just watch it for the commercials, right?"

"All I know about football is 'The players tried to take the field / The marching band refused to yield' and Refrigerator Perry because they made a GI Joe out of him you had to mail-order out for."

"Like the Emperor. I had both of 'em."

"Totally, me too. Oh, and, I know this too," singing, "'Aaaall my rowdy friends are *here* on Monday night,' and, 'Are you ready for some *foot*ball!'"

"Okay, boys." Maggie holds two of her Dust Bowl dresses up to the light and looks them over. "Mrs. Joey you get the . . . red one. Mrs. Ben Frank gets the *white*."

Ben Frank and Joey step out of their pants and take off their shirts and put the dresses on over their boxers.

"Perfect. I'm going to take a picture of—oh *wait*, shit, shit, shit! You guys need to see the photos of me losing my *virginity*!"

Joey's head says yes, but all he can do is smile and nod. But of course, yes, why not, yes.

They sit cross-legged on the bed, Ben Frank and Joey in their dresses, Joey with the comforter wrapped up around him, Maggie in a short blue slip. Joey looks down at her legs, pale, white and new. He looks away.

Maggie opens a red shoebox labeled "$tupid $hit" and lifts out a Polaroid camera and then a stack of photos.

"Here's . . . uh, I don't know what's happening in this one," she says and hands it to Ben Frank, who hands it to Joey. "This one I think is my back or it might be the wall." She laughs. "I forgot how shitty these were."

They look through the photos but you can't see much. A leg in grainy black and white. Patches of gray that might be body parts. The side of an arm or possibly a leg. A black gloss of hair, hers; blonde, his.

"Oh, wait, check *this* out," she hands Joey a Polaroid from the bottom of the box. "I had Cecilie take this when I was sixteen to give Tyler for Valentine's. I stole it back when we broke up."

In the photo, a younger Maggie is in her bedroom wearing red flapper beads down her chest and a white bandanna pulling her hair back. She's topless, but she's covered up with tiny butterfly decals she's stuck over the photo. "Look," she whispers and peals one of the stickers off—a nipple, a brown spot barely there in the blur. "The stickers were scratch and sniff. They smelled like rosewater a million years ago but the smell is gone. You can try to smell them if you want." She scratches at one of the stickers and holds the photo up to Joey's face. "Here, smell it. Roses? Nothing, right?" There she is, and Joey yanks the comforter up around his lap and leans forward, and all he can see is her body in that photo and he tries to push it away and think of awful things. *A dead seal on the shore. Aunt and uncle opening Christmas presents in their sweat pants and Disney pajama tops. "It's a juicer! Just what I wanted! How did you know? Wow. Thank you. Meh-erry Christmas, merrrrry Christmas." A cheering crowd at a Padre game, Steve Garvey running the bases and everyone standing up and shouting and losing their minds with joy. Cartoons. Sitting cross-legged in front of the TV, the coyote after the roadrunner, the cat after the mouse, a team of ducks dressed as explorers rowing a canoe down a river, and "Life is like a hurri-cay-ay-*

ane." Eighth-grade Spanish teacher Mrs. McCarren—her tube body and clown makeup, the gray-red hair, the mole on her cheek with orange bristles coming from it—Mrs. McCarren saying, "Cambio, say it with me, caaaaaambio. Like change for money. Caaaambio." An old TV ad, Channel 8 station identification, "Makes no difference where I go / You're the best hometown I know / Hello, San Diego, Hello, San Die-eh-eh-GO / Channel 8 loves you."

They've run out of photos. Maggie shrugs and laughs. "Theeee end," she says with a happy nod.

Joey laughs uncomfortably and Maggie shrugs again and smiles. Ben Frank picks up Maggie's Polaroid camera and turns it to face him, clicking the flash up and down. "This have film?"

Maggie nods. "I put a new one in."

"Can I use it?"

"Course."

He aims the camera at Joey and Maggie. "Do something interesting! This is getting boring! Fix it!" He takes a picture and the photo slides out. Joey grabs it out of the camera and looks at it, white, milky, opaque, darkening, changing to colored shapes, faces, eyes, the shapes of Maggie and him sitting together, smiling. He slides it under the pillow to take later and his hands start to shake. *I'm Henry the eighth I am, Henry the eighth I am, I am? I am.*

"Fix it," shouts Ben Frank.

Maggie grabs a jam jar of pennies from her bedside table and throws it out the open window into the side yard.

Joey hears the glass smack the fence and the pennies scatter and it makes him feel wild. He stands up on the bed, bouncing on the bedsprings.

"Yes!" says Ben Frank as he snaps a photo. "Fix it!" The photo slides out of the camera and he throws it behind him. It wings left and spins out the window.

Maggie laughs and steps up onto the bed next to Joey and flaps her arms slowly like they're wings.

"Fix it!" shouts Ben Frank.

Joey, bouncing on the mattress without knowing he's moving. "Flash us!" he shouts.

"Spring Break 2000!" cheers Ben Frank.

Joey embarrassed now. *Flash us. Or don't. It's too much. Really. It is. No, please. Please do it. But she won't do it, will she? But there—look! And leaning forward, pulling the front of her slip down, laughing, smiling, and they're perfect and stone white and full and beautiful, oh god, and now the universe and everyone in it, all the people, buildings, pets, streets, cereal commercials, hills, valleys, all the farms, mice, schools, factories, energy drinks, fruit stands, porn videos, t-shirt printers, rocking chairs, toddler shoes, chests of drawers, pickups, race cars, fire trucks, vans, buses, sports cars, low-riders, cop cars, classic cars, muscle cars, cars driving with three good tires and the one tiny spare wheel (and you look at it as you drive by and go "Awwww, baaaaby wheel!"), all of it, every stitch, brick, and log, all the nails and boards, all the jails, rivers, lakes, churches, laptops, chicken coops, skateboards, plates of noodles, railroad ties, the whole lonesome, quaking, wonderful, jittering, warmongering, bitching, hooting, coughing, eyeballing, moneygrubbing, flea scratching, silly-headed, dead-serious, rowdy, terrible thing goes lopsided, sloshing to one side, tossing, churning blue liquid for a quick snowy instant, the* Titanic *breaking in two K-RACK, the* Mayflower *fighting to stay afloat, the waves crashing up its bow with a great K-PRFFFFF! The* Amistad *full of slaves, "Give us us FREE!" And sea spray! PAAAAAA! The rigging strained in long grrrroans, crrrrreeks, wood cracking, splintering, oh! There she is! Maggie! The Liberty Bell! A trumpet! A freight train! Plymouth Rock! A thousand jet planes in Vs! Zzzzzsssjjjoooom! Pawww! Fuck the Blue Angels for ruining our picnic, darling. Breaking the sound barrier and all the windows of the world shatter inward! Ksssskk! A thousand wars and 200,000 thousand years of big white bones in the earth! Clap clap clap! Names on graves! Ho ho ho! Dancers on the floor twirling and drunk and everyone in love, 1920! You'll pat everyone's heads once as you walk by and utter a loving 'Fuck you' which is really 'Love you', this time, not always, love now, for now love. Fuck you, everyone at the wedding. Fuck you to the uncles outside fighting and they're wearing belts and they've got mustaches as big as a rat and they're shirtless as uncles always are! Fuck you to the mustaches! Fuck you to the bride in the back crying with her sisters. Fuck you to funerals! Throw me in and cover me up! Ha! A toast! A wake! Fuck you, Irishmen drinking. Fuck you, birthday party clowns! Blow out the candles make a wish about money! Births! Fuck you . . . the crying red, you, new and breathless in the new air with a new face like a pinched-up new onion! Education! Taxes! Divorce! Health insurance! Dentists drilling like a symphony, fuck you! Bakers baking in steaming rooms with flour like stage makeup, fuck you, fuck you, fuck you! Fuck you, corporate raiders raiding corporate! Fuck you waiters smoking butts in alleys, shaking their heads, and "ahhh," "gad dam't," "ugh," "fuhhhhhck" and bartenders wiping counters with a rag saying, "Hey now. Slow down, buddy" and fisherman in yellow slickers hauling nets and the wave breaks on the bow BAAAGGGGHHHHHHH! Fishsticks all around for dinner tonight but it better not be minced this time or there'll be hell to pay, don't make me tell you again! ("Pass the tartar sauce, baby." "Uh, please?" "Please." "I'm kidding." "Thank you." "Lovely weather tonight.") Fuck you, politicians stumping wildly with a lone finger raised, eyes closed, sweating, "Aaaaand another thiiiiiiiiiing! Not only will I—" wild promises! Soldiers crying in hospitals, fuck you. Fuck you, hustlers on street corners showing some leg. Fuck you, work crews building roads! Work crews building dams! Building apartments and tract housing and libraries and fisheries and tanneries and paper mills! The slaughter* *of slaughterhouses! The dull hours in banks! Fuck you to the bodies in front of TVs watching* M*A*S*H, *laughing along with the track, waiting for Klinger to do something cute, and what?! Fuck you, girls saying, "I'm so bored of everything. I wanna quit my job and move somewhere new." Fuck you, guys saying, "She's the one. I know that sounds cheesy, but she's the one." Fuck you, parents saying, "I'm so scared/proud/worried of what he/she's/they (are) becoming." Fuck you, teachers saying, "Got it?" Got it! Fuck you, breakfast! Lunch! And Dinner! Lunchables! Snack! This! Everything! Fuck you! Everything!*

And Maggie yanks her slip back up, laughing with tears in her eyes, delirious, shrieking, and Ben Frank snatches the Polaroid as it comes out of the camera and waves it dry in the air.

Maggie: laughing, trying to talk, tears in her eyes.

Ben Frank: "More! Fix it! Maggie, punch Joey! Knock him out!" Aims the camera.

Joey: "Take a picture of Maggie and I while we make out!"

Who are you? So awkward like a dog standing up and speaking People on a flea collar commercial, "Rrrrye rrrov rrrue!" "While we make out"? How could you—but Maggie pulling his hair and kissing him dramatically. Her tongue fighting in his mouth. The taste of her mouth, cigarettes, girl, wine. The flash goes off, bang! and their teeth conk together.

"Ow!" she laughs and falls off to the side, on her back, bouncing with the mattress springs, knees bent, legs spread and her slip pushed up around her thighs, red panties with . . . watermelon print? Strawberries! "Ow!" Holding her mouth. "Ow! That was a *terrrrible* kiss!"

Maggie slips off the bed, falls to her knees, scrambles up and ducks out the door, running.

What? Joey turns to Ben Frank, who's lying on the floor now, arms and legs spread. "What?" But she's back with a baguette and another bottle of wine.

"It's my mom's. She doesn't give a fuhhh-uhh-uck."

They pass the wine around until it's empty. Ben Frank bites the wine cork in half. Spitting one piece at the wall, ptooo! The other half falling onto the mattress. *Pick it up and throw it at the door.* They tear the bread up and eat it like wild animals, put music on and scream along with the angry fast songs on Maggie's stereo. They jump on the bed until they fall down and get up again. *World's a mess; it's in my kiss! World's a mess; it's my kiss!* Maggie jumps on the bed in front of Joey, screaming along with the song, her big, luminous eyes, her body moving under her slip—slow motion—and Joey screaming back at her and reaching out to her with nothing but the ugly, clumsy force inside him. Arms at his sides. Hands clenched in fists. *Like in kindergarten, "Keep to yourself, hands to yourself, sit on your hands during the lesson, quiet, quiet, quiet, bah bah, good, good, good, yes, good work, Joseph C."* And she shoves him hard and he's falling back onto the mattress and she keeps jumping, jumping over him now, laughing and screaming, her legs, thighs, jumping, further, strawberry print, and he's dizzy with love. He wants to cry. He wants to pull her down to him.

But . . .

But?

Ben Frank loading more film, taking pictures and they pile up on Maggie's bed in a stack of white bands framing blurry colored images—one, two, three, four, five, six, seven, eight, eight, eight, eight, eight!—the record skips, the singer shouting, "Can I have a taste of your ice cream cream cream cream! cream! cream! cream cream cream cream cream cream!"

And then, at some point, they stop.

Or Joey does.

At some point, Joey wakes up in the dark.

Outside, the dawn is coming and it's bird-sounds like some soft, dreamy cartoon and the night fading to purple. The clock next to the bed is flashing '12:00!' '12:00!' '12:00!' in red numbers. Maggie—lying between Ben Frank and Joey, and Ben Frank is asleep.

Joey rolls onto his side and props himself up on one elbow and Maggie's looking at him in the dark.

"Hi Joey."

"Hi Maggie."

Joey leans over her and they kiss. It's a hard, sloppy, bad kiss. Their teeth knock together again, but this time they keep going.

Joey grabs her waist and pulls her on top of him.

She sits up, and lifts her slip over her head.

BOOK THREE

GHOSTS AND THE AMAZON

"They hung the deserter from the tree. In the morning the body was gone. Nothing but his fingernails and toenails scattered in the grass. He'd left them behind and walked home."

—Ed Distler, *Fall*

1979

DECEMBER 1ST

Channy's book is called *Youth is a Wolf Dark and Golden*. "Today was my best day working," she says. "As soon as he was down for his nap, I did twenty pages handwritten, then looked them over and it was about ten pages of usable material, which is good. I don't know . . . I'm really *seeing* it now. I can feel the story. Feel it . . . like, *working* in me when I'm not writing. Sandra's fourteen and her inner-life is really enjoyable to write because I'm speaking in the voice of a child—of me—I'm writing the fourteen-year-old me, and the deeper I go, the more I remember. It's like how you can tell someone about a dream, and the more you tell them, the more it comes back to you. You know what I mean?"

"I don't know. Kind of. I only remember sex dreams."

"Really?"

"Only the bad ones. Embarrassing ones."

"Anyway, what I meant was the dream . . . or the story or whatever just *develops* in front of you and then it's like you're chasing it, trying to keep up before you run out of steam. Today's work was nice. It was *satisfying*. I felt like I had done something even though . . . I mean even though I really *hadn't. Done anything*, I mean. It's not exactly curing cancer. It's . . . I don't know. *Yyyeah*. Look at that *sunset*."

"It looks like the inside of Jake's abalone shell ashtray."

"That's a good thing?"

"Not the ashes and the butts, but the shell itself, all the colors and the silver part."

"I've never seen an abalone shell."

"Yeah, you have. Like the inlays in Issy's banjo."

"Oh yeah. Right, right. I get ya. I've seen that in jewelery too."

"Hippies."

"Right. Hippie jewelery."

We sit out on the back deck and the fields stretch below us, dry-yellow and tawny with the setting sun, patches of snow around the pine trees in the valley, the sheep and goats eating what's left of the grass, calm and serene and still.

"This *view*," says Channy. "If we ever move, we're taking this view with us."

"Deal. So . . . right, yeah, you were saying?"

"Saying?"

"Saying. Ten pages. The book."

"The book." The boy sleeps in her arms. She tugs the quilt up around his face and rubs her cheek on the top of his head. God, she's beautiful. (If there were ever a face to look at that made you feel proud of the species . . . how natural and animalistic we can look—catlike, lionish—and at the same time refined and wholly human, symmetrical, the high cheek bones and the nose red (the tip) with the chill, the red childlike pucker of the lips, her eyes so dark blue. Her face is very un-American. Not politically . . . that's a bad way of saying it . . . more so, a face you don't see out here. You see her face in movies about Holland, Russian Olympic athletes, in old paintings of German aristocracy. I wish she could see what I see. She told me last week, "Merc, I look like a sick twelve-year-old these days.")

"Today was good?"

"Yeah, it was really good. Okay, so, right . . . so what I've been writing is about when Sandra's living with her parents in the trailerpark. She . . . she spends all her time down by the bayshore, in the marsh. It's all sand-flats . . . mud hens, seagulls, dinghies or rowboats or little sailing ships tied up to the dock, the estuary, briny, quiet, golden sunsets . . . you know, easy, *pleasurable* things to write. It's summer and Sandra's off in her head, daydreaming, staring into the water, drawing in the sand with a stick, skipping rocks, praying over the bodies of dead birds, collecting shells. It's all very idyllic and peaceful and solitary. What she wants is what I want, so it's easy to speak through her. She wants to be kind and to be around animals and she wants to be away from the city and she wants to dream and let the dream last forever. She wants a life without conflict. She's . . . she's happy, but her parents aren't having as easy a time. Her mom's in beauty school out in Linda Vista and her dad's working at the shipyard. Her uncle's just out of the army and he's trying to find work and having a hard time with that and it's the four of them, all cramped into one shitty little trailer. They have a car—a baby blue Volkswagen van—but between school and work and job-hunting it's a mess for the adults and everyone's arguing and her dad's drinking too much and her uncle's depressed. Which is why . . . which is why the marsh is so comforting. She gets up early before everyone's awake and walks through the trailerpark to the bayshore. Five minutes and she's away from . . . from civilization altogether, away from the *city*, the *country*, modern *times*. Down at the bayshore . . . amber light, bronze color in the sand, the sky a big vast painting. When she's there, it's a thousand years ago and she lets herself forget about the world and she goes off into her imagination and lives in it until it's time to go in for supper. It sounds nice when I say it now. I mean, kind of sad, but nice. Like sadness you're *okay* with . . . because . . . because it's in your *past*. You've dealt with it and you've passed through it, and even though it's very real, it doesn't have any effect on your current, y'know, day to day. Does that make sense?"

"It does."

"What I wrote today is her end-of-summer scene. All summer she's been having these strange little fairytale adventures; sand castles, clam shells arranged to spell words, a funeral for a dead beetle she found by the pool, little spears sharpened with her uncle's penknife, a daisy chain woven through with marsh grass. It's the end of the summer and in a few weeks she's going to be starting high school. She's turning fourteen but she's immature; she's still a child, still living up in her head. The day Sandra turns fourteen, her family forgets her birthday. She wakes up early and everyone's gone. No card. No presents. No cake in the fridge. No ice cream in the freezer. Her uncle—who has the van, I explain this part better in the story—comes home at noon and goes back to bed. He walks past Sandra sitting at the picnic table in front of the trailer and he mutters something like, 'Hi, hey, babygirl,' and goes inside to sleep. An hour later he gets up, smokes a cigarette at the picnic table without saying anything, and then leaves again. He's looking for a job. Or so they all think. What he was really doing, they didn't learn for years, after he died up in Canada alone in that cabin."

"Whoa, *what*?"

"Another time."

"Come on, Channy."

"Seriously. Later. I'll . . . later."

"Okay, sorry. Go on."

"So . . . uh . . . where was I . . . uh . . . I lost my train of thought . . . um, yeah, okay, two . . . two hours after that he (her uncle) comes back with Sandra's mom and they've got groceries and neither one mentions her birthday. They go back inside and from outside Sandra can hear them arguing. A little later Sandra's mom comes out—she's been crying—and she takes the van to pick up Sandra's dad at the shipyard. An hour and forty minutes pass and meanwhile Sandra sits at the picnic table waiting, a watch with a broken band sitting in front of her, ticking away. After a while the van pulls up (a cloud of brown dust around it, the light from the sunset coming through the dust) and Sandy's mom and dad get out and she knows they've been fighting. 'Hey, baby, hey, Sandy,' says her dad. 'Hi, San,' says her mom. By then she's sure they've forgotten her birthday and she decides to cut her losses and head down to the marsh. She goes back inside the trailer, gets her sweatshirt and the penknife and her lunchbox (for collecting weird leaves and mussel shells and whatnot) and she walks down to the marsh feeling like the last girl on Earth. She's fourteen. Summer's gone. Nothing has changed. So . . . so she's down there in the weeds, crawling around, looking through the brush, thinking about horses, talking in her head to God (which she does a lot), not really praying, per se, just talking to him like . . ."

"Like an imaginary friend?"

"Yeah. Like an—"

"Sorry that sounds mean. I didn't—"

"No, it's okay. That's . . . that's pretty close to . . . anyway, she's . . . she's digging in the sand, gathering acorns and maple leaves and pigeon feathers and dark purple crab shells—*tiny* ones, like little coins—when she hears the sound of someone in pain. *Muffled*. Not close but not far away. It's a girl's voice. Sandra gets really . . . really *still* and lays there on her belly in the bramble and shuts her eyes tight and listens until she knows where the sound is coming from. Then, as quietly as she can, she crawls on her hands and knees through the brush in the direction of the sound, pushing her lunchbox ahead of her."

"This is turning into Nancy Drew."

"Shut up."

"I'm kidding."

"I know."

"Just . . . yeah, sorry, Channy, go on."

"For that, I'm not baking you any cookies tonight. I rescind the offer."

"I hate you. You know what right? You'll be seeing divorce papers tomorrow from my attorney."

"Who's that?"

"Issy's goat Dixon."

They laugh.

The sun has disappeared behind the hills and in the valley, Channy's cousin Issy is leading the sheep and goats to the barn, swishing a branch in front of her, calling out, "Sheep, sheep, sheep! Sheep, sheep, sheep!" while a tiny white kid-goat (Dixon) trails at her feet like a puppy.

"So, what I was saying before I was so rudely interrupted, in the story Sandra creeps through the brush until the sound gets louder, and then the sound stops. Sandra keeps crawling in the same direction until she comes to the shore and sees movement and color through the bramble. She lies there in the sand with her chin propped up on her lunchbox and . . . slowly . . . very slowly . . . she *draws* the branches of the brush aside, and it's the kids from one trailer down. Travis and Luna Gable. They're older than her, but not much, seventeen, eighteen, and they're on a beach towel and Travis is on top of his sister and he has pants at his ankles and Luna's dress is pushed up to her belly and his hand is over her mouth. He's thrusting into her—over and over again—and then he shoves his hips into hers one last time and looks up to the sky and makes a painful grunt and he's done. Of course she's never seen anyone have sex before, so she's not entirely sure what happened."

"Jeez, Channy. Did you really see that?"

"Shush. Just listen, okay? So, Travis rolls off her and lies there on his back and pulls his jeans back up and says, 'Well,' and his sister laughs and says, 'Boy, you doan know nothin' about *nothin'* do you?' and Travis says, 'You shut your mouth or I'm goan *drown* you.' He sits up and digs a finger in the sand. 'Luna, you're just the pot callin' the kettle black.' Luna lies there, legs bent at the knees and thighs spread off to the side like a frog, dress up around her belly, her pubic hair wet and shining, eyes closed, a satisfied, flushed, comfortable look on her face. 'C'mon, let's get goin' 'fore it's dark,' says the boy, dusting himself off. The girl stretches her legs out straight in front of her and points her toes and then settles down into the sand with a quiet grunt. 'Travis,' she says, 'You go and tell 'em I *drown*. I ain't goin' back there never again. Bobo can go fuck hisself.' And then a dry leaf cracks under Sandra, and Luna sits up, fixing her dress down around her lap. 'Travis! What was *that*?' The boy stands up and turns a circle, 'Who's out there?! C'mon out and we won't do nothin'. Show yo'sef.' Sandra stands up from the brush and the boy says, 'Sandra *Lynn*, how much you saw?' 'None of it.' 'None of *what*?' says the boy. 'I didn't see nothing.' 'Thas *right* you dihn't see nothing,' says the boy. 'You tell anyone anything and I'll . . . I'll cut your *throat,* Sandra Lynn Fainey. I'll kill your parents, *too.*' The boy drags a finger across his neck in a slow, horizontal line, his eyes small and hot and mean and Sandra turns and runs. She cuts through the marsh, around the sand-dunes, across puddles from the tide, and doesn't stop until she's safely home."

2000

MAGGIE'S BEDROOM, 11 A.M.

In the morning, Ben Frank's asleep next to Joey with his mouth open and his glasses off, flush-faced, childlike. The room is sunny and a breeze moves the curtains in a billowing wave. They're in their dresses from last night. Maggie's nowhere to be seen.

Ben Frank wakes up. "Where're my glasses?" he says, yawning. "Where'd they go?" His big sightless eyes blinking. "I think I lost my gl—"

"No, no, no, here." Joey reaching over to the bedstand where Ben Frank left them. Two empty wine bottles. Breadcrumbs like sawdust. A chunk of baguette stained with wine. A Polaroid of Joey flipping off the camera with both hands, mouth open, screaming, red eyes like demon orbs about to shoot streams of flame. Joey rubs the lenses with the front of his dress and hands the glasses to him. "Here."

"Too kind." He puts them on and yawns again and settles back down in the bed. "I'm going back to sleep . . . just a couple more . . . minutes. The first . . . real bed . . . I've slept in . . . in months. Hold my calls for later." He pulls the comforter up to his neck and turns over with his back to Joey. "Wake me up . . . if anything important—" and he's out.

Joey settles back into the blankets. Ten minutes pass and then he hears the sound of dishes clanking and he sits up to see Maggie pushing the bedroom door open with her shoulder and walking into the room sideways holding a TV tray. She turns around, braided, smiling big. Pancakes, orange juice, scrambled eggs with cheese, sourdough toast. “Breakfast in bed!” she says happily.

FREEWAY, 5 P.M.

Los Angeles—“Lahs Angelis,” says Joey—two lanes to four lanes to six, towers of interstates looping above interstates (and interstates, interstates) while factories and movie billboards pass by the window and then car dealerships with red, white, and blue balloons tied to new cars. The endless gray overhead, glare through the windshield. Sooty smog hanging over the brown hills and telephone lines over palm trees and Chinese diners next to donut shops and dry cleaners in strip malls, a thousand Chinese restaurants with temple facades and gold-lettered signs and names that blend into a blur of Panda Garden China Ming Peking Jade Mandarin Emperor Empress King Golden Express Dragon Dynasty Bamboo House Inn. (Hungover Joey dreaming of peppery fried rice with pearl onions and carrots, snow peas and broccoli in a clear garlic sauce, wontons swimming in mysterious soup bowls with oversized spoons, steaming tea, a fortune cookie.) Ben Frank in the passenger seat with his big shoes up on the dash, his best friend Nate Houck driving with one hand, sticking the other out the window, feeling the air. Maggie, Joey, and Ben Frank’s unofficial girlfriend May, wedged in the back. Cars pass. Pennsylvania plates. Virginia plates. Michigan. Vanity plates that say nicknames. Inside jokes. They read them out loud.

“You know what’s a funny word when you really think about it?” Joey says as they pass the sign for another Chinese place.

“Cheesecake?” Maggie says quietly.

“Chop suey.”

They’re barely whispering.

“Oh.”

“Have you ever had chop suey? I don’t even know what it is.”

“I haven’t had egg fu yung either.” Another whisper.

“I always get sweet and sour pork.”

“I get chow mein no meat,” she says. “Or lo mein. Which is the one with the wide, fat noodles?”

“I think that’s lo mein.”

“Oh, okay.” A sigh.

Something happened last night. Or it didn’t. There are pictures in Joey’s head of Maggie and him together but they’re the same pictures from a thousand fantasies he’s had. If something did happen, Maggie isn’t letting on. Lo mein or chow mein. Fat, wide noddles or the skinny ones. License plates. Puns. Funny words.

In the front seat, Ben Frank is drinking a beer and smoking a cigarette and singing along with one of his tapes, shouting the chorus, "Are you out there?! / Do you hear me?! / Can I call you?! / Do you still hate me?!"

He turns to Nate, "Hey Nate . . . did you know . . . have I told you that—" (laughing, then speaking the lyrics) 'I have a picture of me and you in Brooklyn / On the porch it was raining / Hey, I remember that day / and I miss you.' You know that, right Nate?" laughing "'I miss you.'"

"I don't miss you."

"You will."

"Turn off this '90s bullshit."

"Bull*good*, you mean."

After the song ends, Ben Frank puts in a tape of a parade from the '30s, marching band music, trombones and whistles, tubas, the clatter of snare drums, crowd noise, a piece of an older time stretching as the tape warps. "Okay, now listen how it becomes white noise when I turn it up loud enough," he says, "The whole song and all the people become one sustained note if you distort it with volume." He turns it up until it's static and a rumble of decaying tune. The speakers are blown. The marching band and the crowd and the road noise and wind as one long and droning breath, sputtering, slapping.

May: "Turn it down."

Ben Frank: "Huh?"

May: "Down. It sounds horrible back here."

Joey: "It does. Just turn it down just a little."

Maggie: "No, I like it."

Ben Frank turns it down and then off. "It's interesting how you can become a second player after the fact by messing with a recorded sound source. It's like you're playing music with people who've been dead for longer than you've been alive. It's . . . it feels sweet, good-hearted. Like you're letting these guys have one last chance to play their songs with someone new."

Maggie: "That is really sweet."

Ben Frank: "You think?"

Maggie: "Totally."

Joey: "Yeah, that's actually a cool way of . . . of looking at it. I like that."

Ben Frank: "Ghost band."

Maggie: "Ghost band."

Joey: "Play it again."

They pass a limo and Ben Frank waves at the black windows.

Ben Frank: "Should I?"

Joey: "Yeah."

Maggie: "You should."

May: "Please don't."

Nate: "I'm with the MayQueen on this."

May: "My name's MayPole."

Nate: "MayDay."

May: "Maybelline."

May Stimson has cranberry hair and big staring eyes and freckles and a rabbit nose. To Joey, she's mysterious—a grubby farm girl from 1901, just in from the fields. With the hood of her sweatshirt up, she snaps photos out the window and stares through the glass. May has a look that's somewhere else, here but not here, daydreaming. She holds her camera careful and steady, moving it gracefully like it's weightless. Her thumbs poke out from holes worn in the cuffs of her sweatshirt. Her fingers are ink-stained. Some of her nails are painted. Some aren't.

"What're you taking pictures of?" Maggie asks.

"Oh, y'know," says May, distracted, pulling her sweatshirt hood down and shaking her hair loose. "Things that fit together horizontally."

Joey's so hungover that it's like he's watching from above, straining to hear, there but disconnected. Nothing happens as he expects it to happen, the chain of events knocked off course—but just slightly. The path newly crooked—but still a path.

Maggie squints out the window at the passing crash barrier, a short metal fence, blurring. "I'd like to see them sometime."

May looks at Maggie, smiles sadly, and says, "I love you." She says this slow and quiet and sincere, and then pulls her sweatshirt hood up and yanks the strings and goes back to her camera. It's what Joey would like to say more than anything. May says it like, Nice to meet you, God bless you, How you doing, You thirsty, Can I see that magazine, Got a light?

They drive and Joey falls asleep then wakes up with his face pressed against the window and he hears the road noise and talk radio. Once when he wakes up, Maggie's asleep next to him and he stares at her hand for ten minutes and forty-five seconds. Sometimes Ben Frank or Nate are talking. Sometimes everyone sits in silence, staring out the window, off on their own. May has put on sunglasses. They're big and round and red-plastic framed. Maggie's asleep with her head on May's shoulder. May's drinking wine from a baby bottle, singing quietly. Joey sleeps again. Then he's awake. Then asleep. Every time he wakes up the car is quieter than before and the breeze thundering through the open windows even hotter.

They get to the club at sundown and sit in the empty parking lot under a dark pink sky and pass around a Big Gulp cup of wine. It's a warm, muggy evening. Sweat soaks through their shirts. May fans herself with a Greek takeout menu she picked up off the ground and wears her sunglasses on top her head and looks healthy and flushed and happy. Ben Frank has found a balloon and now it's tied to his wrist and it strains away from him in the breeze. On the balloon, the words 'King Jeep Dodge Chrysler' are printed in big black letters. The wine (stolen) is dry and strong and expensive and everyone's talking and laughing and beaming at each other.

"No, you know who she is," says May. "Albertine Lebon. French girl. They called her Fat Albertine."

"Oh, right, but she wasn't actually fat."

"No, not at all. They liked the nickname. That was it. They liked saying it."

"Fat Albertine. She moved to San Francisco, right? She was dating that girl Andrea from Tulsa. Worked at Arby's."

"She came back a year later."

"How long is she in for?"

"Three years but who knows. She'll be thirty-one when she gets out."

"Three years would feel like forever."

"I bet she'll get out earlier. She's super nice."

Joey sits cross-legged and drums his fists on his thighs. "So. Last night. It was *fun*." He sets it out there. He wants Ben Frank or Maggie to bring up what happened. Just a hint. "It was good times," he tries again. Nods of agreement. Nothing else.

May hands him the Big Gulp cup and talks in a vampire voice, "Drrrink of my blahd, Joey Cahhrr." When she does this, he sees her dog teeth and they're long like fangs. Her teeth are white, blue white, and he feels old.

"Cool. Thanks." He drinks and then wipes his mouth. "This wine is great."

"Forty bucks," says Ben Frank. "Free for us."

"Last night," says Joey, "I hardly remember anything." He looks around. Nothing.

Ben Frank leans forward to take the wine and his balloon dips down and then lifts back up.

Nate is lying on his back on the warm asphalt, asleep, arms outstretched in a T, a lit cigarette between the fingers of his right hand.

"Hey. Look." Ben Frank juts his chin out at Nate and smiles. "Look at him. Awww. *Cuuute*."

May leans over Nate and plucks the cigarette out of his hand. She takes a drag then puts it up to his lips and then back between his fingers and pats his chest affectionately. "Thanks, sweetie."

"Is it time?" Maggie nods at the club. "Showtime?"

The club is a house, an old yellow Victorian on a weedy corner lot.

"Showtime." Joey says.

Inside the club, Maggie and Joey stand in the kitchen doorway looking into the living room. They balance together on a milk crate to see above the crowd. Below them, leaning against the wall, is Jared Brown-Berkowitz, a PR agent Joey knows through Yesenia. Jared looks up and nods and smiles and Joey nods back.

"Hey, Carr. Fancy meeting you here," he says playfully.

"Hey, Jared."

"You got the new record?"

"Not yet."

"Soooo good. Dude, *so* good. He's gonna be huge. Festive Show is doing his press on this one. We're all stoked on it."

"Oh, cool. Nice. I can't wait to see him play."

"Wait 'til you hear the new ones." Jared turns back around.

"I think I can see him," whispers Maggie, craning her neck and gripping the top of the doorframe. "By the drums." She leans back against Joey. They're almost touching. "Yeah," she says. "It's him."

Joey stands up taller and looks out across the sea of heads. The singer, a teenage kid from the Midwest, frowning down at the acoustic guitar he's tuning. His bandmates—a drummer sitting behind a small kit bending forward and stretching his back, a Korean girl holding a flute in front of her, eyes closed, mouth open, clicking the keys, and a bassist who Joey can barely see—are set up in front of a bay window in the living room, cramped together on the same level as the crowd.

The singer test-strums the guitar, then leans it against the wall behind him. He sits down on a stool, picks up a Casio keyboard, sets it on his lap, and begins to play a song. The crowd is silent as he taps out the opening notes of the song. He messes up and stops, swears under his breath, then starts again. His bandmates stand behind him, waiting, looking down at their instruments while he plays through the song on his own. He hits the keys and shouts in a trembly bark. His voice shakes. It's not a good voice but it's a voice that Joey is sure is telling the truth.

Jared looks back at Joey, eyebrows raised twice in quick succession.

Joey smiles and gives a nod.

"God, he's *so good,*" Maggie whispers in Joey's ear. Her hair against his face, unbraided and spun out into tumbling black curls. Joey can smell her—the fresh laundry smell of her dress. She presses against him and she's soft. "I'm so glad we did this."

"Yeah. Totally." *Tell me what we did.* "Me too."

The singer screws up the keyboard part. He stops and then starts again, closing his eyes, nervous.

Halfway through the next song, he breaks a string and gets frustrated. The set falls apart fast. One of the keyboards goes dead in the middle of a song.

The drummer drops a stick then ruins the beat while he scrambles for a new one. People begin to talk and laugh in the back during the quiet parts.

"I'm sorry, you guys. Um, I'm sorry. Okay, uh, here we go. This is the last one. I promise, this is it. Okay, alright," he says and begins plucking the strings with his fingers, then singing, and this one's a story—a suicide attempt, a vision of the future.

Joey looks at Maggie. She's mouthing the words, smiling, swaying just barely to the song.

The set ends. Applause is meek and the crowd thins out fast. After the show, the singer is nothing bigger or better than what he was before—a teenage kid from a flyover state, unknown and tired and kind of drunk, coughing and chain-smoking, packing his gear and joking with his band. Joey and Maggie watch him lay his guitar in its case on the ground. He snaps it closed and shakes his head and laughs at something Jared says. The singer makes the time out 'T' with his hands and Jared laughs and gives him a thumbs-up and walks away, tall and confident with expensive sneakers and a rich guy's taste for cool clothes, a man on the inside of things.

Maggie and Joey follow the crowd out the door.

In the parking lot, they sit on a curb and share a cigarette and watch the club empty.

Joey takes a drag and hands the cigarette to Maggie as a crying blonde girl stumbles past, held up by two friends. Then she laughs and breaks away from them and bolts across the parking lot yelling, "It doesn't even matter!" She turns around and runs backwards, arms spread out, shouting at her friends, "It doesn't matter! It doesn't matter!" Flocks of kids pass by, drunk, flirting, laughing, yelling, girls in tight jeans with sleeveless shirts, guys with arm-length tattoos, jean jackets, scarves, a girl with a bloody nose holding a tissue to it saying, "Dude. You're tellin' *me*."

"Joey, will you ask to drive if Nate's too drunk?"

"Sure."

"Pinky swear?"

"Course."

"I wouldn't say anything, but—"

"No, no, no, it's cool. It's alright. So what did you think?"

"Of the show? So good. I'm really glad he played some of the ones from the tape you gave me. It was perfect."

"Right? I met him last time they played San Diego. There was nobody there at the Casbah and he came and bummed a cigarette off me."

"Did you guys talk?"

"Not really. He was like, 'Hey, do you have an extra cigarette?' and I said, 'Marlboro Reds okay?' just to prolong the interaction, and he said, 'Totally,' and I gave him one and said, 'When you guys playing?' and he said, 'I dunno, soon? Twenty minutes maybe?' and I said, 'Cool, lookin' forward to it.' Still it was enough. I was so hero worship-y that it's good it ended fast. If he was a dick, it would've ruined everything for me."

"I totally understand that."

In the parking lot, Ben Frank is lying on the concrete, drunk and shouting his own name. The car dealer balloon has popped but it's still tied to his wrist, limp and busted and dirty at the end of its string. May stands over him and snaps a photo.

On the way down The 405, Nate drives fast and reckless, sharing a forty in the front seat with Ben Frank, who is nodding in and out of sleep.

"Joey, this is really, *really* freaking me out," Maggie whispers. She sinks into her seat. "I'm way too sober for this right now. He's gonna kill us. I need . . . *fuck*, man. I dunno. I wish we had a *game* or something. I need something to take my mind off this."

Joey looks over at May, sleeping against the window with her sweatshirt hood up. In the front seat, Ben Frank, half asleep with a Mexican blanket over him. Nate has the forty between his thighs and he's singing along with the stereo. "What a beautiful face I have found in this place / That is circling all 'round the sun / What a beautiful dream that could flash on the screen / In a blink of an eye and be gone from me." Nate cuts in front of a semi-truck, the big headlamps of the rig blinding white as it rushes up behind them. Nate laughs and steps on the gas and they pull away from it. He swerves into the left lane and guns it up to ninety. And Nate singing, "And one day we will die / And our ashes will fly from the aeroplane over the sea!" Now one hundred and five, one hundred and ten. "But for now we are young / Let us lay in the sun / And count every beautiful thing we can see."

"Okay," Joey says.

And he leans in to kiss her.

1979

DECEMBER 1ST

"Okay, I've got one for you," said Channy. "Five friends were going to church one morning and it began to rain. All five got there at same time. The four of them that ran got wet and the one who stayed still sta—"

"I've heard this one. A body in a casket and four pallbearers."

"Right. Okay, you won't get this one. I am the beginning of sadness and sorrow and the tail end of sickness. You can't show happiness and satisfaction without me, yet I'm in the midst of crosses. I am always in risk, chaos, and strife but I am never in danger. I am in harm's way, but not in the way of harm. You may find me sitting in the sun, but I am *never* outside of darkness."

"Heavy."

"It's really not. Just think."

"I have no idea. Channy . . . I don't know. Tell me."

"The letter 'S'!"

"The letter 'S' how?"

"The letter 'S,' think about it."

"Oh. I guess so. Right, right, 'S.'"

"Oh's right. C'mon, dumbo."

Her hair is so blonde that it's nearly white. I want to wrap it around my hand and smell it. I know how her hair smells—piney, a forest smell, coconut and guava when it's washed—but it looks as if it would smell like frost, ice crystals, a long winter. Maybe a winter in the fairytale.

Dear Son,

After I came back from Mexico, the three of us holed up in the house and your mother and I fixed things between us. It was the first real time she and I had spent together since we met. With the last of our money—my job at the paper long gone—we spent a glorious three weeks in the house in La Jolla, talking all night and playing with you and cooking meals and eating dinner on the floor amidst the ruins of our previous life. We didn't leave the house except to get groceries, and we didn't clean, and we didn't let anything in from outside. It was a closed circuit. Me and you and your mother and your sister on her way. I learned all about your mother's childhood and I told her mine. We listened to Elton John's *A Single Man* on repeat and she read me riddle after riddle and showed me the journal of riddles she's been collecting from books since she was a girl. That was when I learned about the book, her childhood memoir; she'd been writing it all along.

Your mother's been reading sections to me for weeks. Reading, or telling me about the story, working out the story in her head, talking it out. It's a big, full thing. It winds me up and makes my heart swell with pain and then pride for her, and then I'm lost in the story (which is like being lost in a dream) and I come out feeling shook-up and worked-over. I've given my heart to her book. I can't wait to see it in print and hold it in my hand.

When we left the house, we took nothing but a bag of clothes, the Elton John record, the typewriter I got at *Midtown,* your plastic dinosaurs ("dine-does") and stuffed animals, and a small suitcase with your mother's manuscript and the riddle book.

Without income, we needed a place to stay, so we moved into a room on your mother's family's ranch outside Julian.

The deal here is simple: I do farm work in exchange for rent, and Channy spends her time with you and taking care of herself for the new one to come. She has the book to finish, but beyond that she needs to stay healthy and not stress.

The ranch sits on eighty-five sprawling acres near the Cuyamaca State Park. Issy—short, strong, olive-complected, black-haired—runs one hundred and sixty heads of sheep for wool and a dozen goats for milk. It's a business and she takes it seriously, but life here is slow and easy and good. We eat well and we get a lot of sleep and we end each day satisfied. (I don't know where we'll be when you're older, but I hope it's here.)

Issy's endless procession of girl cousins come in from all over the country—stopping to help with the harvest or sheering, hiding out from bad boyfriends, shacking up to weather a cold or a broken heart or a busted rib. The farmhouse (it's called Rose Morning Manor) has been in the family since the Depression.

Rose Morning Manor has nine bedrooms spread across three stories. It has diamond panel windows and rosewood glass cabinets and a steeply gabled roof. Outside is an elegant wraparound porch, which extends into a teakwood deck (both of which are new additions) and the deck has Adirondack chairs and chaise lounges and a covered gazebo. The sitting room just inside from the deck is dark and wood-paneled and comfortable, and its wall-size windows look out over the barns and fields and smoky woods. (As I write this, a thick fog creeps out from the woods and rolls up over the fields; a mist of rain falls and the sky is dark and low and heavy. It's like pictures of the Scottish Highlands that I've seen. Beautiful. Usually, it's sunny and dry and hot. Today is different.)

Rose Morning is a constant hub of activity. Cousins Denice and Mona, back from school in Providence, fixing the parlor floor with cousins Carly and Morgan (who is eight and lives here full-time). Issy's stepsister Pilar, fresh out of the Peace Corps, sleeping off mono in the back room. It's a productive place, as restful as it is:= Issy building a chicken tractor down by the lower barn; Channy typing her book on the old Underwood in the library; you in the kitchen learning about order and balance by emptying cabinets and piling the skillets and pots together. (You have toys but sometimes I think you'd rather play with a plastic ladle and a salad bowl than anything else.)

Meals at Rose Morning are impressive. Last night began with French onion soup with provolone-cheddar croutons, great slabs of fresh-baked rosemary bread with honey from Issy's bees, a jar of currant preserves from last year's harvest, and a bowl of berries from the new greenhouse. The main course was a pork roast and a big pot of stew in the middle of the table—a Russian potato and fish stew with vegetables from the garden (the fish, rainbow trout, caught from the stream below the fields). Dessert was apple-raspberry pie made with apples from the lake orchard.

After dinner most nights, Issy brews coffee and serves honey mead from a few seasons ago and Denice and Carly smoke cigarettes on the porch with Farmer Johnston's boys and Channy puts you to bed. In the late evenings, Carly plays piano and Denice—trained by their aunt Siobhan—sings traditional Irish songs.

The song that I like best tells the story of a ship crossing the Atlantic from Dublin to New York. It's a bright, hard, sad lament, a dozen verses. It begins with the story of young girl on board the ship who is in love with the captain, who doesn't know she's alive. In the first few verses, she pines for him but he's busy with the ship, and she knows that once they get to port, his job is to sail right back. He can never be hers and she can never be his. Halfway across the Atlantic, the boat goes down in a storm and only the captain and the girl survive. The last verse of the song is them clinging to a plank of wood with the big, gray, freezing sea all around and the wall of fog and no ships for miles. It's clear in the song that the girl and the captain are going to die, but the girl has never been happier because now they're alone together, and together they'll be until they're no more. Denice sings it nearly every night, her voice breaking with sadness, and each time it gets to me and I have to go out to the porch and clear my head.

In the mornings, I let you and your mother sleep and I put on my red and black checked Pendleton and a pair of gloves and I do the first round of farm chores. Open the chicken coop and let them out into the yard; toss layer feed and whole corn and dinner scrap on their scratch dirt; refill their water and rake out their straw if it needs cleaning. After that, I gather the eggs and bring them to Issy who, by then, is beginning the breakfast preparation with Carly and Morgan and Denice. (The eggs will be your job some day. I can't wait to see you waddling around carrying an egg basket half your size.)

The chickens taken care of, I let the sheep and the goats out of the barn and onto the pasture. I sweep the hard-packed dirt floor of the barn and spread handfuls of "fines" (dry sand) on the damp spots, then clean and fill the water drums and measure out a cup of red mineral into three bins. The last thing I do is feed the sheep and goats. I climb up to the hayloft for timothy and brome, and drop bales down to the barn floor until my arms ache (there are two sheep barns, so this happens twice).

When the hay and the alfalfa are spread out and ready, I call the animals back to the barn by tossing handfuls of dry corn into their metal trough.

At the sound of the corn, the sheep and goats come up from the field.

Son, it's the happiest thing in the world—the mass of white at a steady run and the lambs and kid goats dancing sideways across the grass, kicking their legs and springing up in step. Your mother has brought you out a few times to see it and you point your little finger and laugh and I feel balanced and good about everything.

Breakfast then. Everyone at the big table leaned forward, cutting ham and passing dishes of grits and chicken gravy, plates stacked high with pancakes and waffles and bacon and fried eggs. Issy was raised vegetarian, but she cooks meat for us. Her plate is piled highest—hashbrowns fried golden brown, toast slathered in Parkay, biscuits with cherry jam, half a grapefruit, grits sprinkled in brown sugar, coffee, orange juice, and a beer. For you, cereal, scrambled eggs, fresh fruit.

Your mother's never been much of a meat-eater, but with her cool older cousin around, she's cut it out completely. These days, she lives off eggs. Poached with hollandaise sauce for breakfast. Scrambled with spinach and onions for lunch. *Ranchero* eggs with a side of corn tortillas, avocado, sour cream, and refried beans. Fried egg sandwiches with Swiss and cheddar cheese on whole wheat bread. Omelets with mushrooms and tomatoes from the fields. Every day it's something different, but it's always eggs. ("C'mon, I'm growing a child and writing a book," she says. "Aren't eggs the perfect metaphor?" And they are.) It's good to see her eat. She's working toward something better. Whatever goes into her, goes into someone else. She still has her figure but she's growing thicker in the hips and legs and it looks good on her. Farm life suits your mother, to say the very least. I've never been more in love with her than I am now. I can say this with confidence: I've gotten to know your mother, and it's a fine thing to see who she is and what she's becoming.

After breakfast, we go our separate ways. Today Denice, Morgan, Carly, Mona, and I helped Issy build a coop down at the lake for the Peking ducks that she's going to raise for eggs. First, the welded wire fence around the structure, then the structure itself, the frame, four sides, the walls (plywood with nice glass windows that Carly's boyfriend found in an alley down in Mission Beach), shelves for supplies, the roof—slanted, tar-shingled, stapled-in, a vent hole in the top like a small chimney.

At noon, we break for lunch and eat together on the lakeshore—today it was black bread with sweet European-style butter, fresh blueberries and cherries, and salted almonds. A good, simple meal, nothing to weigh you down. After lunch, we dug a square trench to sink the ends of the coop—a foot down to keep out the coyotes and foxes and raccoons—and carried the four sides of the structure to its spot.

Tomorrow's work will include nailing it all together, fixing the roof (with help from one of Johnston's boys) then oiling and hard-beating the dirt floor until it's like stone, and building a nice hatch-clasped door. Issy is going to Santee for the ducks. Nine layers and a drake.

Once I've finished the afternoon work every day, it's time for my evening farm chores and I take the sheep and the goats out into the field again. The land isn't fenced, so by day the sheep and goats stay in a large cattlegate paddock. Issy's plan is to fence a good portion of the lower acres and buy another group of sheep—a dozen at a time until the flock is substantial enough to turn a real profit. Everything is paid for—the wire, the t-posts, the concrete, the seven gates and an assortment of braces and brace accessories. All that's left is for us to lay the fence.

For most of its life, this was a working farm, but when Issy's father came back from the war, he turned it into a summer retreat and he took to drinking heavily and it fell to waste. Eight years ago, he shot himself by the lake after cutting off all communication with the family and holing himself up in the tower bedroom for a year. He didn't leave a note.

After the funeral, Issy took over the land and vowed to bring the place back to its former glory. It's going to be a lot of work, but she's capable and no one doubts that she'll pull it off. You'll like Issy. She's smart and determined, and that's high praise for anyone.

So, that's how we're living these days. You're happy and you're growing fast and I think any day now you'll be running the place.

Your father,
Merc

DECEMBER 2ND

The more I write to the boy, the less I want to write about my life. Looking back on this journal, big blocks of time are missing, huge events in the timeline, our reunion, the wedding, the birth. At one point in my life, that would've bothered me. These days, I don't care. The letters feel more important. The *boy* is more important. I feel myself, my ego, my identity, whatever you want to call it, slipping away. Sometimes, the inner dialog that used to push me through my days is a murmur at best. I like this. Most people you meet, whether they know it or not, consider themselves the center of the universe, the main character in the movie. I know I'm not. And it's good. It's good to live and not think so much about yourself all the time. I'm nothing, and I say this in a positive way. I'm alive and I'm here, but I'll pass from this life and be forgotten, and that's not a bad thing. What's important isn't *you*, but what you do while you're here. "Identity" (as a thing to search for, to worry over) is for the unfulfilled. When you have what you want, you can enjoy living in the moment and not beat yourself up (so much) about "who you are." Who you are is nothing. This is a good thing. The future doesn't exist. "Right now" does.

DECEMBER 3RD

Issy's boyfriend Gus is coming in by way of West Texas to help out with some projects. Gus has been splitting time between here and San Angelo for months now. When he's here, we don't see Issy for a day or two, and then they're out working side-by-side, morning to night.

Gus comes from a long line of cowboys. As he says, the Texas-to-California migration is second-nature; his family has been doing it since the Gold Rush, driving cattle across the desert and plains, there and back again, 'The California trail.'

Channy wants Gus to teach her to shoot, but Gus says she'll need to wait until the baby's born, which is good advice.

DECEMBER 4TH

This trip to the ranch, Gus is helping Issy get set up with horses. She wants to start small. Two and a comfortable stable (built up from the structure and foundation of the old stables). Gus, Carly, Issy, and I are going to build the stable with help from Julius Johnston, the man who runs the next farm down. It's funny, if you would've told me a year ago I'd be off in the country building stables and coops and laying fence, I would've laughed in your face. But, my god, it's a good way to live.

Johnston and his two boys are bringing wood (their own lumber) and helping out with the building in exchange for wool from Issy's sheep and a case of her famous blackberry honey.

Gus and Johnston's families have been working together for generations. The Johnstons came to California for the Gold Rush. Gus's family (the Moores and Holmeses) brought cattle up north for the mining camps. At some point, they joined forces. It's a system and it works.

DECEMBER 14TH

Well, we did it. A fenced-in property and a rebuilt horse stable. I've never felt so good working as I have here. You finish a day and you're calm and sore and tired and you feel like you've done something. I don't make a penny, but the work is something beyond money. Working out here, close to the land, eating what we grow, all the people you love around you, it's the way we should be living. Nature didn't give us cities to live in. *We* did that.

DECEMBER 15TH

The preparations for Christmas are underway. Channy is making everyone hand-bound photo albums. She has taken a break from the book ("To let my subconscious work on it, like Hemingway said.") and she's holed-up in our room listening to the Elton John record and cutting black paper and painting borders in gold and letting the glue set on the bindings.

I'm off with the boy, carrying him around the farm, showing him things. A while back he started to point, and when he points at something, I tell him the name. Point. "Those are hummingbird feeders. Look." I take one of the feeders down from its black plastic chain and let him touch it and he smiles and slaps his little fat hands on it. "Hummingbirds drink this red sugar water. It looks good, doesn't it? Like Hawaiian Punch? Kool-Aid? You're not supposed to drink it, but you're gonna want to. I tried it when I was a kid. It's not what you think it is." He smiles and shows his big front teeth and his tiny lower ones—four of them in all—and says "Gee!" and I say, "Good answer!" and we move onto the next thing.

The boy is curious and open to everything and whatever I show him makes him happy. It's a good thing to see. When I'm around him, nothing bothers me. With the boy in my arms, I can let it all slip away.

The boy is at my feet as I write this, crashing two wooden train cars together. I reach down and rub his little head and he looks up and smiles with his big teeth and his eyes crinkle up and he says, "Ah-goo," and goes back to his trains.

DECEMBER 25TH

We have a full house. Gus and his brother Jack and their sister Nell. Nine of Issy and Channy's girl cousins. Later, an aunt and uncle and their three boys are coming by for Christmas dinner. Issy is making a Yorkshire pudding with beef from Johnston's cows. Johnston will be there, too, with his private-eye pal, Manny Partridge. Johnston's sons are off with their wives' families in Lakeside and Ramona but they were by earlier to bring presents for the boy and little Morgan.

This morning was the boy's second Christmas but it was his first time opening presents on his own. He likes it—even if sometimes he's sidetracked and sets a half-opened package aside to beat his milk cup on the floor.

Today he got three wooden tractors, a wool blanket, a wild assortment of baby clothes and hats and socks and shoes, and a handmade wooden pop gun (from Gus). The thing he's most pleased with is the box Channy's new typewriter came in. He takes the lid off and looks inside and when he sees that it's empty he begins to fill it with things around him—silver and red stick-on bows from packages, balled-up bits of foil from chocolate Santas, his tractors, Morgan's plastic farm animals and their tiny green fences, candy canes, pennies, whatever he can find. When the box is full, he empties it again and starts over.

JANUARY 2ND

Well, it's 1980: a new decade. How strange to have made it here. New Year's Eve was just an extension of Christmas; everyone stayed over and five of Issy's college friends arrived (by way of Detroit, Chicago, London, Florida, and Morocco). We sat up playing cards in groups and then we went out onto the deck to watch Gus and his brother set off fireworks in the valley.

As we began to count down, Issy gave out sparklers and Denice lit them, and we held them up—"ten, nine, eight, seven, six, five, four, three, TWO, ONE, *HAPPY NEW YEAR*!"—and the fireworks hissing off in trails of flame and snapping in the distance, and sparklers spitting out silver, and lighting up flushed, smiling faces.

Channy and I kissed and then we kissed the boy's head and I held them both while everyone ran through an excited version of "Auld Lang Sang" with Issy on the banjo and Carly on dulcimer playing accompaniment.

I think this will be my last entry. There are so many better things to do with your life than write about it. I don't know. We'll see. Regardless, I'm going to put the book away for a while.

2000

DOG BEACH, AFTERNOON

Nicole and Joey sit on the sand by the jetty and watch the waves roll in. "So, Maggie and Tyler and I were down on Newport walking around yesterday, y'know, like, looking in the stores or whatever, and a car in the street next to us is stuck in traffic and we hear 'Tiny Dancer' on—"

"Love that song," (Nicole singing) "Blue jean *baby*, LA *lady*, seamstress for the bah-hand."

"—on . . . on its . . . like, on its car radio. It feels really good to hear it and Maggie and I are singing along as we walk (Tyler was grumpy, as per usual) but then the station wagon in front of it turns right at the stop sign and the 'Tiny Dancer' car drives off—"

Nicole singing: "Pretty eyes, pirate smile—"

"—down Newport and without even saying anything Maggie and I start running after it on the sidewalk and when we catch up we run alongside it so we can hear the song all the way through and we're singing and running and, god, it was *great*. It was like some kind of movie scene."

"So, it's good?"

"Yeah. Totally. It's *really* good."

"I'm glad, Joey. You deserve it."

"I don't know about *that*."

"You do, after putting up with my crap while we were together, and *afterwards*."

"*Come on*."

"No, really. You don't have to be chivalrous anymore. I gave you a rough time and you know it. Be honest. You deserve to be happy," (singing) "Blue jean *baby*," (stops, shakes her head) "It's stuck in my head now, jerk."

"Everybody deserves to be happy."

"Sure, everybody does," she says. "I guess what I'm saying is that I want *somebody* to have a good time. *For reals*. You can't be happy when everyone around you is miserable, and that's how I feel sometimes."

"You're hanging out with the wrong people, Hale-Bop."

"I'm hanging out with my mom, my brother, my sister, her fiancé Bobby, and his friends from GD. They're all depressed. Every single one of them. They hate their jobs and everyone's got the flu or a cold or a sprained wrist or a toothache or, like, effing carpal *tunnel* or they're drinking too much or they're going to effing *AA* and they've lost their mind about it. I'm sick of it. I wanna live in *Mr. Roger's Neighborhood*. Just me and the Speedy Delivery guy and Trolley and the little . . . mewly little kitten."

"You'd be a great Lady Elaine. 'Boomerang . . . *toomerang* . . . zoomera—"

"I'm being serious, Carr."

"You need to hang out with me more often. I'm a ray of sunshine. I'm a ray of sunshine moonwalking on a cartoon rainbow covered in My Little Pony unicorn fur spraying pure heavenly goodness out of—"

"Carr. Come on now. You're getting crazy. You see the paper today? The headline was 'San Diego Says C-Ya to Centennial Summer.' So cheeseball. Don't you wanna kick the newspaper's *ass* sometimes?"

"You're changing the subject."

"It's alright, it's a defense mechanism."

"I guess that's okay."

"Look at the clouds, Joey. It's like when you break a piece of styrofoam in half and you see all the little round parts that make it up and some of them stick to your hand with static."

"That's exactly what it looks like."

"Don't tease."

"I'm being serious. That's a perfect way to say it. You should write children's books."

"I should," (sarcastic) "I'd be great at it, Carr. What are you even *talking* about?"

"I love you, Nicole. You're a good egg. I'm glad things are . . . better. I'm glad you're better and—"

"Whatever. 'You don't love me, you just love my doggy style.'"

"*What*?"

"It's from a song, Carr. It's from Snoop."

"You should hear Tyler do that Dre and Snoop song from last year. He's all, 'Still hittin' the corners in the lo-los, girl' and it sounds exactly like him."

"I don't think it goes like that."

"I don't care. It does now."

They sit and watch the ocean. Seagulls glide and coast on currents of air above the water. People run their dogs along the shore. The sky is pale blue and full of pebbly clumps of white cloud. The ocean—dark and flat and wind-chopped.

Nicole looks older. Her hair is cut short and it blows around her face as she tries to gather it into a ponytail. "Have you guys talked about it much? What it means and all that?"

"We say things when it's happening, but we don't ever talk about it when it's *not*. And besides the car ride home from L.A., we've never gotten together when we're sober. We always make an excuse to hang out as friends and then one thing leads to the next and we're drunk and hooking up. And it's *great* . . . it's great, but it's like the first time she and I got together and how I wasn't even sure it *happened*. When you're always drunk during one particular thing, it makes that thing seem . . . I don't know, seem less *real* because the memories you have are full of holes. I guess that's overstating the obvious, right? But like . . . like, the fewer memories you have, the less it exists. Does that make sense?"

"You're kinda overthinking a simple thing, but . . . yeah, yeah, it makes sense." She takes a silver and orange packet of airline peanuts out of her hoodie pocket and tears the top open with her teeth and offers it to him. "In-flight snack?"

"Sure, cool, thanks."

"Oh, wait, are you allergic?"

"No . . . but . . . what was I saying . . . that's pretty much it. I'm still trying to figure us out."

"You sound like such a girl, Carr."

"Whatever."

The breeze picks up from the west and ruffles their hair. Nicole zips her hoodie to her chin.

"You and her do the dirty deed yet?"

She empties the peanuts into her hand and picks through them until she finds the one she wants.

"*The dirty deed*. Where do you come *up* with this stuff? No, we haven't. We haven't really done anything besides . . . which one's first base?"

"I think first base is when you've made out and maybe had your shirts off. Nothing below the belt."

"We've done more than that. I mean, obviously I want the whole thing, but this feels okay right now."

"Does she want more?"

"I don't know. It's complicated. She's into it, whatever it is. Like she's really vocal."

"Vocal?"

"She says stuff when it's happening and the stuff she says is super crazy and nothing I'd ever be able to say out loud."

"That's great. She's *down*. You're *lucky*."

"Only thing is, I feel like such a *prude*. I can't talk *dirty*. Even if I want the thing, I wouldn't be able to *say* it, and I think because I can't *say* it, she thinks I don't want it—as much."

"Let's practice talking dirty. Pretend I'm her and tell me how much you want to lick my—"

"Nicole!"

"I'm only effing with you. Lighten up. You *are* a prude. You're an adult, dude. Adults can say this shit without getting all blushy and wimped-out."

"I guess." Joey squints up at the sky. A seagull. Then two. One moves to the left, the other stays where it's at.

"Is she still a virgin?" Nicole asks.

"When did I ever tell you she was a virgin?"

"I don't know. She's young. I just figured . . . I don't know. Sorry."

"No, not anymore. She's seeing somebody."

"Right. *You*. What are you *talking* about?"

"I don't know what she and I are but I'm pretty sure we're not *seeing* each other. It's somebody else. One of her—one of our friends. My friend, too. I don't know him that well."

"Do you want to?"

"Do I want to what? Know him well?"

"No, *see her*. Be her *boyfriend*."

"She's got that guy . . . and he really wants to be her boyfriend and they're seeing each other whether she calls it *official* or not. He keeps trying to get her to be more, like, *serious* about everything. They go out on real dates where he pays. He gives her *gifts*. Not expensive stuff, because he comes from a poor family, but *romantic* gifts, thoughtful stuff. She'll tell me about some present he gave her and I'll be like, *What a great idea. Man, that guy really loves her.* She's super blasé about it but it's still going on. And she's still messing around with Tyler."

"What are you gonna do about it?"

"I don't know. When it comes down to it, I'm not sure what her and

I are all about. I mean, she's my favorite person in the *world* and I'm more in love with her than with anyone I've been with, so much that I'm not even sure the rest of them were actually love or just . . . ugh, sorry. I shouldn't even—"

"No, it's okay," Nicole says with a sad laugh. "The past," she picks up a handful of sand and lets it fall through her fingers, "doth not exist."

"But yeah, it's complicated. If I were to be, like, oh, '*Be with me only*,' that would call into question the fact that we're *being* at all. It's just so good and fun and exciting. I don't want to impose myself as some kind of *boyfriend* figure. Hey gimme a cigarette, okay? Like, I don't want to push her into something I *know* she doesn't want. Because I *know* she doesn't want a boyfriend. She hates the idea of having some stuffy-ass douchy quote-unquote committed guy floating around wherever she goes telling her what to do, what not to do, treating her like . . . like some second-class citizen. Tyler got that way and that's one of the reasons she broke up with him."

"Are you still . . . I mean, I'm *sure* you're still worried about how Tyler'll take it when he finds out, right?" Nicole pulls two cigarettes from her pack, sticks both in her mouth and cups them against the wind. She lights them and hands one to Joey.

"Thanks." He takes a drag and blows the smoke out. "Yeah. I am." Smoke gets in his left eye and he shuts it and squints the other. "I *really* am. It makes me *sick* when I think about it. I'm stressed the fuck *out*."

"What are you gonna do?"

He shakes his head. "I have no idea. None at all. If you've got a plan, please enlighten me."

"Come on, Mr. List-Maker."

"I really . . . I really have no idea. I'm at a total loss. It's freakin' me out."

"You should probably figure that out soon. Friends don't do what you're doing to Tyler. This is a total dick move, Joey."

"I know."

"*Do* you? Because I don't think you do. I think it's comforting for you to think you care . . . I think you want to *think* of yourself as someone that cares but . . . I don't think you really care."

"I care."

"*Prove* it."

LATE AFTERNOON

After he drops Nicole off at her apartment, Joey takes a drive on the I-8 East to be alone and give himself time to think before taking Maggie to the bonfire party.

Outside El Centro, the highway is bordered on either side by sand dunes that stretch off as far as he can see. The sky is clear blue and hot air comes through his windows and blows his hair and makes him sweat, and it feels good to sweat.

He pulls off for gas and gets an orange Fanta in a glass bottle and a ham and cheese sandwich in a plastic triangle box.

At the gas station, the desert is silent: the wind whistling around the pumps and over the station roof, the banging of an old, metal 'Drink Coca-Cola!' sign against the siding of the garage; sand and rock all around, skyline in all directions, a rust-blacked '50 Chevy behind the bathrooms. Joey takes a piss and then stands out on the desert floor and looks at the Chevy. No tires. No glass. Bullet holes in the passenger side door. He sticks his finger in one of the holes then walks to his truck.

Back on the road, the radio stops picking up stations and the numbers on the dial spin and cycle as it fights to find a signal. Driving with his knees, he opens the sandwich package and drops the ham slice on the floorboards of the truck. He drinks some of the orange soda and eats half the sandwich and leaves the other half in its package on the seat. When he's done with the soda, he holds the bottle out the window and the wind blows into its mouth and whistles a slow, deep drone. The radio dial spins. The sun bakes his arm until it hurts.

Near the state line, a country station picks up and it fades in clear and strong. The static becomes a woman singing, "Like straaawberry wine, seventeeeeen / The hot July moon saw everythiiing." Tapping a finger on the steering wheel to the beat (unconsciously), Joey exits the freeway and pulls into town and stops at a red light. Empty streets like a movie set back lot, no one out. Old West facades. Dusty neons of bar signs. A junk store with a headless mannequin in the glass display. A pet shop with a woman in the window turning around the 'Open' sign to 'Closed'.

The song ends and the DJ says, "KTTI, Yuma, Arizona! This is Karen Kay with the Drive at Five. We're playin' today's best country and yesterday's favorites! More of your KTTI Country after the break!" and then a car commercial with the announcer singing that if you wanna buy a truck, you should go see Cal.

The stoplight turns from red to green and the breeze moves it on its wire and it sways forward and back. Closed-up diners. The First Chance Saloon. Ruby's House of Ribs. A gas station with blacked-out windows and gutted pumps. Astro Mart. A few cars on the street, parked. Everything dry and still and bleached-out by the sun.

The Colorado River runs alongside the town and Joey pulls off at a park with grass and picnic benches and a public restroom.

He leaves his shoes on the front seat and walks across the grass toward the sand.

The sand is hotter than the pavement, but when he reaches the shore, it's cool again.

The sun is setting. It boils up orange and fiery over the hills and then it slips down and everything is golden and dark.

Joey dips his foot into the water.

It's warm.

Enough for a swim.

The river is shallow and clear and it moves fast to the west. On the opposite bank stands a wall of cattail reeds and they rustle with the breeze. Up river, the freeway overpass crosses the water and two Mexican men fish beneath it, the swish of traffic and the sound of the moving river joining together as one.

Joey's eyes are tired and he shuts them and listens to the sound of the freeway, the cars far off then closer, then racing away. *You could have been one of them but you stopped and now you're here. You're here because you made the choice. The other drivers are there not because they didn't choose, but because they made a different choice.*

He rolls up his jeans to his knees and wades into the water. The river moves around him and the wet sand is disappearing beneath his feet and in his head it's Maggie Tyler Maggie Tyler and he slows it down and cuts it in two until it's just Maggie. Maggie, Maggie, Maggie, and then he adds his own name. Joey Carr Maggie Harker. The shared sounds, Carr, Harker, one word, a breath.

There's a hot, dry breeze coming from the south and it smells like sage and rain and dust.

Joey sits down in the water and then he lets himself float on his back, his ears under the surface and the sound of the sand and the river stones grinding, the big sky overhead, clouds pulled up around its western edge, pink and red.

OCEAN BEACH, NIGHT

The moon is out and they walk across the sand to the bonfire, which is gushing smoke and sparks up to the sky. The sand is dry. Here and there: dried kelp as a black stain on the sand. Everything gray and colorless under the moon.

Maggie walks next to Joey, barefoot in a blue and yellow flower-print '40s dress and a denim jacket with a brass sheriff's badge pinned above the pocket.

"*Aliens*, you know," she says. "I just hate that they're even *up* there. I don't ever want them to come and *do anything* to me." Her hair is blowing back in the breeze and Joey can't take his eyes off her.

Tyler, walking to the left of Joey—tall and narrow and leaned forward against the wind like it might blow him over if he didn't—quiet, moody, sullen. "I don't think you have to worry about aliens."

"No, aren't aliens the *worst*?" she asks. "Besides E.T."

Joey laughs. "I always thought E.T. looked like a piece of poop."

"E.T. was sweeeet, no way. It's the rest of the aliens that I hate."

Tyler has a six-pack of Sierra Nevada held by the cardboard handle. Maggie is hugging a brown paper Ralphs bag with a bottle of red wine, a mason jar of blackberry jam from Joey's apartment, a butter knife, a wedge of cheddar, and a giant loaf of French bread. Joey has a Ralphs bag with a pint bottle of Jack Daniels, a family-size bag of Ruffles, and a box of peanut butter Ritz crackers.

Closer to the bonfire they hear a stereo. The sound is thin and drawn out in the distance, a bouncing rattle of drums and voice, then louder until they recognize the song, a rap song, and the rapper says, "I see no changes / All I see is racist faces."

Ben Frank jogs across the sand, waving a pirate sword in the air. "You guys made it! You're here!" He drops his sword in the sand and it sticks upright and he throws his arms around Maggie, spinning her in a circle. The grocery bag drops and the contents spill across the sand. "I love you guys so much! You're here! This party's *boring*. Fix it! Maggie, you're my only hope."

"Ben Frank," says Maggie, on her knees, gathering up the groceries. "What's this I hear about you burning all your things?"

"I want *nothing!*" he shouts defiantly. "Joey Carr!" He bearhugs Joey and Joey's breath goes out of him with an *Oof*. "Joey Carbuncle Capture the Flag *Carr*! Back from the dead! And Tyler Monopoly Seaquest Baywatch Monahan!" he shouts and Tyler sticks his hand out to shake but Ben Frank hugs him anyway. "Tyler, you look like a ghost! You look like a ghost who's just seen a ghost of a ghost!"

Ben Frank turns back to Maggie and takes her grocery bag. "Let me carry this. Here. Let's walk. Maggie, I'm burning all my things because I'm exorcising nineteen stupid years of growing up in this shitty surferdude fratboy dickhead beachtown. I want *nothing*! When I get on that bus Tuesday, I'm taking *nothing*. Besides my sword. Check this shit out, I got it at Con." He hands Maggie the groceries and picks up his pirate cutlass and swings it over his head and it catches a red glare from the firelight. "I'll protect you guys tonight. One for all, etc, *et al, ad nauseum, in omnia paratus.* Let's go get warm! You guys need a drink? May and Nate brought forties to celebrate my whatever this is. Mickey's. Mickey's, okay? Mickey's is always okay; what am I saying? Oh! You should have some pizza before it's gone. Cheese and black olive. You guys don't eat meat, do you? You shouldn't, the revolution's on. Did I tell you that I'm on acid? Me and Leroy are. His is working. Mine's not. I can't believe you guys are *here*! You look like ghosts who saw a movie about a ghost! You look like an audience full of ghosts who saw *Ghost*."

They walk to the fire where May is snapping photos of a tall, wolfish black kid in an eighteenth century sea captain's uniform. He's barefoot and the pants of the costume are rolled up to his knees and his curly beard and hair grows in a stormy fire-lit halo around his face.

"Joeymaggietyler," says Ben Frank, "This fantastic Zeus-ian character here is one of my nearest and dearest, Leroy Harris. Joey and Maggie and Tyler, meet Leroy. General Leroy Caesar Augustus Patrick Swayze Garbage Pail Kid Johnny Utah Tank Girl Casper the Friendly Ghost Gary Busey . . . Billy the Kid . . . Gumby . . . Galapagos . . . Master Splinter . . . John Galt . . . Pregnant Guppy . . . uh . . . *Harris*. He's burning my stuff for me. He and I are on acid tonight. Mine isn't working yet. Did I tell you that already?"

Leroy picks up a wooden model ship. He looks at it, his eyes dark and high and swimming, and says, "Up next, we have a ugly-ass worthless model . . . uh . . . is this a . . . a *sloop* . . . with . . . what . . . *Sea King* painted on the back, a ugly-ass worthless *ship*." He turns it in his hands and drops it into the fire.

"Nooo," Maggie says under her breath. "Oh man, no."

Leroy takes a painting from a stack of framed art in the sand. "Up next, a ugly-ass worthless painting by Ben Frank of a whole mess'a baby turtles eatin' a anchovy pizza. *Entitled*"—he turns it around and squints and holds it at arm's length and reads off the back—"*Everyone's Hungry*" and into the fire goes *Everyone's Hungry*.

Up next Ben Frank's entire DVD, laser disc, and VHS collection. ("Ugly-ass worthless buncha films.") VHS: *Back to the Future Part 3, Corey Haim: Me, Myself, and I, Stalker* (Tarkovsky, 1979, bootleg bought in Astoria), *Stand by Me, Point Break, New Kids on the Block: Hangin' Tough, The Truth about De-Evolution* (bootleg, taped with May's double VHS set up), *Labyrinth,* and *The Last Unicorn*. Laser disc: *Tron* and *Braveheart*. DVDs: *The Big Chill, Do The Right Thing, Grand Canyon, Buffy the Vampire Slayer* (1992 film version), *Bill and Ted's Bogus Journey,* and Ben Frank's prized trio of Schwarzenegger comedies, *Kindergarten Cop, Twins,* and *Junior*. On the sly Joey grabs a lesser-known Schwarzenegger classic, *Stay Hungry* (VHS, 1976), from the pile and slips it into Tyler's messenger bag.

After that, a pair of dress shoes ("ugly-ass worthless clodhoppers"), a Nintendo cartridge (*Mike Tyson's Punch-Out*), handfuls of colorful clothes, more art, a giant '80s camcorder, a wooden pirate pistol from Disneyland, a jar of marbles (which snaps into pieces and startles Maggie), a medical encyclopedia from 1913 (*Davil-Emerson Medical Encyclopedia, C to F*), a box of horribly water-stained music and literary magazines (various issues: *Hit It Or Quit It, Muddle, Maximum Rock 'n' Roll, Punk Planet, Flipside, Typewriter, Cometbus, Absolutely Zippo, SCAM, The Poetry Conspiracy, Burn Collector, Actress Magazine, The Word*), a box of moldy, water-stained comic books (*Wolverine* #10 and *Transformers* #5, three graphic novels, *Gotham by Gaslight, A Death in the Family, The Killing Joke,* a book-bound collection, *The Greatest Joker Stories Ever*

Told, assorted *X-Men, Rock 'n' Roll Comics, Action Comics, Real Stuff, Archie, Artbabe, American Splendor,* and *Love and Rockets*), and then it's done.

Maggie and Tyler stand off to the side of the fire. Tyler has an arm around her shoulders and she's leaning in to him, holding a silver can of beer in one hand and saying something too quiet to hear, something just for him. Her cheeks flush and glow red with the fire. She's smiling. And now her eyes are closed and she's resting her head against his chest.

Joey watches them. *They look good together*. He looks back at the fire. *Stares* into it.

3:51 A.M.

Ben Frank and Joey say goodbye in the parking lot. The wind has picked up and brought the clouds with it and the moon is gone. Now the only light comes from the streetlamps that run in a row down the middle of the empty parking lot. The asphalt is sandy, damp.

May and Nate's cars are parked on either side of one of the streetlights, and Tyler's Mazda off in the corner of the lot in the darkness. Maggie and Tyler are halfway there, walking away from them, holding hands. Nate's car is covered in ice cream truck stickers and it has a dog skull and crossbones painted on the hood. May's car has eyes painted on the side and a mouth across the bumper like a WWII fighter jet.

"So, yeah," says, Ben Frank, "once I'm settled and squared away with school, I'm gonna write you at *least* once a week. And *letters*. No more of this *email* bullshit."

"Letters. Good. No more emails."

"Right."

They hug goodbye.

"*Letters*."

"Letters."

They break away from each other and stand in the yellow light. Ben Frank has an empty forty of Mickey's in one hand, but he holds it to his chest like it's full. "Fuck emails," he says, distracted. "Fuck the Internet." As he squints off into the night, he shivers and pulls his t-shirt sleeve up and rubs the scarred mess on his shoulder. "I never want to go online *again*," he says, distant, his mind somewhere else.

"Ben Frank, *take care of yourself*. Don't do anything crazy."

"You know *me*."

Joey feels a splash of water on the back of his neck. Then another. "It's raining," he says.

Ben Franks leans in and whispers, "The thing that happened with you and Maggie, are you happy about it?"

"It's complicated," he says, looking back in the direction of Tyler's car. "It's really . . . complicated." Maggie and Tyler are standing next to the car, arguing.

"Yeah, but are you *happy*?"

"I'm really happy. Despite everything."

"I'm glad," he says, nodding matter of factly. "*Good.* None of our friends are happy anymore. It's stupid. I don't think we know *how*. Did I tell you my acid never kicked in?"

Joey laughs. "Like sixty-five-hundred times."

"Okay." He laughs and looks down at his feet and scratches the back of his head. "Okay."

"Alright, Ben Frank."

"Alright," Ben Frank looks up at Joey, frowning again. He lays a finger on the nosepiece of his glasses and moves them back into place.

"You okay?"

"Yeah," he says, "Yeah, I'm okay. I should get going. May's car has no wipers."

"Right. Yeah, you should get going. Alright, Ben Frank, see ya."

"'San Diego Says C-ya Centennial Summer!'" he says and gives Joey a sloppy, left-handed salute and breaks into a grin.

Joey laughs. "Later on, Ben Frank." He turns and walks away.

When he gets to the parking space, Tyler yawns and asks if he's okay to drive.

He nods yes.

Tyler tosses the keys over the top of the car and Joey grabs them as they hit his chest. When he looks back, Ben Frank is staring out toward the black void where the ocean is, hands shoved deep in his pockets, looking lost and small under the big yellow cone of streetlight, the rain falling through it, a steady drizzle.

Leroy Harris is lying on the roof of his car, tearing at his sea captain's costume, kicking his feet, anguished, shouting something Joey can't hear.

May is on one knee, taking photos of something on the pavement, and a few kids stand off to the side laughing and drinking forties. Someone rides a skateboard past Ben Frank, ollies up over a beer can, and lands again and one of the kids shouts, "Ha!"

Ben Frank turns and gets in the car.

Joey does the same.

SEA WORLD DRIVE, 4:15 A.M.

Joey—driving Tyler's car and Tyler asleep in the seat next to him, his white sweatshirt hood over his head, talk radio playing low ("—asked about the September 16th disappearance of Ukrainian journalist Georgiy Gongadze, President Leonid Kuchma had this to—"), the windshield wipers plipping back and forth. As they pass the lights of the SeaWorld tower, Maggie's hand comes from the backseat and rests on Joey's hip then tugs at one of his belt-loops. ("—regarding the opener of the 2000 Summer Olympics in Sydney, Governor-General Sir William Deane and—") He bends his left arm back (awkwardly) between the door panel and seat and she takes his hand and holds onto it. They say nothing.

1980

JANUARY 5TH

Channy told me this one the other day. "What lives without having a body, hears without having ears, speaks without a mouth, and air alone gives it life?"

"Singing? Laughter?"

"Close. Think about it." Her eyes went narrow and sly, enjoying the game.

I wanted to grab her and pull her into me until we passed through each other on the opposite end. My brain said, "Fuck," but in a good way, a pleased, content, surprised, in-love way, "Fuhhck I love you because you amaze me every day and I can't wait to see you whenever we're apart." But I said, "Come on. No one knows the answer to a riddle besides the one who tells him. It's unfair."

"No, you'll know it if you think about it."

"I give up."

"You *can't* give up."

"I have already. It's done."

"The only mercy comes from me." She pulled her winter coat up around her neck.

"Oh yeah?"

We sat in our deck chairs overlooking the snowy field.

"I'm the *mercyholder*. Witness my mercyholding *power*!"

"Oh yeah, I bet."

"Is my nose red? I hate when my nose gets red in the cold."

"I love it. On some people it looks sickly but on you it's . . . it does well by you. I still don't care about all this *mercyholding* B.S. I like your red nose because you look even Russianer than ever."

"I'm not Russian."

"You are. Bring me some vodka and a saber."

"Stop trying to distract me from my mercyholding."

"Zip it. *Zip*. Zzzzip."

"I hold the mercy and you're my prisoner. Get used to it." A strand of white-blonde hair had fallen in front of her left eye. She puffed air up at it and it lifted then settled back down again.

"I love you, Channy."

"I know. I love you, too."

"No, I mean I don't say it often enough . . . and I've done some . . . I don't know . . . never mind."

She took my hand and brought it to her mouth and kissed it. "It's an echo," she said.

"What's an echo?"

"The answer. Don't shrug. The answer to the riddle.

"I don't even remember the riddle."

"You remember everything."

"Except the riddle."

We held hands, and when the sun began to set over the hills to west, we went back inside.

JANUARY 6TH

The best thing is watching the boy dance. He stands in front of the record player, holding onto the side of the table and his little baby hips knock back and forth to Elton John's "Return to Paradise," especially when Channy sings along. "Good-BYE / Doesn't mean this HAS to be the END / Fading dreams go cold as ice!" That stupid awful song, the worst song on a damn good record, but when the boy is loving it, I love it, too. He can make you change your mind. If he likes something, that means that thing is pure and good and how can you not love a pure and good thing? When he's really feeling the music, he shuts his eyes and shakes his little head side to side like Ray Charles and does this move that's like The Twist. At that point, everything bad doesn't matter. It doesn't *matter* that I'm going to die someday. It doesn't matter that my mother looks less and less alive each time I visit. It doesn't matter about me and Sorel and about the lies I've told and that the child to come isn't mine. When the boy is happy, I'm caught up and carried away in his joy. I'm sure that it'll be the same with his sister. This is what I was meant to be—here for him, for them.

Of course, when I'm away from him and outside of his spell, I worry all the time. He's so small and clumsy and there are so many terrible things that could happen to him. With Channy due in April, the worry doubles. Something could happen to Channy and the new baby together. That, or we could look away for a second and the boy might take one wrong step. I think this is how you get old, all this worry. I'm twenty-one in five days. Is that old? God, no. But I feel three times that. When I go to town, I see people my age and I think, "I'm not that. I was that once but I'll never be that again."

My only solace is that we're here on the farm most of the time and that keeps us off the roads. Moving out here, we sold Channy's Buick and my trusty old Datsun dropped its transmission before Christmas, so until we can get a new one put in, we rely on Channy's cousins to drive us around or loan us cars.

Most of the time we stay put and that's fine. If there's a trip to town for groceries, I ride along and Channy and the boy stay at the house. When Carly is here, I have access to her beautiful 1941 Willys MB Army Jeep and that's pretty cool. Besides me and Channy, Morgan's a third baby-watcher and Gus is here for good now and I know that as long as Gus is watching over them, they're in good hands. It's reassuring. Still, there are so many awful things everywhere.

Now Channy's sitting on the floor next to the record player watching it spin and her gaze has gone inward because her favorite song, Elton's "A Song for Guy," is playing. The boy's asleep in a nest of afghans on the sofa. I'm sitting in the chair by the fire and I'm trying not to cry. My nerves are raw and when you feel this way and you hear something like this song, you've got to fight to push the tears back.

My defenses are down. The wall's been pushed over.

2000

CLAIREMONT, 10 P.M.

Maggie takes a housesitting job a few blocks down from her mom's. Saturday night, a party. Sunday, three '80s teen movies in a row until everyone's asleep. A week later, the wine glasses and soda cups and beer bottles cover the dining room table until they're forced to eat dinner on the floor. Bread crusts and orange peels on the linoleum, magazines in a stack next to the bathtub, soup cans for ashtrays on the front and back porch. The Blockbuster boxes in a pile on the couch. (In order of watching: 1) *Better Off Dead*, 2) *Sixteen Candles*, 3) *Harold and Maude*, 4) *Romeo and Juliet* [1996], 5) *Trainspotting*, 6) *National Lampoon's European Vacation*, 7) *Moll Flanders*, 8) *Where the Buffalo Roam*, 9) *Uncle Buck*, 10) *Space Balls*.)

Joey comes by after work and spends hours in the upstairs jacuzzi bath, reading the family's Christian Armageddon novels, laughing and shuddering and dropping them over the side in disgust, then picking them up again. At night on the couch, they watch endless TV until they're alone. Maggie and Joey become nocturnal, and when they become nocturnal, Joey doesn't sleep at all. Off to work at seven and back at the house by dark, up all night waiting for Maggie's sister and her cousins to sleep and Tyler to leave so that he can be alone with Maggie. Four a.m., five, six, watch the sun rise from the backyard picnic table where he keeps a pint of Jack Daniel's under a flower pot. (Sitting on the picnic table, shivering, barefoot in jeans and a t-shirt, smoking cigarettes, then a celebratory slug of whiskey when the sun shows over the fence. And off to work.) Sleep in his truck on his lunch break. Two-hour lunch breaks. His boss Rob is quitting soon, and Rob doesn't care about anything. Go home to sleep. Drink margaritas at the chain Mexican place in the strip mall he's guilty about going to. *As long as you get the work done*, he tells himself. On Thursday, he drives to work drunk from the night before and throws up in the parking lot while his coworkers walk past him, carrying laptop bags and briefcases. The rest of the day is a week long and he decides to quit drinking and start "dressing older" and "blend in."

Tyler is moody and distant. While they watch movies and eat popcorn and talk, Tyler studies physics. When he's not doing schoolwork, he drinks, and when he drinks, he gets loud and excited, but it's not a good excited. He's pushy and it makes the rest of them nervous and they talk about it when he's not there.

"Tyler doesn't believe in depression," says Maggie.

Joey and Maggie and her sister Jolie and her cousins Molly and Cecilie sit on the living room floor listening to the family's Disney soundtrack records on the wrong (slow) speed (Maggie's idea) and eat take-out Mexican from El Cotixan (and "Onnnnnnnce uponnnnnn a tiiiiiiime therrrre werrrre tehhhhhn lit-t-le cannnihhbaaallls swinnngin' frrrom ahhhhhh viiiiiine / Wwwwwuh-one trrrrried tahhhhh pahhhht a bigggg wiiiiild caahhht aaand thennnn therrrrre werrrrrre nihhhhh-ne," and cousin Molly giggling, looking at the back of the record sleeve.)

"Whatever," says Maggie's cool, tough sister Jolie, tucking a strand of dyed blonde hair behind her ear. "What does that *mean*, he doesn't *believe in depression*? That's like not believing in *burritos*." She shows them her dinner as evidence. "Like, *dude*. It's *right here*. You can *see it*. It's delicious and it's full of *chicken*." She rolls her eyes and shakes her head and then bites into her burrito like a shark.

Cecilie stares at them, her food in front of her, untouched. She sits with her arms wrapped around her knees, sad and hardly there. "How does he not believe?" she whispers after a while but no one hears.

Molly coughs through a swallow of soda. "What does that mean?" She stares up at Maggie, big-eyed. "I mean, I don't really know what it *means*." She shrugs.

"He doesn't believe in depression. He doesn't believe it's real, that people get depressed. When Tyler and I were seeing each other and I got super, *super* depressed—I know the girls remember—the doctor gave me Paxil. Tyler never understood. He *still* doesn't. He was all upset with me for *letting* them put me on it—like I *failed* myself."

Jolie: "Whopat dop-oes Jop-o-opey tho-pink . . . uh . . . op . . . abop . . . out thop-is?"

Maggie: "Op-I dopon't knopow."

Jolie: "Whopat dopo yopu mope-opan?"

Maggie: "Wope nopevoper top-alk opabopout opit."

Joey: "What are you guys doing?"

Jolie, Maggie: "Nothing."

Jolie: "Yopou gopuys oparope wopeopird. Yopou shopould topalk abopout opit."

"Maybe Tyler's just . . . I don't know," says Cecilie. "I don't know." She gets up and drifts off into the kitchen. They hear the faucet turn on and then it shuts off.

Joey says nothing while he pretends to inspect his *chili relleno* burrito. He opens up the tortilla on the yellow paper and silver foil it came in. Cheddar cheese, breaded Anaheim pepper, refried beans, sour cream. No rice. "They forgot the rice again. It's always something."

"Yeah. Tyler's totally depressed," Maggie nods.

Joey looks up and Maggie gives him a stare that tells him what he already knows. *It's us*. Her big, shimmering eyes, darkening, going soft, wider, sad. *Even if he doesn't know the whole story, it's enough*.

"Yeah, no rice. Somebody give me a reason that I shouldn't take this back."

When Maggie and Joey are alone and the house is quiet, they lie together on the couch with their hands down each other's jeans. After she comes, she laughs. She tells him she laughs because she's happy. At first he thinks she's laughing at him, but she says, "I'm not laughing at you. I'm happy," and Joey says it back, "I'm happy, too." When he comes, it's fast and it takes him by surprise and he has to lie still and catch his breath. When things were happening with Nicole, he thought about Allysia or Kate Lewellyn in order to finish (Kate, whom he never even liked for the three months they were together. The fantasy Kate, the better one). With Allysia, he thought about girls he knew from school. Girls who wouldn't talk to him. Getting off to the ones then felt guilty and horrible because he knew they'd be disgusted by the thought of it. When he's with Maggie, he thinks about Maggie and that's enough. He wants to tell her that, but it feels like he's giving too much away. He still needs to say the important thing, but he chickens out.

Even if she doesn't know that he's in love with her, Maggie and Joey are moving to bigger things. They're pushing forward but slowly. Maggie and her boyfriend are moving faster. Joey tries to ignore this. He tells himself that everything outside the house happens along an inconsequential timeline. Out there, it doesn't count. Here's where the "real now" is—the wasteland of bottles, the smell of night jasmine and honeysuckle through the window. Mornings—overcast, fog from the sea. The sunset—a neon blast from a comic book, purple sky fading to dull red or Tropicana orange crisscrossed by telephone lines, blocked out by the shaggy heads of palm trees. (You fool yourself long enough and you can forget that your truth began with a lie.)

The day Maggie leaves the housesitting job is the day that Joey sees them together for the first time.

Joey's in the health food store on Garnet Avenue. It's a Thursday, late afternoon, sun through the big windows, blocked out in places by handbills and fliers on the glass. The lights are off in the store and reggae music plays on the boombox by the register. The girl behind the counter is talking on the phone, leaning on her elbows, wrapping her finger in the cord, saying, "Yeah, yeah, *I know,* yeah, I know. *Right*? Dude, oh, *totally*."

From the store's backroom juice deli, a blender starts up, whirls angrily, sputters, then stops again. Something plastic (the blender cup) knocks against something hard (the counter edge). Knock, knock, knock. And then the blender again.

The girl behind the counter says, "Dude, you don't have to tell me, *I know*. When I win the lottery, I'm *totally* moving. I don't care *what* my sister thinks. I like girls. Girls who like girls go up north. You don't stay in San Diego. Facts of life, yo."

The smell in the air is carob and black licorice and vitamins. It's a good smell and sometimes Joey comes here to shop because he misses the way it smells.

And then he sees them through the windows. Walking past. Holding hands. The guy talking. He points at something in the sky and she squints as they walk and blocks the sun from her eyes with her hand. He's so tall. Taller than Joey. Big like a man should be big.

And then they're gone. Joey gives up on the rest of his grocery list and takes his carton of raspberry kefir and Fig Newtons to the counter.

WORK, 10 A.M.

The next day at work an instant message pops up from Yesenia and Joey looks to the left of him and she's sitting one cubical down, typing. He looks back at his screen and clicks on the message. It reads, "joey whatd u do this wknd what happened last week you were gone wanna go outside & smoke w/ me? OMG today SUX so much dick! im getting a migraine WTF i can totally feel it coming on NOOO."

Joey writes back and tells her about housesitting with Maggie and how happy he is with her despite the mess with her boyfriend and that he'd love to go smoke a cigarette. He hits Send before he remembers what happened with Yesenia at his apartment. But it's too late. Her typing noise stops and she gets up from her desk and walks past his, the spikes of her shoes clicking on the floor. He imagines the knife game where you place your hand on a table and try to stab the spaces between your fingers without hitting your fingers, the faster you go the better you are. It was in a movie. *Rambo*? No, *Alien*. Yeah. Maybe. He laughs at how long he spent thinking about it, and then remembers Yesenia and thinks, "Ugh."

On his lunch break, Joey sits outside the building on a park bench and smokes with Marcus Riggs. The team that Marcus is on has something to do with sporting events. They type. Joey's side types. Their side looks tired in the morning and deflated by the end of the day and so does Joey's.

Marcus' side is managed by two guys with the same first name. Jeff Zeffirelli and Jeff Taylor, also known as 'The Jeffs.'

"Marcus, I hate the fucking Jeffs."

"Why? They're good dudes."

"The name. The fucking *Jeffs*. Fuck the Jeffs. Makes me want to smash my face in with the side of this bench. Like wham, ugh, crush, splat, dead."

"That's not their fault, Carr."

"But, Marcus, *the Jeffs*. Everyone's always, like, 'the Jeffs did this,' 'the Jeffs did that.' People are *obsessed* with the Jeffs. They fucking *love* the Jeffs. The Jeffs even *look* like 'the Jeffs.' Arrrrgh, I hate them."

Marcus laughs loud and his eyes crinkle up and he shakes his head. "So you hate the name. It sounds like you got nothing."

"Nothing?"

"The Jeffs aren't the enemy here. It's *nada*. You vote?"

"Yeah. Fingers crossed on keepin' Number Two out, right?"

"What do you mean?"

"I don't know. Nothing."

"So, what's going on, Carrlile?"

"What do you mean what's going on?"

"I mean between you and Yesenia. What's up?"

"Nothing's up. Why would anything be up?"

"I just saw Yessy crying in her car. I figured you guys had a fight."

"A fight?"

"You guys're seeing each other, right?"

"No. *No*!" Joey laughs. "No, we're really *not* seeing each other. *At all*. Dude, yikes."

"Were you?"

"Never. We were *never* seeing each other. I mean, we're *friends*. What are you, a journalist?"

They laugh.

"I just figured—I think *a lot of us* figured—you guys were at least fucking. She's cute. Kind of. Her ass is a lil' slow-down-wide-load for such a short little girl but I could . . . I could see being into that ass, liking that ass. It's big but I bet—"

"Noooo, no, no, not at all. I'm seeing somebody else. Kind of. Not officially."

"Good, because, Carrso, Yessy's a *nightmare*. Everybody from our side is *terrified* of her. When she walks by all stomping mad and P.O.'d about something fantastically minor, we make the train noise. Woo wooooo. She's a runaway train. Woo wooooooo, woo wooooo. McMartin—you know Mickey from I.T., right?"

"Yeah, McMartin's a good guy."

"He's the *best* guy. Totally. Mick calls her the Crazy Train."

"She's kind of intense, but she's not—"

"Dude, Joey, *kind of*? She's a *homicidal maniac*. She'll rip out your spine like Predator if she's on the rag."

"'The 'rag'? That's a horrible . . . awful thing to say. That's not cool."

"Oh, hey, Joey, I owe you . . . I owe you from Sushi Deli last week." Marcus pulls his wallet out of his back pocket and opens it and then stops. He holds his driver's license up to his face and squints at it. "Dude, wow, *wow*. Carr, I look so *young*."

"So what. I look younger in mine too. Everybody does."

"This was taken *six months ago*. Right before I got the job."

"Can I see it?"

"It's a free country."

"What does that even *mean*?" Joey takes the ID and holds it close to his face. In the photo, Marcus is smiling and bright-eyed. The date of birth says he's thirty-six but he looks twenty. Now, six months later, he's pale and his hair is thinning and he has shadows under his eyes and lines around his mouth.

"This job is making me *old*. I'm too young to look like this." Marcus takes his ID back and slides it into the window slot of his wallet. "I don't know. If this is my life, I want a do-over. 'M.G.,' she says, 'hey, by the way—'"

"Hey, M.G."

"—Always tells me we need to quit our jobs and fuck off and move out to the country."

"You don't look as old as you think, Marcus. Don't worry."

"Yeah, whatever. Hey, Carrmine, you wanna smoke another cigarette?"

"Sure. Course. I'll smoke *ten* more."

After the cigarette, Marcus gives Joey his pack and tells him he's quitting. Joey takes it happily and sticks it in his front pocket and calls Marcus "a good egg."

"You're a good egg, Marcus."

When Joey gets back to his cubical, Yesenia is at hers. She's typing something fast, leaning close to her computer and squinting down at her keyboard and up at the screen. She picks up her coffee cup and blows on it and takes a sip.

Marcus sits down in his chair and swivels it left and then right and leans back. He sighs and clicks his mouse to turn the screen on and stares at his monitor.

MISSION BEACH, 4 P.M.

A week before Halloween, the air gets cool and the leaves begin to turn. On Monday, Joey calls in sick and he and Tyler smoke crystal in Tyler's family's garage and then drive down to the boardwalk with their hearts fluttering and a thousand things to say. They sit on the seawall and watch the last of the diehard sunbathers on their towels fighting to catch what's left of the sun. Girls with brown skin on green towels, yellow towels, black towels. Old men, shirtless, in folding chairs next to coolers, their skin red and creased. Joggers on the shoreline. Girls with long peach-colored limbs in gray running shorts and gym shirts, flush-faced, sweating, arms and legs pumping. Speed-walkers. Guys with sweatpants, baggy t-shirts, headphones, armband radios, water bottles in hand.

From their spot on the seawall, the ocean looks different than it did all summer. It's bigger and darker, tousled by wind and new autumn swells that come in jagged over the sandbars, cut up by riptides, pushed by storms a thousand miles away. Now the surfers wear thick black wetsuits and struggle with the waves, paddling into them, standing up, hacking big white fans of spray with every turn, racing along the tall, gray faces of the waves, climbing and dropping and slashing turns until the whole thing comes over and down and bursts into foam.

Joey looks up in time to see one of the surfers launch himself off the lip of the wave and fly up above it. In the air, he grabs the rail of his board with one arm and then lets go as he lands on the breaking crest and drops back into the wave again.

"I bet he's a pro," says Joey.

"I wasn't watching." Tyler holds his cigarette out for Joey, but Joey shakes his head and squints at the horizon-line, watching it move and warble.

"I'm good."

"You quitting again?"

"Maybe . . . I want to."

"I don't."

Joey—breathing in deep, and the air has the sweet and tangy smell of rotting kelp—beyond that it's the following three smells in descending order: 1) Sea air (briny, an after-smell of smoke from beach fires) 2) Vanilla from the waffle cone hut by the Banana Cabana Hostel, 3) Tyler's cigarette, which smells like Joey's aunt's Honda Civic.

"I can't tell if the horizon's moving or if it's just me." Joey sticks his thumb out and shuts one eye and centers his gaze on the top edge of the nail, balanced along the dimming line of sky and water; in the far distance, a Navy battleship sits heavy and low beyond the kelp beds.

"It's you . . . you and the horizon working together . . . like the A-Team."

"Ebony and ivory."

"'Together in perfect harmony.'"

They laugh and their minds race and they talk about work and friends and Labor Day parties and Halloween candy. Joey tells Tyler that he wants to quit smoking cigarettes by eating candy corn. Tyler tells Joey a dream he had about a girl and how, when he woke up, he felt like he knew her and, more so, that he loved her. Joey tells Tyler a funny dream about beating a screaming Regis Philbin with a shovel and Tyler stops listening halfway in. (No one brings up Maggie.)

Tyler looks thinner than normal, birdlike shoulder bones, veins, gristle. Joey tries to ignore this, but he can't. Around Tyler, he's forced to see the product of his actions and he tries to think it away, change the subject, ask questions he knows the answers to, bring up disconnected things (TV commercials, magazines, weather, movies, school, MTV, dogs, Michael Jackson's nose, money, the Wild Animal Park, the ironic charms of *Coyote Ugly*, the meal he got Thursday at the Fishery [breaded scallops, fries, sourdough bread, a lemon slice, a Dr. Pepper], different types of marbles: [1) Cat's Eyes, the classic, his favorite 2) Clearies, 3) Doughboys, hard to find, usually in pre-War collections 4) Steelies, aka ball bearings, the large ones called "Steely Saturns," 5) Hazels, 6) Empress Hair, the rarest, 6) Ruby Drops, 7) Tiger Eyes, 8) Dixies, 9) Milkies, 10) Bumblebees, and 11) Caramels.] He goes on to talk about his grandfather's marble collection and the giant, golf-ball sized Cat's Eye he kept in a sock.) But then, changing gears: "Hey Ty, you still have that Vick's, right?" Tyler nods and digs into his messenger bag and pulls out a green and white plastic jar of Vick's Vapor Rub. Joey, staring at Tyler's hands, big veins, bony, the hands of an old woman. "Thanks." He dabs his pinkie finger into the Vick's and rubs it inside each nostril. "There we go." The menthol and eucalyptus burn and Joey breathes it in and his high comes on stronger. "Wow, that gave me the chills," he says, rolling his neck and stretching his arms out in front of him. "I love crystal. That's a dumb thing to say, but I do."

"You've got chills?"

"Yeah. The chills."

"Would you possibly say that . . . they're maybe . . . *multiplying*?"

"Huh?"

"Nothing."

"Oh. Right. *Grease*. Good one."

"Not really."

"But still."

From behind them comes the sound of someone walking past carrying a boombox. A song done in tribute to the rapper who was killed a few years back and the story on the news and all the stars getting together to sing at the VMAs. "Seems like yesterday we used to rock the show / I laced the track / You locked the flow." Tyler starts to nod his head to the beat and then the song has passed by and Joey turns to watch the boardwalk—people on bikes and skateboards, rollerblades, rollerskates. A pretty girl carrying a white plastic laundry basket on her hip, her plaid shirt buttoned once at the bra-line and blowing open in the breeze, showing her belly and neck. A man with a stroller watching the girl walk past. Bums and college kids. Surfers carrying boards.

Joey turns back. "Tyler, I tell you my friend Marcus from work quit?"

"I don't know who that is. I only know Yesenia. And the Jeffs. By reputation."

"Oh. He was just a friend from work. He got me the job. Married a distant relative of mine who I haven't seen in 200,000 years back in April. Really cool, really solid and nice, older guy but super down. Used to say his job description was 'nothing but good old-fashioned barbarism and materialism.' Couple days ago he just up an' quit without telling anyone. Left all his stuff in his desk. Didn't even take his coat. Left it on the back of the chair. Can you believe he left his *coat*? I kept it. I might run it up to his place in La Jolla tonight."

Tyler shrugs, bored. "I'll come with if you want."

"Sure. That'd be cool."

"We could go look for Munchkinland afterwards."

"Anyway, you'd like Marcus. He and I used to get bagels together. This little Mexican woman Hilda would come into the office in the morning with a basket of bagels and muffins and walk through the cubicles saying, 'Muffeens? Ceenameen tweest?' He'd buy them for us one day. I'd buy for us the next. Sometimes, she came after lunch with tamales. I wish I could leave just like . . . I don't know, I guess . . . never mind. It doesn't matter. I need the job."

"What? I'm sorry. I wasn't listening. Sorry."

"Nothing. Not important."

A man in a gray sweatsuit and headphones walks along the shore with a metal detector, swaying it back and forth over the sand. The man stops, kneels down, and sets the metal detector next to him. Out of his tote bag he takes a pink, child-size plastic shovel and begins to dig in the sand.

"Joey, what are you going as for Halloween?"

"I guess I'm gonna go as a tree."

"What kind?"

"I dunno. Palm?"

"Really?"

"Yeah, hang a bunch of coconuts around my neck, dress in brown, get . . . like, get a bunch of fronds and make a hat out of them. Maybe have a monkey stuffed animal stapled to my leg like he was climbing me."

"Did you just come up with that right now?"

"Yyyup."

"A palm tree." Tyler laughs happily and goes back into his messenger bag and pulls out a pack of cigarettes. "Menthols aren't technically cigarettes, so you can smoke one with me." He pulls two out of his pack.

"Okay."

Tyler drops one of them on the sand and hops down to pick it up.

"Party foul," Joey says as Tyler pulls himself back up.

They light up and sit, dangling their legs off the seawall, and watch the gray mess of the ocean. The wind has picked up from the west and it blows their hair back and makes the sleeves of their hooded sweatshirts flap.

"God, I love smoking," Joey says.

"Yeah, don't quit. We can die together."

"How 'bout you, Tyler?"

"How 'bout me what?"

"Halloween."

"I don't know. Maybe a girl from the Middle Ages," Tyler says. "A slovenly *wench*."

"You'd be a good Middle Ages girl."

"I guess when it comes down to it, I'm like a girl, anyway." Tyler stares straight ahead, jaw tight, trying not to smile.

"You're like a girl how?"

"I just wanna have fun," he says, grinning proudly.

"And that makes you a girl? What are you *talking about*?"

"You know, like 'girls just wanna have fuh-un / They just wanna / They just wanna-uh-uh,'" he sings the song and Joey gets it and they laugh.

"Good one."

"Who are you hanging out with on Halloween?"

"I don't know." *Maggie*.

"Really? It's *Tuesday*."

"I don't know." *Maggie*.

They watch a surfer take off on a big, stormy wave. He stands up and drops down the face of it and then falls off his board with a great splash. The wave comes down around him and erupts into a wall of whitewash.

When the wave's passed, the surfer is separated from his board and Tyler and Joey watch him swim to shore, the board washing in with the wave, broken in half. "Party foul," says Tyler pointing to the board, and they laugh and climb off the seawall and walk back to the car.

WORK, MORNING

At work, the next morning Joey reads a letter from Ben Frank. In the cubical next to him, Yesenia is training the new temp, a short blonde guy, who's come to replace Marcus. "You got it. You got it. Don't worry. You're gonna do *fine*. Oh my god, you're *way* too smart for this job. Haha. I like your *tie*. Wow. Where'd you *get* it? It looks *so good* with your shirt. Is it silk? Can I touch it? Really? Can I? Wow, you can *tell* it was expensive. Do you mind me asking how much? Ooh!" she does a campy, high-pitched Jersey accent, "Mistuh *Money Bags* hee-uh. Hahaha. I'm kidding, I'm kidding. Okay, now click on that hyperlink right there. Yeah, good. We need to get a jpeg for this."

Joey,

It's Ben Frank of Chicago, your weary and consumptive champion of justice, your burrito Supreme Court judge. Next week is Halloween and I'm going as a dinosaur. My costume is green plush and its tail drags behind me and my Neanderthalic four-eyed face looks out from the gaping, fanged mouth. Chicago, Chicago, Chicago, pissy bricks and industry, drug dealers and Persian goons with horrible lisps. I hate it here. I hate it everywhere. Says Melville about another such barren American waste-scape, "Such dreary streets! Blocks of blackness, not houses, on either hand and here and there a candle like a candle moving about in a tomb." It's butt-cold here and the wind rips bricks out of buildings and the bricks whip past at Mach 2 and if they hit you they tear your head off and you walk around bored and frozen and headless in your long coat and you hold it closed because the buttons are gone and you think obsessively about pizza, golden swords, and the guillotine. My only chair is a stack of oversized art books (do you know about Henry Darger?) and my room has a pile of blankets on the floor and a French-Canadian girl practicing violin in the corner, sawing on the thing stupidly. Her head is huge; she's top-heavy. I can't stand to look at her. And now, because I'm drunk, some truth from your favorite malingering fungus on the tip of a narwhal spike, *in vino veritas*: I miss you. Come visit before I wise up and cut this shit out. My plan is: Portland by May (the month) with May (the Stimson). James Bozic and Frances Alicio are moving up there in January so that James can write a book. I think it's time to get out of here and cut my losses (of which there are many). Regardless: Exert yourself and be a real person for once, because I'm starting to believe I made you up. I'm bored with invention and I have no follow-through. I think I have a plan to take over the world, if only because that means all the pizza I can eat until the day I die. Oh, the French-Canadian is squawking at me, Chicago-style: "Ben Frahhnk! C'mere, sit by me while I play. Write yuh lettah over *here*." The horrorscape of this stupid shitty Jungle Chicago! Get me out of here, Carr. I'm too conspicuous. They all want a piece of me. I come home from parties like some henpecked rooster who's dulled his talons scratching the cement (whilst trying to believe it's dirt). I won't pussyfoot anymore: If you don't visit me, we're no longer friends. Request extended. Limited time offer. Recurrent wishes of love sent to you and Maggie. Write soon. Save me from these fur-coated, ham-starved pigs. Visit sooner. I hate you,

Benicio del Franko

1980

JANUARY 26TH

"Your mother's dying," the doctor says. "It's a matter of time. You and your brother should work out the details before it happens, because you never know how you'll take it. People think they know what to expect, but grief will surprise you."

Jacob and I meet at a diner in Ramona. We sit and eat our steaks and then we split a piece of apple pie with vanilla ice cream and a chocolate malt and when we're done he says, "So?"

"So, what's so?"

"What are we doing about this?"

"I don't know what we're doing about this, Jake."

"Merc, you know what Mom always wanted."

"Yeah, Jake, I know."

"Buffalo," he says, shaking his head. "Of all places, *Buffalo*. Jesus, Mom."

"Yeah."

"Merc, we don't have to go."

"We do. Jake, of course we have to go."

"We don't. We can get her shipped out there and have them put her in the family plot. As long as we pay the money, we're fine."

"Jake . . . there's no one to . . . I mean, *sure*, of course, they'll bury her out there if we . . . if we *pay* them, but someone needs to be there when they put her in the ground. She wanted a family funeral and you know Roy's family's in no shape to go out now that he's sick. We're all that's left on her side. *Someone* has to be with her at the funeral. She's our *mom*."

"I swear," he shakes his head. "I swear, baby brother, I never thought this . . . you know . . . this whole—"

"I know."

The waitress walks by.

"Hey, excuse me," says Jake, "You serve beer, wine, anything like that, cocktails?"

"Nope, sorry, hon."

"It's alright." Outside the diner the sky is dark and copper-red to west. A silver Greyhound bus pulls into the parking lot, the air brakes hissing. Jake yawns and rubs the back of his neck. "What do we do about the money?"

"I don't know, Jake. We pay for it, I guess."

"You know Mom has money saved up."

"Do we use her money to pay for her own funeral? Doesn't that sound kind of . . . I don't know . . . insulting? Jake . . . shouldn't *we* pay? Isn't that *our* responsibility?"

"A funeral's not a birthday present, Merc. Hey, hey," he says to the waitress, "Can we get our check and a . . . and a doggie bag?"

"Course. You want a fill-up?"

"Just warm it up."

"How 'bout you, hon?"

"I'm good, actually. Thanks, though."

"No, prob. Be back with the bill in a sec."

"Thank you. Jake, I don't know. It feels wrong to use her money."

"What does she care? Merc, she's not Mom anyone. She hasn't been Mom in years. Mom's been dead since Dad was killed."

"Jake . . . I don't know. I just . . . I feel like Mom's still *in there* . . . that she's there somewhere, she just can't *tell us* she's there. We can't just let her—"

"Let her what? She's dying. She's not in there. That's a *body*. Look, I've . . . I've gotta get back to P.B. before nine. Here's five for mine."

"Jake—"

"I'll see you later, okay? I've gotta go." He taps his watch. "It's late. I'm sorry."

FEBRUARY 1ST

The day my mother died, I knew. I was in town with Issy shopping for Valentine's Day presents and I knew.

We got back to the house at dark and Channy met us on the porch. Her face was red and I could tell she'd been crying. "Merc? Baby? I just heard from the hospital and—"

"I know."

"Oh baby, I'm so sorry," and she wrapped her arms around me and held me and she cried.

I didn't.

I'm not sure why.

It's been twenty-four hours and I still haven't.

FEBRUARY 2ND

Jacob and I are holed-up in a crappy little motel in Lake Havasu City. The plan was to leave early and get here in time to see a guy who owes Jake money. We took the I-8 to the I-10 and Jake drove ninety the whole way here. The drive was uneventful—no traffic, no cops, a clear shot across, the desert still locked in winter, rocky hills and snow in the ditches. It was wasteland and I stared out at it and I tried to remember Mom. After twenty-one years, I should have a whole list of things to look back on. Even with a memory like mine, I don't, and each one is isolated in time—a gray strip of memory, with flat patches of dark on either side.

The first I can remember: Four years old in the back of Dad's beautiful old '49 Chevy Deluxe ("High Vanilla Crème" paint job, bright red upholstery like a piece of red velvet cake). Mom's brother Carl in the front, smoking and ashing into a Folgers can on the floor, drinking a bottle of Coke. Mom and I and Jake in the back, no seatbelts. We're driving down the east coast to Jacksonville and I remember a line of cars in front of us and green on each side—twin walls of jungle, alive, mysterious. It's humid and the windows are down and the smoke is blowing from Carl's cigarette into the back seat. (Carl, who would later die in a mine collapse in Pennsylvania with his cousin Jace, after running off with Mom's money.) Mom's talking to me, but the hot air coming through the windows is blotting out her voice. What I remember is this:

"Honey, we're in *South* Carolina now. Say South Carolina. No, Care-oh-lina. Say it."

And:

"Baby boy, promise me you'll never *smoke*."

"Okay."

"Honey, I don't want you to smoke. Promise Mama you'll never smoke." She never said why I shouldn't smoke.

"Okay, Mama."

"Mercander . . . please be healthy and happy for me. Don't be sad like cousin—" (she said a name, a woman's name, but I've long since forgotten it. Some wild family tragedy, forgotten, long since dust or wilting in an old folks' home, strapped to an air tank, gray, gray, gray).

"Okay, Mama."

Later: I'm seven and we're upstate on vacation at the lakehouse. Jake and I are running the length of the dock and diving into the lake, over and over again. We race down the plank boards and cannonball into the water then climb back onto the dock and do it all again.

We're never out of breath.

We run, we jump in, we sink to the bottom, kick hard and swim back up, climb onto the dock again, and we do that over and over. The water . . . I remember the water more than anything . . . warm and dark and clean, a good smell to it, like tree bark and stones, smooth stones. It's a beautiful, sunny day, the woods curving around the big, open cove in a sheltering wall.

At dusk, there are bats in the sky and the sky is a bloody, mellow red. Red and light blue, the blue hanging in patches high above us, the red absorbing the rest, but slowly. Everything is slow—even when we run fast, it's slow.

Mom comes out and calls us to dinner. She looks young. She has long black hair held back with a white plastic headband and she has a tall crystal glass of something in her hand and she's wearing a long white dress.

Jake and I swim up to the edge of the dock and hold onto the side, out of breath finally.

"It's suppertime, boys."

"We're not hungry," Jake says speaking for both of us.

"It's on the table. Your dad's waiting."

"Can't we stay out here?" (Jacob again.)

"Don't you guys want to eat? Susan made a venison roast." (Susan was the cook and head maid. A big black woman who lost her husband in the first World War and never stopped working after that. She cleaned and cooked and fixed the cars and watched after us from morning 'til night. At bedtime she sat up with her books and read until she slept. Susan loved the Greeks . . . all the great philosophers she'd quote back to us, Dostoyevsky too, and Turgenev, Pushkin, Gogol, even Chekhov—she loved the Russians, like Channy—and Proust, the old Testament, Joyce, Countee Cullen, Shaw, Woolf, Jessie Redmond Fauset ("the Midwife"), Du Bois, Ben Franklin, Douglass, Dos Passos, Nella Larson, Zora, Jean Toomer, old issues of *The Crisis*. Her life was reading, and she passed that onto us. "Boys, one of the greatest pleasures you'll get from life is wasting the day away with a book and losing yourself to the story." Jake and I loved Susan. Her grandfather was a slave who killed his master's hound dog and was hung from a tree then burned in front of his family. The stories she told were from another world. Brutal, painful, sun-baked, sweaty, transcendent. She kept a diary—she wrote all the time—but they buried her with it a few years ago. She was eighty-five. What I wouldn't give to read about her life. My god. Goddamnit.)

"Boys, Susan . . . she worked hard to—"

Jacob interrupting: "I'll drive me and Mercander into town later and get some hotdogs at Oat's. We'll go see a movie."

"A movie?"

"Yeah, a movie."

"What movie?"

"I don't know. Whatever's there."

"Nothing with killing and guns, okay?"

"Mom."

"Promise me."

"Mom . . . we're . . . ."

"Nothing with killing."

"Alright."

She's quiet for a while and then she gathers up her skirt and sits down on the dock with her feet in the water, stirring. "Okay, you can stay. No more splashing, alright?"

"Okay."

"You can swim, but no more splashing."

"Okay, Mom."

We kept swimming and she stayed with us until dark.

When the sun went down, I thought she'd call us in but she didn't.

After a while, it was clear that she wasn't going in and that Dad wasn't coming out and it scared me and I felt like things were changing.

There are smaller memories between that, but the next clear memory is Dad's funeral. The soldiers taking the flag from his coffin, folding it into a triangle, and handing it to Mom. Everyone in black and my dad's Army buddies in uniform and my cousin Pete nudging me and whispering, "Your mom's *smiling*." And she was. She held the flag in her white-gloved hands and there was a terrible, crooked, watery grin on her face and her light eyes were dancing. After that day I remembered everything. From then on. That's when it began.

FEBRUARY 3RD

Jake's plan was a bust. In the morning, we drove out to the trailer park in the desert between Lake Havasu and the hills and the white-trashy guy in the manager's trailer said that Jake's friend had left the night before. "*Yup*. Took all his stuff and that boy *left*. I sees him drivin' out the gate and that pickup was all full of furniture. Me and Cecil McBride, we was standin' out here drankin' some beers and shootin' the breeze and that Injun's truck rumbles by and stops at the gate. Cecil's his friend, Cecil he says, 'Tommy, you leaving?' and that sonofabitching Tom Bluefeather he says, 'Goin' to the dump.' It was ten at night and I *knew* they weren't goin' to no *dump*. People 'round here knows that damn Injun into some bad bus-i-ness with the Cubillos and Jap Waterhouse so's I let 'em pass. Him and his squaw and their boy just drove right off and left me with a trailer full of Indian garbage and a broken septic system and two month' unpaid *rent*. Listen. Listen. You sees that sonofabitching Squanto Geronimo Cochise sonofabitch and you tell him he owe me two hundred dollars. Tell him Jimmy

Ray Kuper don't forget a *debt*. He don't forget *nothin'* at all. Jimmy Ray Kuper, he *remember*."

It was early, so we went and got breakfast at a cafe by the London Bridge that was full of old people eating plates of pancakes and eggs and grits, then hit the road for Albuquerque. The I-10 East, eight hours of Jake driving the speed limit, cops all around.

Albuquerque was nice. Red-rock desert on the edge of town, then a sleepy main street where we found a place to get steaks. The Alby Eat House. I got a strawberry milkshake and played some old doo-wop songs on the jukebox ("The . . . ten . . . commandments of luh-luh-love / Love, oh sweet love") and Jake sat low in the seat and smoked cigarette after cigarette and drank his rootbeer float and wouldn't talk.

Jake and I aren't speaking much in general. He asks directions and I read the map. He pulls over for gas and tells me to wash the windows and check the oil. Nothing else. He drives. I stare out the window.

The plan was to stop for the night and get an early start in the morning. I found a motel in the yellow pages—the Big Comet Inn—but Jake wanted to drive all night, so that's what we're doing. If we keep it steady, we'll be in Oklahoma City by morning. Jacob is playing the country music station and I'm writing this by flashlight. It's black all around, our headlights on a yellow-gray strip of road in front of us, but nothing beyond that—great, deep, inky black night and the green lights of the console and the flashlight in my lap.

"Merc, why don't you turn that thing off?"

"I'm bored, Jake. I'm just trying . . . I don't know . . . it was your idea to drive all night. Let me drive. Let me do *something*."

"Merc . . . just . . . just keep it *low*. Don't point it up."

"Alright, Jake."

There's a song on the radio that I know for some reason. Jacob knows it, too, and now he's turning it up and singing along with the woman: "Now someone else will hold you / Just the way I do / How can I face tomorrow / When I know I'm losing you?" Jake has a nice voice. It's been years since I've heard him sing.

"Jake, *Mom* sang that to us, didn't she?"

"I don't remember."

"Do you remember much about her?"

"No." He turns the dial and it's a late-night church show, the organ swelling in a great shuddering roll behind the preacher and the preacher saying, "Gaaaaaather them peoples AROUN', gather them together! Them mens and them *womenses*! Them *childrenseses*. And thy straaaaanger that is within thy gatesssssssss . . . that they may *hear* . . . and that they may *fearrrrr-uh* the Lohhh thy Gaaawd," and a woman somewhere in the congregation shouts, "Gawwd!"

and the preacher says, (stomping the stage below him) "The Loh thy Gaw-ww-aaw-aw-aw-aw-aw-*awd*!" and voice in the crowd says, "Yass. Gawwwwww awwww awwwwwwwd!" and another, "Praise!" The preacher: "Because Gawd gots a *plan*!" Audience: "Yes!" Preacher: "Because he know he *can*! Because he understan,'" breaking into song, "Lo-oh-oh Jesus / Walkin' right down the street, oooooh! / Lo-oh-oh-oh Jesus / Standin' right on your feet / He does a dance and he sings a song / Do what he want / Do what he *can* / Lo-oh-oh Jesus, sittin' on top of the world, ooooh! / Lo-oh-ord Jesus, yeah, he sittin' on top of the world / Talks to me / And he talks to you / Talks to your mama / And he—" Jake groans and turns it to the news ("—Ali's tour of Africa with the President's envoy today met with—") and then an oldies station, and Del Shannon singing, "Aaaas I walk along I wonder a-what went wrong with our love / A love that was so strong / And as I still walk on I think of the things we've done together a-while our hearts were young / I'm a-walkin' in the rain, tears are fallin' and I feel the pain / Wishin' you were here by me to end this misery / And I wonder, I wa-wa-wa-wa wonder / Why a-why why why why why she ran away / And I wonder where she will stay, my little runaway, a-run run run run runaway," and then the organ solo, shrill and high and ghostly.

FEBRUARY 5TH

I woke up in the backseat in Oklahoma City. Jacob was asleep in the front and the windows were fogged.

Six-thirty in the morning. The glass was cold to the touch.

I pulled the blanket around me and swept the fog from the glass and saw the empty parking lot.

Above us in the mist—a billboard for a car dealer. J and L's Toyota Town and two smiling women twelve feet tall, one with a set of car keys in her hand, proud. 'Your Place To Save Big in OKC!'

As soon as I was awake, I was hungry.

Breakfast.

Pancakes.

I tore a page out of my journal and left a note for Jake and walked around the city by myself.

It was quiet and the air was wet and the place felt dead. That's the best way I can explain it. The whole city felt like the Russians had dropped a bomb that left the houses and buildings and cars and trees but wiped out all the people.

It was horrible. At some point in my life I would've liked this feeling. Not now.

I found a newspaper box and read the headlines through the glass, but they were all a day old. Killings in the New Mexico prison uprising. Congressmen under investigation after a two-year FBI operation. National Security

Adviser Zbigniew Brzezinski touring the Pakistan-Afghanistan border. Larry Holmes TKOs Lorenzo Zanon. West beat by East in the NBA All-Star Game.

Seven in the morning, sleepy dead OK City. A gas station with dripping pumps. Parked cars on the street. The smell of diesel. Not a pancake to be seen.

From there, we drove clear to Memphis in the crazy rain—Jake passing semi-trucks on blind turns, headed straight into a wall of water, the rain spraying our windows in a wild downpour, the sound on the car-top deafening. It was a total whiteout, but Jake leaned forward in his seat and pushed his old '57 Bel Air eastward and we made Memphis in six hours, 460 miles by the map.

"Hey Merc, you love '50s crap, right?" Jake asked as we drove down the main drag. "You wanna see Graceland?" He had his flask between his knees and it was open and you could smell whiskey in the heat and he was smoking and ashing out the window. "You wanna see Elvis' house?" Johnny Cash was on the radio singing, "I taught the weeping willow how to cry, cry, cry" and Jake turned it up and asked about Graceland again. "Graceland? Yeah? You wanna go?"

"Not really."

"Me neither."

But we drove by anyway.

There was a gate and a few people taking pictures in front of it and setting out flowers, but that was all.

Memphis was downright hot after all the snow and rain and sleet across the country. We had lunch at a diner a few miles from Graceland. Raymore Slim's Silver Dollar Dine-In. Southern food. Collard greens and fatback. Fried potatoes and biscuits and gravy. Jake got a beer. I had a Cherry Coke. Best Cherry Coke I've ever had. Syrupy, aching sweet, three maraschino cherries instead of one.

"You believe how much *gravy* they gave me?" Jacob said, mopping up the gravy with a slice of white bread. "Look at this. This is totally insane. Who eats this much *gravy*?"

"You complaining?"

"God no."

Each time he finished his portion of gravy the waitress, brought more.

"Darlin' honey, you need 'nother gravyboat 'n' some white bread?"

"Yes, god yes."

It was the first I'd seen him happy in months.

He leaned over the table to me and whispered, "Merc, how long can this go *on*? This is *absurd*."

I laughed and said, "Let's find out," and he laughed too and it felt good to laugh with him.

"Alright, baby brother, let's see, let's see."

Jacob ate biscuits and white bread and gravy until he was sick and we went out into the streets of Memphis to walk it off.

What a great town, Memphis. Pretty women. Kids running everywhere. Men who looked like country stars with big, gray mutton-chop sideburns and fancy boots and cowboy hats with decorated bands around them; everyone content and talking and laughing and easy with each other.

A few blocks down, we went to place called Pence and Brogin's Country Store and I bought a pair of used cowboy boots.

"You look good in those things," said Jake as we walked out of the place.

"Yeah?"

"Yeah. I think it fits you. You out on the farm and all. Farmer John."

"More like Clint Eastwood."

"That'll be the day."

"I think you're jealous."

"Maybe I am."

"You could always come on out there and stay for a while. I'll teach you to ride. You used to ride at Roy's when we were kids. Those summers out there . . . ."

"Me? No, you know me. I'd go crazy on a farm. I wouldn't last a day. I need a bar and a TV and my own bed."

"You might be surprised, Jake. It's healthy . . . you'll feel . . . like a better version of yourself."

"A better version of myself?"

"Yeah."

"You sure you aren't in a cult out there?"

"A cult?"

"You sound a little brainwashed, baby brother."

"No, we're not brainwashed."

"You sure?"

"Yeah, no. We're just happy."

"That's what they said down in Guyana."

"Yeah, yeah."

"I'm kidding, Merc. I'm glad you're happy. I haven't been happy . . . I don't know . . . in *years*. I don't *remember* the last time I was happy."

"You gotta do something about that, Jake."

"Yeah, what?"

"Barbecue?"

"Huh?"

"Across the street."

"Across the street what."

"Mikky Jikky's House of BBQ."

"B . . . B . . . Q . . . I can't believe you're *hungry* again. Really? Alright, hell, alright, let's do it. But you're drinkin' a beer with me."

"Deal."

After Memphis, Jake finally let me drive and I took it from there to Cleveland while he slept in the backseat. Memphis to Cleveland was a fourteen-hour shot, the I-40 East toward Nashville into Kentucky, then Ohio on the I-70. Small towns passing like a blip on the screen. Billboards with faded images of grinning doctors in lab coats holding toothpaste tubes and women with boxes of laundry soap and a baby on one hip. I drove and watched the world pass by. Cattle. Tobacco fields and yellow expanse of grassland. Trucks with big loads of hay and straw. An abandoned gas station with a sign reading, 'Dane and Dee's Gas and Go! Side Show Out Back Fifty Cents! We Have 'George The Lion' In a Cage! Come By And See Him!'

FEBRUARY 10TH

This last week has been a blur. From Cleveland, I drove straight to Buffalo. The map said two hundred miles, but we were stuck in traffic half the time, a six car pile-up on the road ahead of us. It rained the whole way there, a steady, gray, lifeless drizzle, and Jacob slept until we pulled up to our motel, The Drive Right Inn.

Good name.

Jake woke up and stretched and said, "What?"

We checked in and went straight to a bar on Marble Street so Jake could get a shot of whiskey.

A shot turned into six and then Jake got in an argument over heavyweight boxing with some skinny drunk woman and I had to pull him out of there and take him home. Driving back to the hotel, he slept and it was so sad to see him folded over in the seat next to me that I cried and had to hold it together and got to the motel feeling low and miserable.

Buffalo was cold and stupid and industrial. Brick warehouses in ruin. Cops everywhere, and everyone gray-faced and bitter and shuffling about with their coats pulled up around them against the wind. Horrible.

It snowed the day they buried Mom. Jake and I stood shivering and watched them put her in the ground and then the man we hired said a few words about the "land beyond" and how Mom will be "waiting there in heaven with a choir on high" and when it was done, we walked back to the car. The whole time my brain was on a loop, "Bullshit," it said, "Bullshit, bullshit, bullshit." No choir, no heaven, no land beyond, no Mom. You die and you're dust. How stupid. Worthless. Gah. Terrible.

On the path through the cemetery, Jake asked, "Hey, baby brother, you believe in God, right?"

"I don't know, Jake. I don't think I do."

"I always have. Never had a doubt in my life. We'll . . . y'know . . . see her again."

"I hope you're right."

"We will. But . . . I don't know . . . I mean . . . what I've been thinking about is . . . I've been thinking about this a lot . . . it's . . . just . . . which Mom will she *be?*" he sounded young when he said that, younger than I ever knew him.

"What do you mean which Mom? *Ours.*"

"No, I mean, will it be the Mom I remember before she started to change or will it be the one she was when she . . . when she passed?"

"I've never thought about it like that. I guess the one you remember."

"Yeah, but who's to say that the one I remember is the right one? Why should she be . . . be, I don't know, *re-set* to that earlier version just because that's the one *I* think is best?"

"Good question . . . I guess."

"I mean, shouldn't it be *her* choice?"

"If you're dead, how can it be a choice?"

"Maybe the choice . . . the choosing . . . happens before you're gone. Like it's . . . preset."

"That makes sense."

"Why not the teenage her, the little kid her, or the one she was when she met Dad? I'm sure she had a best possible version of herself . . . we all do, right? Best . . . like, the best time period of herself."

"Jake, you said 'the one I remember,' do you remember much about Mom?"

"Yeah . . . yeah, baby brother, I do."

"Will you . . . I mean . . . could you *tell* me about her?"

"Sure," he smiled sadly. "Where do you want me to start?"

On the way out of town, Jake's faithful old '57 blew its engine and we've been stuck on the outskirts ever since.

Jake's plan is to find someone to buy the car for scrap, then use that money and what we have left from the funeral expenses to get two plane tickets home.

As of yet, we have no options. We've been at the motel this entire time. The TV's sound is busted, so Jake and I sit in our beds with the screen playing the Olympics. He's been telling me about Mom for days and it's good to hear him talk.

Slowly, painstakingly, there's a picture of her developing—how she lived, what she loved, how she was when Jake was a boy, the things she and Dad did when they were young.

When Jake sleeps, I pour a bath and lie in it with the book that Channy lent me for the drive. It's Tolstoy, *War and Peace*. Her favorite. I've decided to read it straight through some other time. For now, my thoughts are too scattered. I'll read for a while and pretty soon I'm just turning pages, looking at the words without seeing them. The book is great. I can tell. And I *will* read it when life is less crazy. What I've been doing is opening it to random pages and reading here and there.

Things like:

"'MASTER NOT here—no understand . . . me, you,' said Gerasim, trying to make his words more comprehensible by saying them in reverse order." God, I did that so many times in Mexico, and now I feel like such an asshole . . . for even being there. What a fucking "ugly American." What a cliché I was. When I think back on it, I get dizzy because I feel so sick. I thought I was Kurtz. I was a leech, a tourist. I never want to be that guy again.

Anyway, my favorite section, the part I've been mulling over all day:

"The uncle sang as peasants sing, in full and naive conviction that in a song the whole value rests in the words, that the tune comes of itself and that a tune apart is nothing, that the tune is only for the sake of the verse. And this gave the uncle's unselfconscious singing a peculiar charm, like the song of birds. Natasha was in ecstasies over the uncle's singing. She made up her mind not to learn the harp any longer, but to play only on the guitar. She asked the uncle for the guitar and at once struck the chords of the song."

Fantastic. I can see how this book means a lot to Channy—Channy the writer, I mean.

I keep coming back to those lines.

FEBRUARY 18TH

Jake sold the car to a man who drove up from the city. The man (Aaron Lankin was his name) paid Jake in cash

and then we rode back with him in his baby-blue Ford convertible and flew out of JFK three days later.

It was good to be back in New York City. Coming to New York felt like closing the book on an old chapter of my life, or stitching a wound I didn't know was open. It was exhilarating to be there and not feel haunted like I thought I would. I was anonymous amongst all the people rushing about and okay with it, safe and untouchable because no one could see me. No one cared. No one was watching. I was poor little Mercander Carr, not a care in the world, beholden to no man, *secure* above all. New York with fresh eyes was fantastic. Walking through Brooklyn I could imagine a century back in time with old borough bosses and clopping horse carts and sooty sky. I saw the whole of the city—history, dirt-marsh-to-skyscrapers—I was a baby walking through these streets for the first time, "What are these ladders to the sky? Is this okay? Are we okay?" I fell in love with the immensity and all the gray stone and fruit carts and racks of sunglasses and closed-down blocks, the old rich neighborhoods gone to ruin—to sod!—the poor neighborhoods thriving with MUSIC, rhythm, sound bursting out from every doorway and each crack in the wall, big radios the size of suitcases. *Food smells*, the kind of food you'd die for, fried, greasy, unhealthy, garlic, onion, pepper, curry, coconut . . . soul food, Indian, Chinese, Greek, Italian, all sorts of mysterious flavors and spices blending together as one big wave of information, the world as cuisine, the stew of LIFE, New York! My heart jumped for it and I promised to move back, to uproot everything and give myself to the city. Of course, I knew it wasn't an option. The country had left its stamp on me. I couldn't talk about "different ways of living" and "a better, smarter life" in the country, then go back to the damn city. Still. *Still*, my heart was alive in New York and I was myself again in a way I hadn't been for years, and wouldn't be again. Two years. God, two years? All this living and just two years? Sorel and I. The exile in Mexico. Long, sad days at the newspaper. The overcast afternoons visiting Mom in the home and sitting in her room watching her stare at nothing, dead-eyed, flat . . . at what? Memories? The past? She was there. I knew she was. Some part of her held on while all the wind in the world dragged her out of herself.

I pushed my luck, of course. I went to the little . . . what would it be called . . . a bodega, sounds so pretentious . . . I went to the little corner store, the market where the boy was killed and everything changed for me. I went in and bought a pack of gum and came out and threw up in the trashcan. That was it. That was as deep as it had me. Residual. Traces. There was a shred of fiber that held me to that store, to that night, but I'd pushed on. I'd moved past it and gotten over it by sheer force of will. Or denial? Maybe some of both. A little denial is healthy. Is it? Sometimes you need to look your troubles in the eye and say, "Tonight, you have no influence over me. For my own sake, I'm choosing to ignore you. I'll deal with it later but I need some REST. I need some time to get better." Recovery is pure *will*. (Will and support, I guess.)

On our last day in town, we took the train out to Coney Island. The ride was long and sleepy and we talked for a while—about Mom, and about the election—and then Jake fell asleep with his head on my shoulder.

When we got there, we bought hotdogs and Cokes at Nathan's then wandered around the amusement park.

Me: "Jake, isn't it weird that your middle name is Nathan and that hotdogs are your favorite thing in the world?"

Him: "Why would that be weird?"

Me: "I don't know. It's weird."

Him: "It's not weird."

Me: "I guess not."

After a while, we walked down to the shore and Jake and I sat on the sand and watched the ocean. It was a cold, breezy day and the Atlantic was stormy and ripped by wind, nothing but dark blue water as far out as you could see.

"Merc, I ever tell you about the club that Grandpa was in out here?"

"Which grandpa?"

"Herbie. Mom's. It's . . . it's another Mom story. Kind of. She told me this when I was a kid. Grandpa was part of this club out here that met somewhere on the island. Anyway, they got together in the '30s and made films recreating their dreams as a form of amateur psychoanalysis."

"Freud came to the island at some point. I remember reading about his visit in school."

"It had something to do with that but the club happened later."

"I think it was Freud who called America 'A giant mistake.' I remember that from school."

"Fuck Freud."

"Seriously."

"Grandpa and his friends made these dream films of theirs . . . this . . . this big group of Freud enthusiasts all working together on their off-time. They met up and talked about psychoanalysis and had parties and made films of their dreams. Y'know, silent movies, home movies, and staged these grand elaborate dream stories for each other. Sixteen-millimeter films. Mom said the group tried to get their own psychoanalysis *theme park* built on the island but it never got off the ground."

"I'd love to watch a film of Grandpa Herbert's dreams. I never knew him."

"I guess I knew him when I was a baby, but he died when I was two and I don't remember him at all. According to Mom, Grandpa Herb was a real character—a real Roaring Twenties kinda guy. He was a playwright, an inventor, an author of books on Darwin and . . . what was it . . . the Indian wars, if I remember right. One day you should ask . . . *wow*, Jesus, I almost said 'you should ask her sometime.' I almost did. Wow. I swear." He looked down at the sand and dug his hands into it and pulled up a double handful and let it drop again. "Goddamnit, baby brother. What's going on? What's happening to us?"

"I know."

"Just . . . ugh . . . goddamnit."

"Do they . . . do . . . do the films still exist?"

"Maybe in someone's . . . someone's garage somewhere? A box of forgotten . . . thrown-out junk? All I know is what Mom told me. She was foggy on the details, but with some of it she wasn't. I remember Mom having just *brilliant*, *lucid*, crystal-clear recall of certain things, just like you. Then being . . . being . . . I don't know . . . *blank* on the rest. She'd tell me something and there would be all these *tiny*, seemingly inconsequential details no one else in the world would ever remember. Like she'd remember what they were eating for dessert that night and how it was . . . what it tasted like, what was on the radio, that sort of thing, but then there would be parts that weren't even there. Important things too—who she was with at the time, what city they were in, what year it was. Like she always talked about us watching the Beatles on *Ed Sullivan* but she could never remember the name of the show or what house we were in or whether Dad was there or not."

"We saw the Beatles on *Ed Sullivan*?"

"Yeah. You were little. I don't think you watched but you were there. Mom loved them. She thought they were nice boys. Especially George."

"Jake, sometimes I wish they would've had me earlier so I could've known them better."

"No one knew Dad."

"I guess but I feel cheated sometimes. You know what I mean, Jake? Cheated?"

"Yeah, sure. I get ya. I'm sorry, baby brother. I wish it would've played out some other way. I mean they're . . . *gone*. *Both* of them. That whole thing, whatever they had together, their own empire, their love and their history, just *dust*. I used to think about them as this big imposing presence, *them*, Monique and Harold Carr, this indomitable head of our family with all their friends and the things they loved to do and they places they went, their music, dad's sports trophies, mom's literary awards—"

"What?"

"Mom's literary awards."

"Really?"

"You didn't know?"

"Mom wrote?"

"She did. She was . . . she's been published in all kinds of journals and magazines. Poetry. She wrote poetry for a long time."

"Wow. I had no idea."

"She never talked about it."

"Wow, this is kinda fucking me up right now."

"Merc, do you remember when the tuna crabs washed up on Kellogg's Beach when we first came out to California on vacation?"

"No."

"Not a good example. I was . . . I was working up to a metaphor. Doesn't work. Anyway, I know God always has a plan for this stuff, but I just wish we had a few more years. Especially . . . for your sake, for the sake of their grandkids. I wish . . . he'd been around. Dad. Our dad. Who was he? I wish I knew. I really do. I don't even think he liked me."

"Jake, there's no way to—"

"Let's go back to that bar by Nathan's. I feel crazy. I need a drink."

"No, you don't."

"Alright."

"You really don't."

"Okay."

"Yeah."

"Okay, Merc. Let's just . . . let's just stay here for a while. On the beach."

"Alright. We can . . . we can do that."

"Merc?"

"Yeah?"

"Merc, there's something I want to tell you."

"Okay."

"It's something . . . I guess I've always wanted to tell you and I've been thinking about telling you all day but . . . but I haven't told anyone and maybe . . . I think I owe it to you because, because, you know, I *changed*."

"Jake, you don't have to—"

"I changed. I was one way and then I was . . . like I am now and I don't think I'll ever be that way again and . . . I don't think I'd want to if I could . . . it's not me anymore or maybe it is, maybe it could be again. I always . . . I think some part of me felt . . . *feels* like I let you down because here I was, this dependable . . . this honest, forthright, stand-up guy. I had a future and I wanted things from the world and I wanted to make my mark and have people know me and I wanted you to look up to me and . . . God, I don't know, but—"

"Jake."

"No, let me tell this. You're my little brother . . . I remember you as a baby and you were so excited about life and so sweet and funny and crazy and perfect . . . so perfect and I wanted to be your hero, someone who'd make you feel safe but when I came back . . . *before* I came back . . . we were . . . okay, okay, it was the rainy season my last month there. We were out on patrol, three, four days in. We'd run into some North Vietnamese the second day but it was nothing . . . them shooting at us on one side of the river, us shooting back at them. Nothing. Nothing happened. The third or fourth day we went into this village on orders to . . . we were told there were . . . enemy combatants hiding out . . . taking, taking, you know, *refuge* in the village. We had tips like that all the time but it never led to anything. We'd go in and ask questions with our translator . . . this nice kid from Saigon . . . we called him Sly . . . and nothing, nothing. No leads. Never. Nothing. So we go into this little village in the middle of the . . . just the middle of deep, deep jungle and our LT, Louie, this young kid from

Vermont, college kid, good family, but . . . he was tough. Jewish kid. Stubborn. But funny, God, he was funny sometimes. And Louie gets rough with a couple guys in the village . . . pushin' 'em around, callin' 'em names they didn't know, but . . . but, you know, they could tell they were being swore at. They knew. You *know* when someone's insulting you even if it's in another language. 'Faggot gooks.' That sort of thing. Horrible things. 'Dirty fucking slope chink cock-sucking slant-eye bastards.' And afterward . . . we did this a few times . . . it was . . . it was kind of the standard operating procedure. We burned the village."

"Jesus, Jake."

"We didn't hurt anymore. We weren't rude or pushy. We asked them to leave the village and then we set fire to the thatch roofs of the huts and let it burn. We did it all the time. Just in case, you know. A precaution. That night . . . that night, it rained. It rained harder than anything I've ever seen. Harder than that time down in Jacksonville with Carl. Harder than those summer thunderstorms at the lakehouse. We sat up trying to sleep under our ponchos and it just came down, the darkest night you ever saw, blackest night, the rain coming straight down, no wind, and we sat there in the middle of the jungle and we tried to sleep and the ground all around us became mud and we sank into it and the rain . . . it was loud, God, it was so loud, all you could hear was the rain. You couldn't even smoke because, because, you know, they'd *see* us. We had to just grin and bear it. I propped myself up, my M-16's butt-stock in the mud, hugging the rifle, arms and legs all around it, the poncho over me like some shitty dumb useless tent and I . . . I missed you and I missed Mom and I wanted to be home and I wanted to take back ever enlisting and just . . . I wanted to wake up and have it all be a dream, something I could do over, start over, not make that big mistake. Of course, I didn't know Mom would be someone else when I got back. We knew she was changing. I did. I think you did, too."

"I did. I didn't understand but I knew."

"I knew, too, but I didn't know that the Mom I'd come back to would be this . . . totally different . . . totally different person. All I wanted was for her to make it better. To do that thing that moms do where they have this *power* to change things, to stop whatever's happening and make it go a different way by sheer *will power* and by . . . the strength of their love. I kept thinking, Why can't my mom be here and change this? Why can't she save me now? Which is stupid, I know, but that's what I thought. Anyway, at some point I slept and when I woke up it was just dawn and the rain had stopped. It was gray and misty in the jungle, mist creeping through the trees, colorless, like smoke, very wet, very damp. It wasn't cold but what with the rain all night and being soaked for hours and hours, you had a hard time getting started, you felt old, creaky, stiff, you know? By the time everyone was up, it was clear that Louie was gone. Not a trace. His pack was there, his gun, poncho, helmet, all of it in a pile, but he'd *vanished*. It was so quiet. So quiet and still and all you could hear was your own breath and the drops of water dripping off the trees to the jungle floor and no one wanted to say anything or even . . . even *guess* what might've happened. We waited a while. Waited in case he'd wandered off to piss or something but we all knew he wasn't coming back. Anyway, a few hours later . . . we were back-tracking now . . . a few hours later we found him. He came out of nowhere, walking toward us, blind . . . his eyes . . . his *eyes* were cut out of his head and he had two . . . square *holes* where his eyes had been, black holes so deep . . . *deep* into his head and blood dried down his face and he was . . . he was walking . . . stumbling, walking alone through the jungle trying to find us and I kept thinking, my God, how *alone* he must've felt out there, alone in the jungle in the morning when he should've been back home in Vermont, getting up to have breakfast or sleeping in or reading the paper with his parents. Louie . . . when we found him, he dropped to his knees and cried. You can cry without having eyes, did you know that? You can. I saw it happen. His body sobbed, he shook. There were no tears, of course, but he cried. Louie lived about twenty minutes after we found him. I'm not sure why he died . . . I guess he lost a lot of blood, but I think it was just the *relief* of being found. I think he'd given up ever being found and once we did find him he just shut down. He just passed, silent and calm on his back with all of us sitting and standing around him and the medic trying to talk to him. He just . . . went. I'd seen a few people die over there. Not as many as you might think. And nothing that close. But I was right *there*. I had my hand on his chest and I was talking to him and I felt his heart beating and then I felt it stop and a breath went out of him and you could tell his life was gone. He died right there . . . right there with me sitting next to him, talking to him, *god*. Of course . . . of course we knew it was someone back in the village. One of those guys he'd messed with had been Viet Cong. I *think* we knew. It seemed . . . God, I'm sorry I'm telling you this—"

"No, Jake, go on. You can tell me."

"We decided it was the village. Revenge for how Louie'd treated them and revenge for us burning their homes. We decided it was the village and we went back. They were there rebuilding. Maybe . . . twenty, maybe less. Fifteen? Rebuilding their huts and we . . . we came back and we killed every man, woman, and child. We slaughtered them, cut them to pieces. I killed an old man. Just this old man, somebody's grandpa, some tiny old man with white hair and the black pajama clothes they all wore, barefoot, wrinkled little man . . . he was so small and thin and he looked so hungry standing there and he shook his head, no, please, you know, begging me, shaking his head and I put my rifle up to my shoulder and pulled the trigger and the bullet caught him right between his eyes and he dropped like he was nothing. He was the only one. After that, I went off on my own and threw up and you could hear the shots and women screaming and the sound of struggling and movement and then after a while it was quiet again. It was over. My God, baby brother, we *did* that. *I* did that. Some days I wake up and I forget about it for . . . for just the smallest second and I feel alright and I'm excited to start the day and then I remember and it comes back over me like a pile of stones and pushes me back down. It's never away from me. It's always there, and no matter what I'm doing, it's like I'm always thinking about it, even if I'm thinking about something else. I can't get away. My God. What did we *do*? What did I *do*, baby brother?"

We sat in silence. The sky over the ocean had gone dark, and far out to sea you could tell by the clouds that it was raining and that the rain was coming toward land.

BOOK FOUR

FALL

"And as the shelling of the 1st Belorussian Front began, the boy found the red glass bottle in the rubble and inside was the stone and he broke the glass on the rock wall and the stone glowed deep red in the flickering light and he held the glowing stone up to the gray and smoky sky. It was 20 April, 1945, Adolf Hitler's birthday. The boy had found what he'd come for. Now everything would change, everything would fall."

—Ed Distler, *Ghosts and The Amazon*

2000
OFFICE COURTYARD, LUNCHTIME

Joey drops the chicken burrito in the fountain and watches it sink and unravel onto the blue tile.

"No, *really*. What are you *doing*?" asks Yesenia, frowning.

Joey takes off his Ray-Bans and rubs them on his shirt and looks up at the sun and the dying trees in the industrial lot's park—all the identical glass and steel office boxes that stand around them in the valley.

"I just quit eating meat."

"Oh yeah? Right now, you did?" says Yesenia, squinting up at him. A scowl. She shakes her head. "What's *up* with you right now? You're being *weird*." Her arms are crossed and she's frowning hard, deeply.

Joey wipes the sweat off his brow with his sleeve and looks at the swipe of dirt it left. "Right now I did. I quit right now. Officially."

"Why?"

"Who cares? Let's smoke a cigarette."

"Alright."

In his truck cab, in the parking lot, Maggie sleeps wrapped in a Mexican blanket. Co-workers walking past the car to and from lunch. Briefcases, laptops, a string of keys. They have no idea.

Yesenia shakes her head and pulls two cigarettes out of her pack of Gauloises and hands one to Joey along with a lighter. He lights it, takes a drag, and then puts her lighter in the front pocket of his shirt and looks back up at the sun. "The sun, Yessy. Look at it. Think about what it is."

"Alright . . . whatever you say, weirdo-pants."

"Don't talk so loud, Yessy."

"You okay? You've seemed really different lately. You've lost a lot of weight. It's not healthy to be that skinny. Girls don't like that kind of skinniness in a guy. Can I have my lighter back? It was a gift from my sister. She got it in Prague. Have you ever been to Prague, Joey?"

"This place gives me the creeps, Yessy. We're standing on a graveyard."

"Oh yeah?"

"It's the graveyard of a place. It's fall—those trees should have yellow and red and brown leaves. But they're dead. Dead as winter in . . . in, like, in someplace cold . . . or dead like the sun fried them, like the sun fried them right where they . . . where they stand. Why are those trees dead?"

"Whatever, psychopath-city. Can I have my ligh—"

"I'm serious. Just stop for a second . . . just stop . . . breathe in and . . . and *think about it*. Look around. A graveyard. The sun and everything dead. What if a giant foot came down and stomped on us, and a voice said, 'My bad,' and then there was a laugh track. What if we—"

"Hey, just give me my lighter and let's go back inside. I'm, like, three days behind."

"I'm going home." Joey puts his sunglasses back on and pats his front pocket to make sure the lighter is still there. He pats his other pocket to feel the bag of crystal. Half-gone. It's his third day without sleep.

"Home? It's not even—" she looks at her phone, "*noon*. You can't just—"

"I'm going home." He turns and walks across the parking lot to his truck.

To Maggie.

1980

SEPTEMBER 23RD

Fall is here and things are changing. Smoke in the air from the chimneys of Rose Morning. Issy, burning a great pile of branches and blackberry vine and scrap wood in the valley, tiny and bundled-up against the cold, Dixon, her favorite white pygmy goat trailing behind, smoke gushing up to the sky. The sky pale blue, the smoke so *black*. The leaves are turning, too. Not much, but enough. The bulk of our crops were summer crops, so the harvest is over, the pantry full of things in jars with dates and names written in black marker. The garage freezer stocked.

Channy and I and the kids spend most of our time together in the sitting room with the fireplace roaring and its big view of the fields and the thick wall of pine trees and the hills beyond. It's good here and warm and I hold the baby and sing to her while Channy makes tea and the boy plays on the floor with his *Star Wars* figures and Matchbox cars.

I'm tired. Something about the cold. It gets into me. Makes me slow. I'm tired, but this is okay. I wouldn't want to be anywhere else.

2000

HOME, DAWN

Maggie gets up and goes to the kitchen. Joey hears cold air rasp out from the freezer and then he hears it stop with a muffled clap. She comes back and sits on the loveseat and slides the yellow wrapper off her Popsicle. "Grape," she says.

Joey cuts a line for himself and hands Maggie the CD case and a rolled-up twenty and she shakes her head no. "No. One's enough."

"You cold?" Joey leans back to the wall and turns the heater up.

Maggie takes the easy chair by the wall and wraps herself in a Mexican blanket and talks while the incense burns down. Joey sits on the floor at the foot of her chair and leans against it and listens. They're afraid to leave the room, so they establish a set of ground rules. The kitchen is safe—a beer to take the edge off. Dr. Pepper. Water, always water. ("You can do *anything* as long as you drink enough water," he tells Maggie, jaw gritting, though he goes days without drinking it himself.) The hallway is a dark tunnel. The bedroom a pit. Sometimes they listen to music. Mostly they talk.

Maggie: "I don't know what I want to be when I grow up, and when I'm around people who've got it figured out, it makes me *super* uncomfortable and I feel really inadequate."

Joey: "It was the fundamental things that they didn't tell me that fucked me up. I feel like I'm years behind people my age because my aunt and uncle never took me aside and told me how it works. Like when you first started coming over here and you saw I didn't use sheets on my bed and I was like, 'Sheets?' They never told me that you use a bottom sheet and a top sheet and you change them regularly. How basic is that? They never told me certain that foods have protein and that you need to eat some of it every day. That's why I ate so white trash for so long. They didn't . . . I mean, they didn't even tell me about drinking *water*. I mean, of course I know about drinking water, but I figured I'd get enough from soda and coffee and . . . and, like, juice, ice tea, whatever. They never . . . they never gave me a set of rules to live by and as a result I'm . . . I don't know, look at me, I lie all the time, I do a ton of drugs, I have no work ethic, I'm not . . . I'm not nice to people. I'm selfish, lazy, I talk shit without . . . you know, without thinking about the repercussions . . . I see that now and I hate it. I hate this shitty, flimsy person I've become. I've got no substance. I'm weak. Weak all around, weak character, weak morally. I want to be better. God*damnit*."

Maggie: (reading out loud) "'A man can live and be healthy without killing animals for food; therefore, if he eats meat, he participates in taking animal life merely for the sake of his appetite.'"

Joey: "It's beautiful out there in the fall. The grain fields between the hills are all golden and there's a place right after you exit for Pine Valley to get soft serve cones with those chocolate-dipped shell things. We used to go out there with my aunt to ride horses when she went through her outdoorsy faze. Best thing was this . . . I don't know, like, this general store or whatever across the street from the frosty place where all the comic books in the rack were, like, ten, fifteen years old. It was like time had stopped. I used to buy piles of them every time I went there. *Fantastic Four, The Amazing Spider-Man, Justice League, Action Comics*. They had no idea . . . but . . . but I don't think they cared. They sold these comics for, like, fifty cents or whatever, and they just did their thing. They didn't give a fuck. You should see my comics collection at my parents'.

All in Mylar bags. I've got Golden Age stuff, a lot of old *Batman* . . . all the first series solo *Wolverines*. I have one . . . one that freaked me out so badly that I had to hide it at the bottom of my toybox. *Arkham Asylum* . . . a graphic novel. All paintings. Really bloody, impressionistic . . . Grant Morrison and Dave McKean. Even if you don't like comics, it's art . . . scary, dark, haunted art."

Maggie: "Tyler and I just looked through the screen door at each other and didn't say anything. It was horrible. If he asks me, I'm going to tell him. I can't lie to anyone. Especially Tyler. If he asks . . . if he asks, I'm telling him. Hard as that'll be. I'm sorry, Joey."

Joey: "I didn't have any friends for the first three years of high school and I used to leave school at lunch and ride my stupid-ass beach cruiser around just so no one would see me eating by myself. I used to ride to am/pm every day and get a barbecue rib sandwich and a Dr. Pepper and sit on the curb and eat it and then ride back in time for the bell. There was another kid who did the same thing and we always managed to show up at different times so that we didn't have to talk. It was weird. He and I just *knew* what each other was doing. He's a pro surfer now. Has tons of friends. I think I'm doing okay too . . . socially . . . I have friends and whatever. Who's calling . . . ugh . . . I'm unplugging it."

Maggie: "I had a . . . really rough year."

Joey: "Like when you spell 'boobs' with a calculator."

Maggie: "When Kurt Cobain killed himself, I went to church that Sunday and in Youth Group there was this lesson about how he was going to hell because he took his own life. That was just *one* of my problems with church. But, I dunno, I still believe in God. That church just sucked. They were awful."

Joey: "I love dogs. I've always wanted a pet."

Maggie: "When I get scared, I instantly go into attack mode."

Joey: "When I was nine, I wrote a poem about Stonehenge for school. It went, 'Stonehenge, people go to see. How did it get there? Oh, gee.'"

Maggie: "It was the best summer of my life. Joel and Callie and Tyler and I just sat around Tyler's pool and listened to Sublime and the Steve Miller Band and Tool and Bob Marley and went and got burritos and hung out in the garage and ate ice cream. Tyler still had long hair and swore he'd never cut it. Sometimes the boys rode skateboards around . . . badly, but it was okay. I felt like anything was possible, that whatever I wanted could come true. I don't think I've ever been that happy or free since."

Joey: "I like that dress on you. You should wear it all the time. You look like you're from another era or something."

Maggie: "I can never work anyone else's remote control. It's always such a mystery, all those buttons and modes and settings. I always mess it up and then no one can fix it."

Joey: "I'm always worried that I'll end up totally unemployable when

I'm old. Like I'll end up being one of those day-laborer guys on the corner by the carwash on Grand waiting for work and nobody will want to hire me. I have nightmares about it all the time. Like being totally *unneeded*."

Maggie: "No way, I *love* your truck. I don't know what Nicole's talking about; it's not boring at all. I feel like it's so faithful and trusty that if you whistled, it would just come from wherever it was, like some kind of brave dog or a cowboy's horse. You should give it a name."

Joey: "When Chente was still here, we lived off *chorizo* burritos. *Chorizo* fried up with egg wrapped in a big tortilla. Maybe some butter in it. Some fresh lime if you had one. Chente always said that the manly thing to do is to go through the drive-thru and say, '*Me gustaría un chorizo burrito sin huevo*' . . . y'know chorizo *without* egg, because the flavor is stronger that way. The voice in the drive-thru would always go '*Siiiiiin huevo?!*' and we loved that because that meant we were tough."

Maggie: "I know it's super dorky and lame and naïve, but I love seeing the Hollywood sign. I always get all excited when I see it and I feel like I've, I dunno, come up to big, wild *Tinseltown* to make it in movies or something. I mean, not *make it* in movies. Not porn. You . . . you know what I mean, Joey. All that *possibility* and the dreams and the places you could go if you were discovered. It's romantic and it's something that'll never exist again. Maybe that's what makes a thing romantic. Unattainability. Is that even a word? Unattainability? It sounds like one."

Joey: "Down by the lake where you'd fish. In a little cabin restaurant with deer heads and license plates and farm tools on the walls. Video poker machines . . . it was on Native American land. Pie, chili beans, cornbread, coffee. The chili was amazing. Cheddar cheese sprinkled on top. I don't miss meat, but I do miss a good . . . y'know, a good, big, hot bowl of chili. It was always so warm in there after being out on the lake all day. Hot chocolate, beef strew, Saltines. My uncle was into fishing for, like, *six months* and then he was over it. But every trip we took is like . . . *emblazoned* in my memory. Some of the best times of my life. For those six months, I felt like he could actually *stand* having me around. I was so proud. I was . . . god, I was, like, six or seven. When he gave up fishing, it was like he gave up on me."

Maggie: (sitting in the chair reading to Joey from Ed Distler's *Fall*) "'Yuri's plane is not a plane anymore. It's a black carriage drawn by horses and they cut through the mist, the reins snapping, damp leather on horseflesh and wood, the cry of the horses. The gypsy witch Moria in a wet flapping slicker, hooded, whipping the horses, driving deep into the black woods. She looks back at them and smiles with flashing white teeth. And the pine trees, a dark wall up against the sky—and the sky purple and gray—the moon a fingernail of bright white. Everything flat and strange like it's cut from construction paper. And where are we going? And to what end? The plane hit the ground like a whale diving back into the sea.'"

Joey: "My great-uncle Roy had these cassette tapes of old radio shows. Most of them were super dated and cheesy, but the Lone Ranger ones were great. Of course it was kind of corny and the moral of the story was always hammered home at the end, but I loved them and I used to sit on his lap in his chair all full of wonder and awe and listen to those stories and imagine myself saving the old woman from the land barons or saving the miners from the band of outlaws. The outlaw . . . what was his name? Butch . . . Cavender, Cavanagh, Cavendish, it was *Cavendish*. The Cavendish Gang. Anyway, but here I am with Tyler, lying, sneaking around behind his back, doing the kinds of underhanded shit that the Lone Ranger's enemies always did. Lying. Hurting my friends. Being a backstabbing, greedy shithead. You can't be a good man and a liar at the same time. The Lone Ranger would've shot me with a silver bullet and the story would be over. No one cries at the funeral of the bad guy. Who wants to admit that if the fantasy stories were true, the hero would *kill* them?"

Maggie: "I got right up in that fucking skinhead's face and I was like, 'You better stop picking on my friends or I'll fucking kick your *ass*.' He looked at me like, 'Who. The hell. Is this crazy fucking baby-sized girl?'"

Joey: "Nicole used to tell me to 'Stop showing off' and she'd say it in front of people. It was so *humiliating*. Ugh."

Maggie: "Ronny? He's a total ax murderer."

Joey: "I think that they're sea lions, not seals. Or maybe they're seals and not sea lions. You know, the ones on the rocks at Children's Cove. It has something to do with the ears. Pinnipeds. Steve's girlfriend Eva gets really crazy when you switch them around. She goes all Russian mafia on your ass."

Maggie: "I'm glad you're nice to me."

Joey: "I'm getting water. You want water? We need water. I'll get you some water."

Maggie: "What? I can't believe you *thought* that. I'm so sorry, Joey. Oh, Joey. No, no, no. Sundays are my most *un*favorite days. On Sundays, I do all the boring shit that I don't have the energy to do during the week. Some people might pick their favorite friends to spend Sundays with, but not me. Sundays are about surviving and getting through until Monday morning."

Joey: "I like the way your hair curls up right there. Yeah, right *here*."

Maggie: "My boyfriend asked me to—wait, whoa, did you hear that? I just called him my boyfriend. Ugh."

Joey: "The harder I try, the worse it is."

Maggie: "You know how you can't imagine some people being old? I can't see my cousin Cecilie as old and it freaks me out. She's like a ghost as it is but there's no way she'd . . . I don't know. It *scares* me."

Joey: "Like on Halloween, how he was just *standing* there in the doorway after we got back to your house, *staring* at us while you and I sat on your bed in our costumes and I could, like, I felt it in his eyes. They were just so *hurt*. He didn't say anything but his eyes were . . . *screaming*. I think when Tyler said he was going back to his house, he expected me to leave, too, like he thought it would be inappropriate for just you and I to stay alone in your room. And I understood that and I felt bad but . . . but at the same time, I didn't *care*. I was so drunk, I just wanted him to *leave* so that I could be alone with you. I *should've* left when he did and then he wouldn't have suspected anything. I just looked at him and he looked at us and he stood there in the doorway all stick-thin and unhealthy wearing the blue wig from his David Bowie costume, looking *so fucking overwhelmed*."

The sun is orange and blazing through the window blinds so they tack up a beach towel to keep it out. It's quiet in the apartment complex all day and then at six o'clock, people come home and it's loud until midnight: fighting, laughing, the neighbor playing the same videogame for hours, dishwashers banging. After midnight, you hear TVs and nothing else; by two o'clock, it's quiet again.

Every morning, Joey calls in sick. "That cold's in my lungs now," he tells the voicemail, faking a ragged cough. "Getting worse. I'll try to come in Thursday," he says. "I'll try and make it in Friday." "I'll definitely be in on Monday." Routine becomes rhythm. Sunrise. Day. Sunset. Night. And then a week has passed and the bag of speed Curt sold him is gone.

When it's empty, Joey cuts along the seams with a pair of mini-scissors from a sewing kit and opens it carefully and licks the inside of the plastic.

Nothing.

Maggie's passed out on the couch.

He calls Washington Mutual to check his balance, then gets on the phone and calls Curt.

TIJUANA, 1 A.M.

At the strip club, they sit at the rail while the dancer walks circles around the brass pole, the red lights low and flashing. She's older than most of the girls here and she has a tall, heavy body—big, thick, but fit and strong. Her dancer name is "Luz." The announcer behind the DJ table says it before every dance. "*Luuuuz! Luz! L-l-luz! Y ahora mismo, presentamos la Luuuuuzzzz. Luz, la brillante estrella de nuestra n-n-n-noche obscura, Luz.*"

Joey and Tyler and Joel Campbell sit between two groups of sailors, their drinks in a line in front of them on the short wooden counter, an ashtray full of butts at their elbows. Luz has been dancing for three songs now and sweat runs down her neck and belly and from her armpits, her red-brown skin shining dark. And now she's on her hands and knees crawling to the rail, her heavy cleavage hanging like udders. When she gets to the rail, she kneels, thighs spread, and cups her breasts in her hands and paws at them to the pulse of the music.

The sailor next to Joey shouts, "Woo! Yeah, girl!"

She pulls one of her breasts up to her mouth and sucks on the nipple, staring down at the sailor, rolling her hips at him.

The sailor pulls a five out of his wallet, folds it longways, and sets it on the stage. He turns to his friend and talks behind his hand, "I wanta *titty fuck* that big ol' Mesican bitch."

"Hell yeah, dawg!" His friend puts his fist out and they bump knuckles.

The song is over.

Luz walks off stage, stepping painfully down the stairs, and the sailors get up and leave.

"*Y ahora, Betiiiiiciaaaa. Beticia bonita!*" says the DJ, his voice booming through the speakers like a monster truck announcer. "*Beticia de sus suuueños! Beticia, la s-s-s-sucia virgin de Tijuana! Sólo diez y ocho años! Betiiiiiciaaaaa!*"

"So, what happened to you at work?" asks Tyler as the new girl walks on stage. "My mom was like 'Tyler, Joey Carr called and said he's quit his job.'"

"No," Joey laughs. "No, no. I left work and went home and I haven't been back. It's been . . . wow, god, it's been more than a week."

"My mom's terrible with messages."

"'*Hi*. You have reached the Monahans,'" Joey says, doing Tyler's mom's voice from the answering machine. "'We're not—'"

"My mom doesn't sound like that," says Tyler laughing.

"'We're not available to take your caaall right now, but we'll get baaack to you as soooon as pawsible. Thaaank you.'"

"Did you call your boss later?" asks Joel softly. He runs a hand over his close-cropped hair and stares at Joey, his big blue eyes sad and piercing and sober.

"I did when I got home. I told him I was still sick."

"And they were okay with that?"

"I guess. I don't know. Fuck 'em." Joey takes a sip of his beer and sets it on the counter.

"You're gonna lose your job," says Joel.

"I don't think they fire people."

Tyler gets up to use the restroom and a short, busty Mexican girl in a black corset and mini-dress sits in his chair and scoots it up next to Joel. She wraps her stubby arm in his. "Hello, my trusted comrade," she says full of campy seriousness. "You wan' to fuck me, or am I to go home and cry?"

"What? No!" Joel tries to pull away but she holds onto his arm.

"My name iss Hermanita, my friend. I am very nice. I win Nobel Prize for to fuck." Her hands reach down to his lap.

"What? No! Wait—" Joel struggles out of her grasp and stands up. The girl slides over onto his chair and straddles it backwards. She leans forward and folds her arms on the backrest and looks up at him, making a pout face. "You are *aller*shic to me?" Her eyes are lined in dark red and her black hair is cut short and slicked back on top and buzzed on the sides. "You don't like me? I am now to go home and commeet suicide." She puts her hands around her neck and jerks her head side to side and pretends to hang herself. "Goodbye forever, Hermanita, forever rest in peace." The girl looks at Joey and winks. "Your friend, comrade," she says pretending to whisper but talking loud for Joel to hear, "why is he so *cru-el* to me, comrade? Why does he want me to cry and cry and cry and cry?"

Joey shrugs. "He's just shy, comrade. Try harder." He hands her one of their beers.

"*Gracias*, comrade. You will be remembered in the revolution." She takes a sip and then another and trains her gaze back on Joel. "My friend, tell me why you don't wan' to fuck me. What is wrong with your good friend, Hermanita? Tell me. If you don't . . . I will cry." She looks back at Joey and winks again.

Joel stands in front of her, speechless. He shakes his head. "It's not . . . I like you . . . as a person . . . I'm just not—"

"My friend, if you like me is fifteen dohlars for the mouth or ten for the hand." She shows him her hand and waves her fat little fingers. "For twenny, ju can fuck me like a real man and I am—"

"No, I mean . . . I don't . . . I wouldn't . . . no thanks, ugh, argh, I'm . . . there's no money."

She takes another sip of beer and sets the bottle on the railing counter. "Okay. For five dohlars and maybe another drink for me it is—"

"No, really, I mean, no, I don't . . . there's nothing. No money. Money all gone. *No tengo dinero*. I'm broke. I don't have any money. Money no have. None."

The girl stands up and straightens her corset. "Okay, my friend, if you change your mind jus send a secret message to me. I am go to the bar. My heart, it is broken; I must drink myself to death. *Adios*." She sulks past him and looks back and smiles and kisses the air and then she's gone into the crowd by the bar.

Joel sits down. "Joey, what just *happened*? Was she a—"

"She was."

"Wow, gross."

"No way, that girl was cool. She was cute. I can't believe you drove her away. She was fun. You should've at least—"

But then the waitress is standing behind them. "Twelve more beers for the three little señors!" she sings happily. She sets an aluminum bucket of ice with a dozen half-size Coronita bottles sticking out and a tumbler glass packed with lime slices on the counter. "Iss ten doh-lars, little señors!"

Joey pays and orders a round of tequila shots and then excuses himself.

In the bathroom, he sits on the toilet and pours out a bump on his ATM card and snorts it and hits the flusher to cover the sound. He rubs his eyes and does another.

In the next stall, a girl is on her knees in front of a guy sitting on the toilet. In the space between the floor and stall, Joey can see her legs kneeling in front of the guy's shoes with his tan slacks bunched up around them. Her legs are bare and she has the tall, exaggerated heels the girls wear on stage. He can hear the sound of it, a wet slurp and squish. Every few seconds, one of her shoes scrapes on the red tile and she adjusts her position. And then the sound is coming faster and the man lets out a gasp and an "Ayyy!" and it's quiet again.

The muffled sound of the music from the club.

The tap dripping and the water in the pipes.

Joey hears her gag and spit and then she's laughing.

He puts his ear to the stall.

"*Tienes amigas?*" asks the man. He wants to know if she has friends.

"*Si, mi amor, millones y millones,*" says the girl. Yes, my love, millions and millions.

"*Bonitas?*" Pretty?

"*Bonitas. Todas. Si, por su puesto.*" Pretty. All of them. Yes, of course.

"*Quanto cuesta por la noche?*" How much for the night?

"*Quantas chicas?*" How many girls?

"*Tú y dos mas.*" You and two more.

"*Yo y dos . . . la noche si? Toda la noche?*" Me and two . . . the night, correct? The whole night?

"*Si, toda.*" Yes, all of it.

"*Con una propina . . . y el cuarto . . . seis ciento cinquenta.*" With a tip and the room, six hundred and fifty.

Joey sits on the toilet and rubs his temples with his thumbs. The door in front of him is etched with initials and poems and drawings. '*Esteban y Lupe '99.*' '*Jesús Cristo Siempre.*' 'Suck my dick!' 'I hav big cock.' 'PB Vermin.'

Just then, he remembers the Sharpie in the side pocket of his jean jacket. He takes it out and begins to draw a picture of a rat. He gives the rat a sword and then angel wings and then he signs it and writes the date. Then he adds shading, landscape, grass, a craggy mountain range, the sun, clouds. Rain from the clouds, slanted.

When he's done with the picture, Joey stands up and makes a point of flushing the toilet, and opens the stall door.

Back in the main room, Tyler's nodding off in his chair next to Joel and the girl on stage is sliding down the pole headfirst, thighs gripping the metal, her hands holding her chest.

Joel is still sober. He sits and inspects his nails, and Joey nods hi and sits down and takes a sip of one of the full Coronitas.

The girl on the pole slides to the floor and lies on her stomach and humps the stage mechanically, slapping the footboards with her hips.

"When did *that* happen?" Joey nods at Tyler.

"After the tequila. He got bored and drank all three shots."

"Whoa, that's so unlike him. He's not a crazy drinker like that. Wake up, Tyler!"

"Where'd you go? You were gone for like nineteen million years."

"Nowhere. You know. The bathroom."

"That long? I was worried."

"Sorry."

The waitress walks up holding a tray. "No sleepings here, little señors. Iss time to go home now."

"Sorry, we were just leaving." Joel nods down at Tyler. "Joey, let's get this poor beast home."

"Poor beast . . . wake up. Wake up, we're splitting. C'mon, bud, c'mon, we're going."

Joey shakes Tyler's shoulder and Tyler sits up straight and looks around, his eyes bloodshot and dark and watery. "What are we . . . where . . . we're . . . wait, *what*?"

Out on the sidewalk, Tyler pukes into a trashcan while Joel walks down to the market. It's a warm night and the streets are filled with drunk tourists—white college girls in loud shouting packs, Navy guys, Marines, a laughing bridal party searching for the bride.

A *mariachi* band in black and gold suits plays a song on the corner. A crowd has formed in front of them and one of the street kids sets his box of Canel's gum down and does a silly dance. The *guitarron* player sticks his foot out like he's going to kick him and the kid picks up his box and runs down the street laughing and shrieking.

The bridal party finds their bride. She's passed out in the alley. A pack of kids have stolen her tiara and are now running down the block with it. On her forehead, they've drawn a penis.

Tyler and Joey stand out in front of an all-night seafood diner. *Los Panchos Super Mariscos*. Four tables inside and a bar counter with stools. A thick, burly man behind the counter is frying shrimp on a flat grill, spraying oil onto them with a yellow squeeze bottle. On his forearm, a tattooed crucifix with a heart in the center wrapped in barbed wire. The place is cheery and clean and bright-lit. People sit at the tables hunched over plates of tacos and big messy *tortas* and drink Cokes from bottles with napkins wrapped around them. Joey leans against the glass and looks in and lights a cigarette. He tries to remember the last time he ate, but he can't.

The cook is making a fish plate. Three deep-fried cuts of fish, shredded cabbage on the side, lime juice and a thin white sauce over the cabbage, garnish of dark refried beans with dry white cheese and a stack of corn tortillas folded in half next to the fish. He sets the plate on the display counter and dings the bell next to the order carousel.

There's a curly-headed girl sitting on a stool behind the register, tall and bony and pretty, slumped forward while copying something from a textbook, her wrist lined with colorful rubber bracelets. It's 2 a.m. and she looks beat. She gives Joey a sleepy smile and Joey waves with his cigarette hand and she does a weary little thumbs down. Joey gives her a thumbs up and she crosses her eyes and sticks her tongue out the side and Joey laughs and she goes back to the book. The cook dings the bell again and the girl gets up to deliver the plate, dragging her feet dramatically and looking back at Joey, smiling.

Tyler is at the trashcan again, holding the rim, breathing hard. Tears roll down his face and he makes a terrible gagging sound and spews out a mouthful of white froth.

"Bimbo Bread!" says Joel walking back to them. He lifts a bag of sliced white bread from his grocery sack and twirls it around by its twisted-up end, swishing it side to side like nunchucks. "Tyler, this bread is called *Bimbo Bread* and it's going to make you feel so much better."

They sit against the accordion gate of a locked storefront. *Zapatos Cathedral.* Behind them, a wall of out-of-style basketball sneakers and dress shoes and high heals in the darkness. Joel sets a bottle of water in front of Tyler and one in front of Joey and opens the twist tie on the bread. "Bimbo Bread," he says again. He brings it to his face and breathes in. "Smells like Wonder Bread. It was, like, fifteen cents."

"Guys, I feel *bad*," says Tyler. "I feel really sick. I don't want to do this."

"Do what? We're going home," Joel tells him, calm and serious. "First, you need to sober up a little and we'll get back safe and sound, okay?"

"And we're going to steal that burro right there and ride it across the border," Joey adds.

"*That* burro?" Tyler says with a shaky smile, pointing across the street to a donkey painted with zebra stripes. The donkey stands on a corner in front of a farm cart and a wooden backdrop of a desert mural with colorful piñatas nailed up in an arc above it. An old man is stooped over a box camera on a wooden tripod and two black guys are sitting in the cart, wearing matching movie prop sombreros and woven blankets arranged over their shoulders. The guy on the left is holding a toy rifle at his side. They look serious and proud and tough. And then one of them breaks into a grin and leans forward and laughs and his friend cracks a smile and the flash goes off.

"That burro. I call him Lil' Tyler and Lil' Tyler loves you and wants you to get home to San Diego and not get us killed. Do it for Lil' Tyler. He's your *son*."

"It's not funny. No more jokes," says Tyler.

"You're just drunk," Joel says, squinting across the street as he talks. "We're all three of us in the same boat, but we need to keep sailing."

"Your boat metaphor sucks," Tyler mumbles.

"It does," says Joel, "but you know what doesn't suck? Getting home soon and going to *bed*." Joel laughs quietly and runs his hand across the top of his head. "Here. Eat this." He gives Tyler a slice of white bread and balls another one up for himself. "See?" he says through a mouthful of bread. "I feel better already." Joel takes another slice of bread, folds it in half, takes a bite out of the middle and says, "See? Easy." He hands Joey a slice. "Joey, show the man how it's done."

"Check this out, the man." Joey mashes the bread into a ball and tosses it into the air and opens his mouth and tries to catch it. It falls behind him and he snatches it up and puts it in his mouth. "The five second rule," he says, chewing the bread.

"*Germs*," Tyler says, with a weak laugh.

"See, Joey's eating bread. Eat some bread, okay, Tyler? I promise you'll feel a hundred percent better if you eat something and drink a little water."

Tyler pulls the crust off his bread, tosses it aside, and takes a dainty bite.

"Good, good. Now drink." Joel nods down at the bottle.

"What about 'Don't drink the water'?"

"It's bottled. It's safe. Both of you should. Okay?"

Tyler unscrews the white plastic cap from his bottle and drinks and makes a noise like it hurts going down, but then he's drinking fast and the bottle is half-full and he looks human again.

"Good work, bud," says Joey. "Lil' Tyler's proud of you. He's writing a celebratory rap record about it."

"No more Lil' Tyler, okay? It's too much. I'm not up for it right now."

"Finish the water," says Joel.

Tyler drinks the rest of the water and hands the bottle to Joel.

"Good work." Joel puts both bottles and the rest of the bread in his grocery sack and tucks it under his arm. "Let's bounce." He and Joey stand up.

Tyler reaches up to them and they each take a hand and Joey says, "Heave ho!" and they pull Tyler to his feet.

Before they leave the main drag, Joey stops and ducks into an alley. "I'm gonna take a piss real quick," he shouts back at them. "Go on. I'll catch up."

Joel frowns. "You sure? Because we can totally wait." He folds his arms in front of him. "It's no problem at all. Safety in numbers."

"I'm fine. I'll catch up."

In the alley, Joey snorts a line off his driver's license. He snorts another one and then decides to finish the bag before they cross the border. It's more than he's used to. Three more lines and then he jams his tongue into the bag to get the rest.

Tyler and Joel cross the street and Joey lets out a thick stream of piss onto a pile of black trashbags.

A wave of pleasure moves up his spine as the warmth drains out of him.

He hears the motorcycle sirens before he sees their lights.

ALLEY, 2:15 A.M.

The first cop stays on his bike in the mouth of the alley while his partner rolls toward Joey and stops. "Geet on thee bike!" he shouts, propping the motorcycle on its kickstand and climbing off. He's a small man and his voice is high and sharp. He has sunglasses on even though it's dark; he takes them off and looks at Joey with a frown and puts them back on again.

The man rests his hand on his holster and takes a wide stance and repeats, "Get. On. The. Bike! This iss *illegal* what you are doing, pissing in public. You are going to *jail* for this."

"I just . . . I didn't—" Joey tries to talk but the speed hits him and he staggers back and falls onto the trashbags; he knows he's done too much. The fall is in slow motion. A long drop through the darkness. It takes a month and then a year and when Joey hits the bags, the soft, rotting trash inside has become bricks.

When Joey opens his eyes, his heart is bouncing in his chest and the cop is standing above him, a black silhouette against the alley lights with a big round helmet. "Stand op," he says. He unsnaps his holster and his hand is on the pistol grip. "Stand *op*!" The cop leans in close and he smells like campfire smoke (the desert outside Tijuana, ten hours past, and the execution of a cartel boss and a local banker. A bullet to each head, decapitation, the removal of the hands and feet, then burning the bodies in the *arroyo*. After that, a drive through the desert to a cafe known for its *nopal* tacos, dust boiling up behind the unmarked van. The cafe closed for the afternoon).

Joey pulls himself to his feet but his knees buckle and he falls again.

Stand up. Stand up stand up stand up. "Just . . . hold . . . and . . . just . . . wait for . . . ." He stands up and holds the alley wall for support. "L-legal," he stutters, his teeth chattering. He's already forgotten what was illegal and why he said "legal."

"*Legal?*"

"Legal." It's all he can say.

"Iss *legal* to piss in public in the States? Don't be silly with me, Mr. Comedian. I don't think your comedy iss funny."

Joey looks past the cops.

Tyler and Joel on the other side of the street. Tyler slumped forward, his hands shoved in his pockets, scared.

The traffic racing past them.

As the panic attack hits—boiling, shouting, gnashing its teeth, riding high a top the speed and sleeplessness and booze—Joey's mind makes words for him to say but they're moving too fast and he's scared they'll hit him and break pieces off his body. He *knows* they'll hit him. *Jail! Yale!* A near miss. *Pees! Pissing! Motorcycles Motorcycle Murder Mutter My Grant Ant An Man Main Mole Moan Moaning Money Money Money Money*. Money? But why money? *There's a reason. Why money, why money, why money?* He fights for it but the reason slips away like the snake that drinks Nicole's blood at night. (It's the fourth worst panic attack he's had. In order of severity: 1) Age ten, up in the middle of the night after a dream about a naked, red-skinned Satan—traditional Satan with pitchfork, pointed beard, and tail—chasing him around a quickly shrinking Earth. Then two hours of death blooming in his head and the world pressing up around him. His uncle standing in the frame of his bedroom door, a black cardboard cut-out uncle, shaking his head, "Go back to sleep, you crazy little faggot. Don't be such a little *bitch* all the time." His uncle with a beer can. Bringing the beer to his lips. Sipping. "Go to sleep *now* or I'll whup your ass." 2) Seven years later, stoned out of his mind on his uncle's stash. Goes out with some kids from school. Falls in the middle of a party, hits his head on the kitchen floor, and when he comes to, he's in a panic and he's sure he's either a) had a stroke, b) broke something inside his head, or c) lost his mind and that nothing will ever be the same again. Two days later he meets Nicole. His prediction comes true. 3) Age twenty, a minor overdose on ephedrine pills, red wine, Vicodin, and hash. In bed alone. A sudden narrowing of the world. In his chest, his organs popping and he can feel them burst and he can hear the sound ("Pissshhhff") and he knows his chest cavity is filling up with bacteria. Calls '911' but stops before the second '1'. Sits in the middle of his bedroom hugging a balloon he found on the beach, the only thing that keeps him positive until the panic attack is over. Talks to the balloon like it's a dog. Gives it a dog name. Puppy Ruffy. Puppy Ruffy loves to play outside and eat peanut-butter-flavored dog treats, which in Joey's mind he feeds him by the handful, handfuls of them, all he wants, whatever he wants, it's on me, here, eat, eat!) *Money. Money!* "Wait!" Joey tries to stuff his hand into his left hip pocket but his pants are too tight. "I have money. Wait. Just. Just hold on—just wait." His hands are shaking and his pockets are sealed up. "Wait, just wait. Why do they even. Put. Pockets in. Jeans. Sorry. Just wait, okay? Wait, I know I have—"

The cop stares at him and then looks back at his partner. He takes his sunglasses off and sticks them in the 'v' of his shirt. His eyes are bloodshot and tired. "Lissen," he says quietly. He looks at Joey sadly and shakes his head. "Lissen . . . you are going to jail and you pay your fine there. Iss . . . iss no big deal. Iss not like the States; we let you out as soon as you pay. You are not in big trouble. Your fine . . . it will be nothing. Jus' a little bit. You pay there. Don't worry. Jus' please come with—"

"*Migueliiito, vaaaamos, carnal,*" shouts his partner. "*Tengo haaambre. Hambre, hombre! Hombre, hambre. El chico esta boracho, es nada. Me voy, Migi.*"

"*Hector, momento!*" he says without looking back.

Joey: "It's okay. Really. Here. I have. Money," and he pulls the wad of bills from his pocket and it falls on the ground. "Wait. Wait." He gets down on one knee. "No, wait."

Joey gathering the bills off the ground, handing them up to the cop, his elbows jerking and his hands shaking. Some of the bills are wet. He tries to say something, but his voice is gone and he smiles and shrugs and then his eyes roll in his head uncontrollably. His mind is alive with information but none of it helps. Numbers: *4.5, 78, 12,010, 3.93, 1.67, 820, 5, 48, 900, 12.5, 457,12.5, 11, 340, 789, 143, 1, 6, 4.5* again. Combinations of letters. *Yook. Bou. Vol. Tes. Ih. Is. Ish. Ishaa.* Disembodied sets of words. *Sugar plantation force ceremony drowsing dogs bath Maggie apothecary carry doctorate matron bishop perspiration mason Bilbo Baggins Jimmy Connors memorial unforgettable teeth machine*. Names of kids he went to middle school with. *Damon Shigliak evil bowl-cutted snake Dungeons & Dragons figurines sweater barf Tate "Tater" Bradley punched you in the stomach the wall-ball courts you cried in front of Sunny and Claire my god Sunny and Little round Osa Nuñez sister of the famous Autistic pianist they made a documentary about*. Names of girls he liked who didn't like him. *Sunny Greenwood and Claire Stoner and Sarah Mary, Sarah Mary Negron the pastor's daughter who died last year in a boating accident in Cancun my god you're dead I used to imagine us fucking*. A list of ways to die. *Shark attack car accident cancer freak accident outdoors fall off a ladder fall off a roof stray gunshot home invasion mugging heart attack snake bite drowning and the worst my god you're standing in the shower in your stupid apartment singing "And the thunder rolls! / The lightning strikes! / Another love goes cohhhhld on a sleepless nigh-igh-igh-ight," and you step back to play air guitar and you slip on a worn-down shard of soap and hit your head and once they find you you've shit yourself and you're bloated and rotting and the shower's still running and you STINK and that's all anyone can think about "This guy sure stinks." The EMT with the mustache: "Fucking gross, we have to clean this up fucking gross disgusting dead asshole, I bet he died singing Garth Brooks."* A breakfast cereal ad and the cartoon ringmaster marching in place, twirling his baton, singing, "*Hello my name is Crispy. How do you doooo? Crispy Critters cereal's entirely newwww.*" And his great-uncle on his deathbed, his voice croaking, *"I shot at the fox but hit the hen he carried in his mouth."* Hit the hen bouncing an endless loop *hit the hen hit the hen hit the hen hit the hen hit the hen hit the hen hit the hen in his mouth. Fox the at shot I I tohs ta eht xof And Money Right On Mister Money Bags Bueno Okay.*

"Okay, jus' . . . okay. Quiet." The cop takes Joey's money in his gloved hands and looks back at his partner and shakes his head.

His partner is laughing.

Joey's arms outstretched. Pushed out into space like satellite antennas. Reaching for something. He can't pull them back. They've turned to steel.

The cop laughs. "You, *gringo*, are fucking *crazy*," he says. "Go home don't drive nowhere take a cab go home to your parents be safe don't come back you drink too mush."

"Thank you. Thank you. Really. Thank you. I really . . . appreciated it. I promise I won't ever—"

"Go home, *gringo*," he puts his sunglasses back on. "Don't come back to Mexico. We don't want you here. You and your money . . . this isn't your playground, *gringo. . . fucking tourists*. Go back to . . . to . . . Naybraska-Ohio-or-what-I-dunno."

The cop walks back to his bike. He straddles it and kicks it started and gives Joey a wave.

There's a *mariachi* song playing in one of the dark apartments above him ("*Volveras / A buscar calor de nido / Que dejaste en el olvido / Nuevamente volveras*"). The cops are gone. Traffic moving past. Tyler and Joel waiting at the stoplight.

Tyler raising a meek hand to wave.

The panic attack fading, fading but still darkening the edges, quivering in the nerves, sick in the fiber.

Joey dusts himself off and makes his way to the crosswalk.

HOME, DAWN

Back at his apartment, Joey drops his keys on the carpet by the door. Maggie's wrapped up in a Mexican blanket, sleeping on the couch and Joey lies down with her and then she's awake and she puts her arms around him and he's warm. "Alive," she says in a scratchy voice.

"Alive."

"I'm hungry," she says.

"Me too."

"Take me to the place where the milkshakes are."

"Okay. I need to get—"

"I'm kidding, Joey. Let me pour you a bath and I'll make breakfast."

"Tomato sandwiches?"

"How 'bout scrambled eggs and quesadillas?"

"When did *you* learn how to cook?"

"Don't tease."

"Is there sour cream?"

"I think you have sour cream. I'll check."

"Lime slices on the side?"

"I think you've got some limes in the fridge. Got any more unreasonable demands?"

"I'll think of something."

"How was Mexico?"

"I don't know yet."

"Was Joel alright?"

"Joel?"

"Joel," she laughs, waking up now. "The Joel you took to watch naked girls, nerd-breath. You know he just came out, right?"

"He came out of what?"

"Joel's gay."

"Oh."

"He told me a couple days ago. I guess I knew already. I think I've known since we were kids. Without *knowing*."

"He took care of Tyler when he was sick. He's a good guy. We need to hang out more, the three of us."

"I thought you'd be back hours ago."

"Yeah."

"You guys have an okay time?"

"No. Not at all."

"You're here now."

"I am."

"And you're okay."

"I am."

Maggie pours the bath and gets him a forty from the fridge and he holds the side of the wall and lets himself ease in. The water steams and burns and all the tension lifts out of him.

"Is it too hot?" she calls from the kitchen.

"It's perfect." He has a hard time getting the words out.

Joey unscrews the cap from the forty and takes a sip. He hasn't eaten anything but Bimbo Bread since Wednesday and he feels the beer cold and twisting all the way down and now his hunger is back and the smell of flour tortillas frying in the kitchen makes his stomach tighten up. He puts the cap back on the bottle and lets it sit on his chest, half-sunk. Silverware tinkling. The faucet. Plates clatter. The faucet again. On the stereo, Maggie's playing a Mexican folk record that Chente gave Joey for his birthday. "*Soy borrrracho y trobadorrrr!*" the singer cries out over the mellow chording of a Spanish guitar. Steam rising from the bath. Sleep coming. Morning. Sunlight from down the hall.

HILLCREST, 6:12 P.M.

The next day, Maggie says she's ready and asks Joey to get tested. "Yeah, of course, sure," and he remembers the magazine story about the man dying of AIDS, his final days, a skeleton with skin over it lying in his bathtub drinking cranberry juice and watching it come straight out of his body as soon as it was in, pissing it out, the water clouding purple around him. Joey was eight when he heard that. It scared the hell out of him.

On Thursday after work, Joey goes to Planned Parenthood in Hillcrest and leaves with a slip of paper that says to call for results.

That night, they fool around until it's too much and she says, "Get a condom."

"Really?"

"Yeah. Really."

"You sure you're sure? The test won't be back for a week. You sure?"

"I am. Get a condom."

Joey finds a condom and she rolls it onto him while he watches her hands move in the dark.

MISSION BAY, DUSK

They were called ghost shrimp and you could make a living selling them to the fishermen at the docks and to the men at the tackle stores. Most of the tackle stores are gone now but the good one was between the bridges by SeaWorld and they sold them in fridge coolers alongside the long white table bins of glittery oiled plastic worms. This was middle school. Me and Travis and Travis' twin sister Meggy and Robby Hakaka and "Tall" Tim Sanders—Sanders, who became a football star in high school and stopped talking to us the day he made the team. After school, we had nowhere to go and nothing to do so we would meet at my house and walk down to the bay and watch the women dredge for shrimp. We would sit by the old docks where you could still smell tar from construction years ago and, when the wind was right, the rotting wood planks above the smell of the bay. There was a rosy dimming sky and the water the same color but darker, a blushing purple-rose, the surface of the water still—not a ripple. It was October. I remember October and that the air had smoke in it from beach-fires and that the sunsets gave the sand an orange tint and we were wearing sweaters with shorts and we had bare feet and end-of-summer tans. Meggy was dressed like a boy in long shorts and big t-shirts with surf company logos on them—Quicksilver, Gotcha, Stussy, Rusty, Jimmy Z's—and only became a girl to us when she turned sixteen and had breasts and long legs overnight. We were all strangers by the time I hit ninth grade. (These days Meggy models for swimsuit ads in surf magazines. She started to at the end of high school and I used jerk off to her bikini ads and feel terrible for it. Her brother Travis is in the Army. He enlisted when he turned eighteen. "Tall" Tim still lives up the street from my aunt and uncle. We pass on the sidewalk sometimes and he doesn't recognize me. Robby? Could be dead for all I know, but I hope he's not. He was nice, a short kid, Iranian ["Persian" he said], loved WWF wrestling shows, carrots dipped in peanut butter, and Legos.) The five of us . . . we sat there and the bay-waters were quiet and still like a lake. Behind us, the weedy dirt cliff with houses, their lighted windows shining like gold, a line of twin-hull catamarans pulled up past the high-tide mark, the big colorful sails wrapped around the mast and tied down. You would sit on the webbing of one of the big 'cats, dangling your feet with your toes in the sand and watch the Vietnamese women in white pajama suits or cuffed-up baggy jeans and blousy oversized shirts and rice patty hats walking along the shore with PVC pipe guns for catching the shrimp. The ghost shrimp guns were a large white tube with a smaller tube inside, a rope handle on the end. They would push the outer tube at an angle into the sand at the shoreline and when they pulled the smaller tube's handle, it made a suction and whatever was in the smaller tube was captured up with it. (The sound it made was just like you might imagine.) The women would plunge the tubes in and pull them up and then dump the wet sand out onto the hard-packed sand and pick out the flicking, jerking shrimp from the rocks and bits of shells. And then they would take their buckets and tube guns and move to a new spot, and the shoreline at the water's edge would be a mess of collapsing, crumbling holes. And then the bay-water would come in (seeping up from below) and the holes would fill up with water and wet sand and the surface of the sand would even out.

HOME, 7 P.M.

After two weeks on speed, Joey goes back to work because the money is gone and somehow in his absence he's been given a promotion which came with a raise. The money flies in and he spends it just as fast. Every fiber in him says, *Stop. You're being stupid. Stop spending money,* but he's given up listening to himself. *What is money? Nothing. Get rid of it.* There are feasts with sourdough bread sandwiches piled high with buffalo mozzarella, pesto, tomato, and basil. Red wine in coffee cups, jars of Kalamata olives. Casserole dishes of hybrid lasagna-manicotti (Maggie invented this and calls it "Maggicotti"). Without speed in his system, Joey's hungry and he wants to taste everything. He and Maggie throw dinner parties for Nicole and Rory and Joel with pots of marinara sauce bubbling on the stove, the windows steaming up against the chill outside, frying pans with mushrooms and onions and bell peppers simmering in olive oil. And garlic bread in the oven—endless baking sheets of garlic bread with Monterrey jack and sharp cheddar melting on top, the great doughy smell filling the apartment, a sink full of ice chilling bottles of Mexican beer. It's a race all week to get rid of the money and then as soon as the next check comes, it starts back up again.

As the company prospers, Joey's co-workers show up in the morning with new clothes and expensive phones and watches. On Monday, one of the Jeffs brings the whole office out to the parking lot to see his new car. A black Lexus. Low to the ground. "Year 2000. New century, dudes. *The man*," he says referring to himself (dramatic pause, thumb to his chest), "needed new wheels. Can I get a 'hell yeah'?" And he got one.

"You know what? *Fuck* new wheels," Joey tells Maggie that night after work. "I want *fun*. Let's go out to eat at Pokez and go see three movies and get ice cream and throw a party every day this week. Let's buy some booze. Wine! A case of wine! New records! Let's go places and buy things!"

"Let's go places and buy things!" she says back to him, wrapping her arms around his chest and stepping up on his shoes with her bare feet. Her hair smells like Jolly Ranchers. She puts her head to Joey's chest and holds him tight.

WORK, AFTERNOON

An email from Maggie pops up: "jc, when are you quitting your job and coming home? quit those fuckers and come now. seriously. i'm at your desk in your room typing this and i just woke up and it made me so happy thinking about you coming home and all the trouble we're going to cause tonight. i need you here. i miss you. come get me and let's go for a drive. let's go places and buy things. come feed me. don't force me to come liberate you and knock over desks and show my ass to people and throw red paint on all the jeffs. do it, come home and kiss me, quit now. come on, you and me. xoxo, miss maggie"

PLACES, THINGS

Gasoline and a pack of Marlboro Lights at Chevron in Pacific Beach. Two orders of fettuccine alfredo with extra sauce from an open air cafe in Little Italy, the big wine bottle of table red, brushetta, Italian bread with a side of warm (seasoned) olive oil, garlic butter, crème brule, and a dish of chocolate ice cream. A box of candles, a blacklight bulb, a book on Haitian death rituals, and a red Bic lighter from The Black in O.B. A mint mocha, a vanilla latte, and a chocolate chip cookie at Java Joe's. Two chocolate chip bagels and an orange juice from Bruegers. Potato rolled tacos, a veggie burrito, and two large Cokes from El Cotixan. Two orders of mock kung po, two bowls of egg drop soup, an order of crispy fried wontons, and steamed rice from Mandarin Dynasty (free soft drinks for you and Joel and Maggie and Rory). Two vegetarian potato burritos and a small Coke to share from Valentine's. Gasoline and an energy drink at Hillcrest Mobile. Chips from El Indio for Maggie's mom. A cup of mango sorbetto to share, a Spumoni milkshake, a scone, and two small cups of gelato (Brownies and Caramel Cream for Maggie, Espresso Bean for you) from Gelato Vero. A grilled cheese sandwich, a veggie burger, two orders of fries, and two Cokes at Corvette Diner. Two movie tickets, two large Cokes, and a large popcorn at La Jolla Landmark. A pack of spearmint gum, Ruffles, a forty of Mickey's, peanut M&Ms, a Mars bar, a Hershey's almonds, and a Milky Way at 7-Eleven in Pacific Beach. A bottle of Jack Daniels, a pint of vodka, a two liter 7-Up, a bag of Swedish Fish, a bag of Peach Rings, a jar of mild salsa, a bag of tortilla chips, and a jar of Queso dip at Circle K in Clairemont. Two movie tickets at AMC 20, large Cherry Coke to share, nachos with jalapeños and extra cheese, large popcorn with butter flavoring, Raisinets, and Red Vines (to bring home for Molly and Cecilie). A wooden Day of the Dead skeleton and a small glass diorama of a skeleton mariachi band at a shop in Bazaar Del Mundo. A plastic cap gun, a pint of Jack Daniels, and condoms from Ralphs in Clairemont. A car wash, the "magic car wash" Maggie calls it, where the soap comes down in colored foamy streams and you sit in the cab of the truck and pretend it's a movie and Maggie gets so happy that she slaps her hands on the dashboard and you say, "There you go again getting slappy" and she says, "Getting what?" A calico Dust Bowl dress for Maggie from Buffalo Exchange. A bag of red grapes, a tub of hummus, a block of Colby jack, a bag of clear cat's eye marbles, two gala apples, and a bottle of merlot from Ralph's in Clairemont. Two cheese sub-sandwiches, a turkey sub to go (for Jolie), two bags of Sun Chips, and a small Dr. Pepper to share (free refills) at Submarina. A stack of books at Tower Records. Tofu fajitas, a rice and bean burrito, two Cherry Cokes, chips and salsa, and a handful of Skittles from the quarter machine at Pokez. Gasoline and a pack of Marlboro Lights at the Mobile Downtown. A potato burrito, a chili relleno *burrito, two quesadillas (for Maggie's mom and Cecilie), "personal chips," a side order of guacamole, a side of lime slices, and a tub of hot carrots from El Cotixan. Two movie tickets at Fashion Valley, nachos, small Dr. Pepper, small Cherry Coke, small popcorn, Whoppers. A pack of Marlboro Lights and a bag of Smartfood from Circle K in Clairemont. Gasoline at a mom and pop place off the freeway. A bottle of Caribbean rum, a six pack of Tecate, a baguette of French bread, a jar of blackberry jam, a block of cheddar cheese, a box of Morningstar Chik Nuggets, a loaf of white bread, a box of condoms, and a family-size bag of Ruffles from Ralph's. Assorted used CDs from Music Trader in P.B. A bag of macaroni noodles, a pound of butter, a block of cheddar, and a box of Ritz Crackers (for Maggie's mom) at Ralph's Hillcrest. A pair of big black sunglasses from Forever 21. A case of Corona, a case of Tecate, three bags of tortilla chips (strips), a bag of Fritos, a jar of mild salsa, a jar of hot salsa, a jar of Queso dip, a can of jalapeño bean dip, a jug of Carlo Rossi red rose, a jug of Carlo Rossi burgundy, a bag of mini pretzels, a bag of nacho cheese Combos, a fifty-pack of red plastic party cups, and a three-pack of paper towels at Von's. A stack of magazines from Off the Record. Spaghetti pomodoro, fettuccine alfredo, two salads, an ice tea, two orders of spumoni ice cream from the Old Spaghetti Factory Downtown. A tub of hummus and a bottle of Two Buck Chuck cabernet savignon from Trader Joe's in Hillcrest. Three rented DVDs at Blockbuster Video. Two fake silver rings from Claire's. A croissant, a baguette, three sugar cookies (for Cecilie, Molly, and Maggie's mom), and an espresso at the French Bakery. Two pretzels from Pretzel Time, one side of marinara, large lemonade. A sticker and a box of Japanese bandaids (for Jolie) at Sanrio Surprise. Two movie tickets at AMC 20, a small Coke to share, Junior Mints. Quesadilla at El Cotixan to share. Gasoline at Circle K in Clairemont.*

1980

SEPTEMBER 25TH

Spent the last few days in bed. It's getting colder (unseasonably) and I can't find the energy to get up and go. The big news these days is Issy and Gus and their "surprise engagement." Of course to all of us it was no surprise, but that's what Issy keeps calling it, the "surprise engagement." The plan is a December 1st wedding. Issy wants to keep it simple but Gus is going all out; he plans meals and orders things from catalogs and spends hours on the phone with Issy's dad taking care of logistics. The idea is to do it traditional. Issy's dad has money, but Gus is chipping in half, so it should be impressive. Channy has taken to calling Gus "the secret Victorian."

"Oh! I forgot to tell you! The secret Victorian ordered two hundred *Russian church candles.*"

"Channy, you're reading into it."

"I'm not. He's the secret Victorian."

"You *want* him to be."

"He is.

"For you, he is."

"Listen, Mercantile, for all your quote-unquote photographic memory and top-of-the-class-ness, you lose out in the most important department of all."

"Which is?"

"You're a *man*. I'm a better judge of character because I'm woman."

"Oh yeah?"

"Don't be sarcastic. Women have to see men for what they are because the process of deciding on a mate is much more complicated for women. Instinctively men are looking for a vessel to carry their progeny and if they had their way . . . well, you know. But women need to make sure the man will protect her, stay with her for life, meet her needs intellectually, hunt, fight off the Huns and barbarians; there's a lot more going into the equation on this side."

"You just set the women's movement back thirty years."

"You know what I mean."

"I guess."

"I'm looking at it from the primitive stance but as a woman . . . a modern woman . . . you still look at men from a dozen different angles. Guys are like, 'Can I stick my thing in this, yes or no?' but women have to be careful. The decision deals with a much more . . . more . . . c'mon Mr. Scrabble, you know what I'm looking for."

"Multifaceted?"

"No, but that works. A multifaceted spectrum of qualifications. So, when I see Gus, I don't see the Texas cowboy who everyone else sees. I mean, I see that, too, but there's a lot more to him than that. You know this: Gus comes from money. His family has had cattle in America forever. But before that, they did the same thing in England."

"I thought his family was some rags to riches American West thing."

"It's bigger than that. His family is old money . . . *old world* old money. See, another thing where girls win out over guys is that we *talk*. We ask each other *questions*. Men don't talk to men. Not about anything important."

"That's not true at all."

"It's not totally true but there's a pretty substantial basis for what I'm saying. Women dig for answers like a bunch of newshounds. We share. Issy and I . . . we have these . . . you should've seen it when you were back east with Jacob, we'd stay up all night and have these big, epic girl-talks and they would last hours and hours and hours—hours on one single subject, archery, politics, shipbuilding, music, chickens, Civil Rights, family—one subject picked apart and examined and autopsied. The point is women talk to each other and we're better off for it. I know *everything* about Gus. Just like Issy knows everything about *you*."

"Remember that thing about me hating you?"

"Listen, you might think me and Issy talking like that is a violation of confidence, but it's not about privacy or . . . or about keeping secrets. In friendships like mine and Issy's, you knock down the barrier and everything is open and available. I know that Gus grew up in these . . . these *candlelit*, cloth napkin, dining rooms with *servants* and in . . . in, like, oil baron cattlemen lunchrooms full of cigar smoke and that he was sent to Europe for school. Of course he can handle himself on a ranch, but he's better read than either of us. Gus studied literature in Oxford and architecture in Rome. He was bred to handle physical work and he can ride and shoot and whatever else, but he was also brought up in the ways of . . . I don't even know how you'd say it . . . which shows how *I* was raised . . . in . . . in, like, high-class-big-money-social-etiquette-land. He's a businessman to the core and he has taste that's *pretty far* on the conservative side."

"Reagan-conservative?"

"It's more than that. It's a basic fundamental set of standards. I mean, it's no secret that Bride Isabella would be fine with a simple, no frills farmhouse wedding, but Gus wouldn't have it that way."

Whenever Channy says the word "secret," my stomach goes tight. I need to tell her about Sorel and the women in Mexico. It's eating me up, but I'm afraid of losing this good thing that we've got. Life now is life as I've always imagined it. What I saw as a boy was school and then work and then a beautiful family life. The school and work part was a bust but I have the important part, and I have it at twenty-one, not thirty or fourty like I imagined.

But Sorel. How do I tell Channy after all this time? I feel like there's a me who has become a good man—an honest, moral, dependable man. And then there's this me who is just awful, a liar, passive-aggressive, weak character. I want to be gallant and self-sacrificing, but I'm lazy. I don't want to deal with confrontation and the repercussions. Maybe admitting that is the first step. Regardless, I need to own up. But how?

2000

FASHION VALLEY MALL, 6 P.M.

In November, the department store windows are full of Christmas decorations, empty boxes wrapped like presents, silver tinsel hanging in metallic waterfalls, cotton snow billowing, animatronic Santa Clauses twisting at the waist and ringing bells, fake trees with white plastic spray. Joey walks through the mall to the sound of holiday songs, the drums slow and snowy: all the standards, jazzy and quiet, the new ones, the holiday pop songs, the kind you hear in every mall courtyard by every mall fountain, in every department store with their big glass gold displays of perfume, the salesgirls in new white starched shirts and sharp collars and black slacks, their hair in perfect dark-blonde ponytails, leaning on the counters to talk to customers. (And over the speakers the Peanuts singing, "Christmastiiime . . . is here / Haaappiness and cheer / Fun for all . . . that children call . . . their favorite time of yeeear / Snowflakes in the aaair / Carols everywherrre / Olden times and ancient rhymes of love and dreams to share." Joey starts to cry, but he's not unhappy. The song gets him. The tenderness in their voices and the innocence, their somber, quiet love for Christmas. *Motherfucking Peanuts,* he thinks. He loves them. Loves the motherfucking Peanuts. Charlie Brown, Linus, Lucy, the boy with the dust clouds around him whose name he can never remember, even Peppermint Patty. He starts to cry but he stops before it's a problem. No tears. He's happy, but raw. His nerves are close to the surface.)

Joey walks through the mall and looks for something to get Maggie, something to reassure her that the fun wasn't just a fluke now that he's broke.

The money is gone.

Gone, and he's out of ideas and the endless party is now a musty apartment with no one in it, Maggie off with her boyfriend for his birthday, and Joey in the mall, thirty-five dollars in cash and fourteen in his checking. It's a cold, clear, sad afternoon.

He looks at a row of silver rings but shuffles off when the salesgirl starts towards him. "Sir, can I show you something? Sir?" (And what a horrible thing to be called 'sir'. It makes him feel weak, old.) Joey browsing racks of new winter coats and tiny colorful sneakers with their plastic-y suede smells and bracelets with fake rubies, the dusky glow glimmering red-black. Thumbing through the DVDs that Maggie might like (a stack in his hands at the gothy teenager chain store. Too expensive and not really cool at all. Puts them all back with a sigh.) None of it means anything to him and it won't mean anything to her. He gives up and takes the escalator to the food court and buys a pretzel the size of a steering wheel with a side of nacho cheese sauce. (The side of cheese is thimble-size, the pretzel won't dunk and it makes him want to throw the pretzel across the court or just get up and leave.) He tells himself things like, *You know she deserves more than the best thing you can find here* and *You know she'll understand that you're broke* and *You know she doesn't care about this kind of stupid materialistic bullshit crap*. He tells himself, *This is not a game plan. This is you being a little bitch.* At his table, an empty seat across from him, Joey tears a tiny piece off the pretzel and dunks it in the cheese sauce and takes a bite and it hits him: *A party. You beg, borrow, and steal to throw her a party, a party to remember. The big one. The blow-out. Your sister's coming to town for the week. Nicole and Rory are back from their trip to Yosemite. You can ask Curt to come and hopefully he'll bring stuff. And you'll invite Ted Boone.*

HOME, 7 P.M.

"Hi. Ted Boone? It's Joey Carr."

"Carr?"

"Yeah. It's Joey Carr."

"*Yes*? Who's this? Carr, is that you? Is that you, Carr? I can hear you drooling on the other line."

"Ted Boone, I'm throwing a party and I need you there to make it special. It's next week and you have to go. Friday night. Tons of people. Food, drinks, music. It'll be fun. I promise."

Silence. "Carr, you caught me napping, and when I wake up from a nap, I'm never sure what day it is. 'What day is it?' I'll shout to no one at all. 'Is it Monday? Did I miss work? Am I late for school?! Is someone mad at me?' Carr, someone is . . . always," Ted Boone yawning, "mad at me. Imagine living with that. Carr . . . this party. Will there be girls?" His voice is a slow croak of a Southern drawl (affected; he's from El Centro like Chente), the sound of a door creaking open, a creaking chair. Ted Boone is a big Orson Wellesian man with long, ratty hair tucked behind his ears. He wears ancient t-shirts that stretch over his potbelly, slouchy pants, and a drooping, sinister handlebar mustache. He's interested in everything and he loves to talk—always slow, measured, drawling. He'll tell you about new-age cults, masonic rituals. He'll give you disproved theories, thoughts on hypnosis, cults of the 1970s (his favorites: the Source Family, Boston Church of Christ, Werner Erhard's Seminars Training, Divine Light Mission, the Moonies, People's Temple, Saul Newton's Sullivan Institute, the Forever Family), UFO cults (especially the Raelian Church and the Unarians), German mysticism, sexual bondage, medical oddities, sadism, mechanical miracles, anything Satanic, anything Russian, or archaic Jewish. (The last five books he read are as follows: 1) *Fighting Mind Control* [Thomas J. Mason Jr., 1971], 2) *Bibles, Guns, and Texas: The Siege on Waco* [Henry Davis Petrus, 2000], 3) *Zoroastrianism and Post-War American Thought* [Patrice Hera, 1945], 4) *The Left-Hand Path and Pentagonal Revisionism* [Cara Gilman, 1978], 5) *Satan Speaks!* [Anton LaVey, 1997].)

Joey tells him that yes, there will be girls and booze and whatever else he might want. He tells him he's the guest of honor.

Silence.

"Weed?" says Ted Boone.

"Weed what?"

"As in, will there be. As in, Carr will there be weed for me at your party because I require weed to be the most realized version of myself."

"If you want weed, there will be weed." Joey grips the phone between his shoulder and cheek and makes a note of it on the back of his hand. 'Curt Weed,' in Sharpie.

"The final request of the weary maestro," he says with a sigh, "is chips and guacamole made from fresh avocados."

"Guacamole. Of course. No problem. I'm great at guacamole."

"No, listen. This recipe cannot be tampered with. There's no wiggle room here. Listen. Chips, yellow corn tortilla chips, restaurant style, strips, rounds, triangles, whatever you can find, not important. Well, scratch that. Not triangles. Triangles break. Go for rounds. Rounds for maximized scooping power. And salted. Unsalted chips are for the dying and miserable. Now . . . now . . . Ted Boone's Famous Evil Guacamole Recipe, write this down. Important—one dozen avocados. A handful of cherry tomatoes. Get the teardrop-shaped ones. I don't know the name. Do they even have a name? The teardrop ones. Not the round ones. Diced. One quarter red onion, minced. You're writing this down, aren't you, Carr? Use all-caps for this: Lemon juice, half cup, fresh, not from the plastic lemon. Don't insult me with the plastic lemon, Carr."

Joey agrees with him about the plastic lemon, even though he likes the plastic lemon.

"Listen, Carr. For the grand finale: the briefest *shake*—sh-sh-shake that's all—of red pepper flakes, then salt and black pepper and garlic powder to taste. You know what that means, Carr, don't you? 'To taste'? Start small; work your way up. A shake, then taste. A shake, and another taste. Little bites. And that part is all-important, Carr. *All. Important. Carr.* You've seen *What About Bob?*, haven't you, Carr? Baby steps. *Baby Steps* by Dr. Leo Marvin, the best-seller to end all best-sellers, the best-seller you keep in your best cellar. 'Baby steps into the elevator.' 'Baby steps onto the bus.' Start small and work your way up. (Underline that, Carr.) The flavor will ride or die on those four basic additions. Can you do that, Carr? This is my binding legal contract. It's a deal-breaker. It's my Famous Evil Guacamole, or no Ted Boone."

Joey tells him that, yes, there will be guacamole and baby steps to make it and that it will be evil.

"Well, Carr," he takes a deep breath, "my requirements are satisfied. As of right now, I will be there. As of—what day is it? Monday?"

Joey tells him yes.

"As of today, Monday, this minute . . . uh . . . it's what, it's 7:03 exactly, 7:04 p.m., I will be there."

Joey starts to give him directions but Ted Boone cuts him off.

"Stop! Stop. I won't need directions. I know everything, Carr." And with that, he hangs up on Joey.

HOME, 7:05 P.M.

As soon as Ted Boone hangs up, the phone rings again and Joey answers it.

"Listen, Carr. Have you heard of Cotard's Syndrome?"

"Hi, Ted Boone. I don't think I have."

"Carr! Hello, Carr?! Are you listening?! Are you awake?!" he knocks on the phone. "Carr, Cotard's, do you know it, are you familiar with the lingo? (You should've stayed in college, my friend.) Cotard's Syndrome is where the stricken believes they are either dead or putrefying. In special cases . . . in the rarest of cases, they believe they don't exist or—and this is my favorite—you're listening, right, Carr? In the rarest of cases, they believe they have become *immortal*. Immortal, Carr! Picture me, Carr. Picture me two weeks ago sitting in my apartment listening to a tape of 'Mr. Tambourine Man' on a loop, loud enough to shake the walls, a head full of cocaine, the book open on my lap and the *joy* I experienced reading about Cotard's. Can you see me? Listen," singing softly, "'Down the foggy ruins of time / Far past the frozen leaves / The haunted, frightened trees / Out to the windy beach / Far from the twisted reach of crazy sorrow.' Close your eyes and *be there*. Picture me."

"I can see you."

"Go back in time. Picture me."

"I am."

"Okay. Now, ask me which one I am," he drawls happily. "Ask me which *Cotard's* patient I am."

"Okay, Ted Boone. Which one?"

"For a while I thought I was dead, walking dead, in that someone had *hexed* me and I was rotting slowly from within, from the gut on out, *bleeeah!* In the quietest time of the night, when I was most alone with my thoughts and senses, after all the clamoring . . . screaming . . . spicy food cooking, drum-beating islanders I share a wall with had gone to bed, I could smell it, *I could smell myself rotting*. My burden for all the years of villainry, piracy, and evil. Just a whiff. It was barely detectable, *barely* there but I could smell the *death* coming from me. *The death*. Picture me. You are me and I am you. 'I am you and you are me and we are all together.' Imagine what it would be like to smell yourself in the midst of decay. Just think of it. When you smell death, it sticks with you and you can't get the smell out of your nose. Then, like all things, it fades. The rot went on until I couldn't smell it anymore. It became such a part of me that I lost track of it, like a person shut up in their house who doesn't smell their own catbox. Later, I decided I didn't *exist* at all, but now—"

"Now you're immortal."

"Carr, last week while researching cannibalism, I happened upon the story of an *in*famous case of Cotard's where the patient (called for the sake of anonymity, Mademoiselle X) first denied the existence of any supernatural divinity. Then, later in her tragic, well-documented decline she disbelieved certain parts of her *body* and then, horribly, her own biological need to *eat*. As her disorder progressed she decided she could no longer be killed by any natural means."

"So—"

"So, nothing. I'm just talking out of my ear, you know me. This means nothing! Pay no attention to the man behind the phone! Carr, you sickening, cowardly, syphilitic deviant, let's go see my favorite naked Russian dance at the nudie bar."

"I can't tonight.

"I'll pick you up at nine in the ever-ready Boonemobile. I'm going to hang up on you now without saying goodbye like people on TV. Don't forget to get ones. Ones, ones, Carr! Okay and—"

The dialtone.

STRIP CLUB, CLAIREMONT, MIDNIGHT

Sophisticated Sam's Gentleman's Club on Convoy Street. A parking lot full of cars and a bouncer smoking out front with one of the girls (their last three topics of conversation: 1) Fish and chips as opposed to Rubio's fish tacos, 2) Which of their shared acquaintances are on drugs tonight [two out of five], and 3) whether the actor from the Quaker Oats commercial is still alive. His verdict: no. Hers: yes.) Ted Boone and Joey inside, sitting in front of the stage, watching the girl Ted Boone came to see. Ted Boone elbows Joey and nods at her and Joey looks up from his drink. The girl grabs hold of the pole and swings herself around it then begins to climb up it like a rope, muscles straining, thighs squeezing the metal. The song: "Sweet Home Alabama."

"Perfect ass, Carr. You have never seen an ass like that. No one has. Alesanda's ass is like Helen of Troy's face." Ted Boone pulls his St. Louis Cardinals cap low over his eyes and lights a cigarette and takes a long, slow drag. "Carr, can I share something about me in the spirit of demystification?"

"Always, Ted Boone."

"The reason, Carr, listen, the reason why people give me whatever I want and why girls sleep with me far and wide is I remind them of the vastly under-appreciated character actor *Philip Seymour Hoffman*. Even if they don't *know* they know him, they *know* him. He's one of those ubiquitous actors who is, as people say, *in everything*. You see him on the screen and you get this wonderful, warm glow inside you, this cozy feeling of security that everything, without exception, is going to be alright. You turn and whisper to your friend sitting next to you holding the popcorn in his lap, 'Oh, it's him! I love him! What's his name? He's in everything.' That's me, Carr. I'm in *everything*."

"I don't think he's a character actor anymore. I think everybody knows him."

"Him but not his *name*."

"No, I think they know his name too. *Magnolia, Almost Famous, Boogie Nights*."

"In what circles? *Certain* circles."

"All circles. Everyone's circles."

"That doesn't matter. Carr, what matters is that people trust me. I'm like a brand that they've been buying all their lives, but a brand that keeps *surprising them* by delivering products that are a wide and distinctive cut above the rest, the next *step*, the new evolution of an already classic idea. Alesanda up there on the pole, she sees it. She *sees* it." He makes a 'v' with his fingers and points it at his eyes and then hers. "She sees it. Every night, I'm in here giving her money and charming her as does the diapered Hindu (flute in hand) to the swaying cobra. We talk. In Russian, in English. We talk a lot is what I'm saying, but nothing more than that. Just talk. That and *only* that because I'm waiting for my *window*. I'll know when the time is right to make my move and then I'll strike and when I strike I will be *impossible* to resist. Mind control, Carr. You need to read Jacques Ellul's *Propaganda and the Formation of Men's Attitudes*. Coercive persuasion. Thought reform. Only, to me, it comes naturally. It's how I roll. That . . . is the web . . . Ted Boone . . . hath *woven*. I move the masses by moving myself. Live by example! Be better and they will bend from your path like long grass! That's how the world sees me. Not larger than life but *better* than life. They see me like they would like to see *themselves*, and that is the world's favorite kind of man. Everyone thinks if they just did this or if they just did that then they could be not just the *better* version of themselves but the *them* that's been waiting all along for a reason to *stand up*. It's a comforting thought while we all wallow in base mediocrity and second-bests and Mom-I-trieds and general disappointment. It's the thought that says: *If only* this, *If only* that and then fill in the blank, I could do whatever I want, I could live up to my potential. Of course, most people never put in the work and because of that they like to live vicariously through the brave hero archetype that people like me represent. Men write books about souls like mine but I'm beating them to the punch by writing my *own* book. The story of Ted Boone, nonfiction, as yet untitled. I'm halfway done with the second chapter. Twelve pages in. I'll show it to you. Someday. If you want I'll sign it. Do you want me to sign it?"

"I guess, sure."

Ted Boone snaps his fingers in the air for the cocktail waitress and she glares at him and walks past without stopping. "*And*," he continues, "*and* people also hate me because I have that kind of coveted, nebulous star quality. I'm the most despised man in San Diego but I could be whatever I want. I could be a newscaster, you know that. I could be the *mayor*, Carr," he drawls, "and I'm not saying that in a boastful . . . hubristic . . . *self-aggrandizing* way. It breaks my *heart*. I don't *like* it, Carr." He frowns dramatically. "I hate that I've got all this inherent *charm* and *talent* and boundless potential. I'd rather be some castoff *bum* and watch TV and eat all day. Sit on the couch, eat fried chicken by the bucket-load, suck it down like guts and slime, put my greasy finger up my nose, squeak, squeak, squeak, watch the news, watch the soaps. I want the biggest part of my day to be when I get out of bed and go to Sombrero's and buy a cup of *horchata* from the white plastic vat at the counter. *Small pleasures*. I want my life to be like driving through an endless orange grove with the windows down and the fragrant air wafting in and the sun flashing through the windshield. I want it *easy,* but it's never easy. You know, when I was younger . . . Carr, you know what I realized when I was younger?"

"No, what?" Joey takes out his wallet and sets a dollar on the stage.

"I realized . . . no, I *decided* . . . no, one day I had an *epiphany* that I would be rich in my golden years. I just *knew* it, and I know it *to this day*." He beats his fist on the rail. "To! This! Day! I knew then and I know now that one day, some day, I'll be so rich I won't know what to *do* with all the money. I'll stack it up tall and varnish it beautifully and then walk on it like stilts, grinning and waving to the filthy plebes as they play their crude fifes and pipes, beating on drums, singing 'Who is this one? / Whose favorite son?' I'll buy rugged stretches of golden coastline, golden beaches to walk meditatively across the heavy grain sand, *brooding* at the roar and boom of the surf, shoeless and bearded and dressed all in white like Christ, hands clasped behind my back. I'll buy an old abandoned beach-house and turn each room into a bathroom. My day will consist of bathing, shitting, pissing, brushing my teeth, flossing, shaving, and looking for gray hairs. I'll buy the Grapevine and bust up the concrete and grow grapes! I'll buy the Victorians in Presidio Park and give them to the mental patients Reagan set free! I'll buy all the graveyards, all the police stations. I'll buy all the Church's fried chicken restaurants and turn them into churches. I'll buy all the Popeyeses and put a cartoon drawing of my face on the sign, saying, 'Come on down to Colonel T.S. Boones, and get yourself a wing and a prayer!' I'll buy exotic animals! Whole city blocks! Famous brands just to discontinue them, goodbye Snickers, goodbye Twix, we loved you so but now we'll love you more because you're dead. I'll buy the rights to songs and have them played on the radio, on repeat, twenty-four hours a day. Carr, have you heard Shatner's version of 'Mr. Tambourine Man'?"

"No."

"It's fantastic."

"I'll have to check it—"

"I'll buy the whole entire species of some endangered . . . some . . . some *ridiculous,* nearly-extinct, bizarre-looking animal just to own it, just to say it's mine and then I'll change its name to *Boonous Villainous Strangous*. I'll buy you whatever you want when I'm rich, Carr. Anything. You should make a list now. Look. There. On that napkin. Right there." He taps the counter with his finger. "Sky's the limit. Your wish is my command. Alesanda here," he points at the girl on the stage, "when I'm rich, it goes without saying that we'll be man and wife, sickness and in health, good times and bad, 'Sunday, Monday, Happy Days,' ring on the finger, third finger of the left hand, sign the papers, kiss the bride, amen, tons of kids with the striking godlike Boone presence (and *prescience*, Carr) and Alesanda's pale, cold blue eyes, as cold blue as a beach agate held up to the flickering, doomy winter *sky*. She'll eat solely from my hand like a trained horse and wear nothing but diamond jewelry and chainmail around the house and I'll take her back to Petersburg twice yearly and buy all her toothless, godless peasant family blue jeans and sugar cubes and radios. They will call me Papa America."

"We call you that already."

"You're teasing me, Carr. I can tell. But you'll see. You'll be there with me, my historian, my Herodotus of Halicarnassus, my records keeper. You will be like the midget *Mini Me,* and I will be The Good Papa America to the town of Petersburg and in the park square the statue of me will be carved from black marble carried up from the local quarry on the crooked backs of Alesanda's people. My hand . . . you'll see it . . . I'll take you there in my steamship and we'll stand in the snow in the shadow of my statue wearing tall boots (our boots crunching in the snow, krish, krash), our fur coats, our big Russian hats and we'll drink vodka from wooden goblets and hot mulled wine mixed with goat's blood and raw egg and you'll see my statue's hand . . . his smooth right hand raised benevolently to the heavens and in my left will be a *flaming sword like the angel of the garden before The Fall.*"

"How."

"How what? How will I get rich?"

"Yeah."

"It doesn't matter. Immaterial! What matters . . . Oh, hello darling, hello sweetheart. Hello, Alesanda."

The pale, blonde dancer crawls up to him and he whispers something in Russian and she smiles. Her smile is a snarl, a sneer. She lies on her back in front of Ted Boone and claws at her breasts, staring up at him, the light in her eyes buried back somewhere deep, a dead flat stare. He waves a twenty in front of her face and she snatches it in her teeth like a fish, turns her head, and spits it out onto the stage, her eyes and earrings and teeth glowing sky blue under the blacklight. He pulls another twenty out of his wallet, offers it to her, then pulls it back, and says something else in Russian. She snatches the bill out of his hand and pulls herself to her feet and stomps off the stage, reaching down to grab her clothes as she leaves.

"Whoa, Ted Boone. What did you say?"

"What I told her was, 'Darling, my darling, how I would love to bend you over this bar and worm my tongue up your little pink—' and then I used a terrible expletive noun for 'rear end' that I won't repeat in polite company."

"You *didn't*."

"I did. Carr, I said this because I'm *paying* her and you can't say things like that to girls you don't pay. She *loved it*, Carr. God she loved it."

"I don't think she loved it. Look at her. She left. She hated it. Ted Boone, Alesanda *hates* you."

"You're weak."

"What?"

"Someone should hold you down and hit you until your skull caves in."

"Ted Boone . . . let's go. This is depressing."

"Someone should smash your head with a brick and eat your brains like a Cadbury Cream Egg."

"Alesanda . . . she *hates* you. You can tell by the—"

"She loved every word and she'll love me once the time is right."

"This is awful. Ted Boone, we should leave. This is bumming me out."

"Women are strange machines, Carr." He waves his hand across the empty stage, the disco lights and spotlights crisscrossing the footboards. "Take my first girlfriend, Suzy. Beautiful yellow-headed Suzy with a 'z'! Carr, I met her in high school at a youth group bonfire on Fiesta Island. It was her birthday party—and Suzy, she said, 'I'm fifteen and I love reading about the occult, petting kittens, and being naked around the house.' Like that. Just like that. Like she was a centerfold in a magazine and that was her one line of life story. Now, this is embarrassing to admit, but I bleeped my own unmentionable to the thought of her saying that for *days*. To the *thought*. Not to her, just the thought, the words, just her voice saying those words, the beautiful monotone enunciation, the moral juxtaposition of ideas. I used to draw her in the margins of my school papers in a fit of *lust*. That awkward little body and those chubby little tits, her huge head and all that yellow hair like something out of Dr. Seuss. But for all her talk . . . for all her talk, there was no walk. Suzy was a virgin and when I broached the subject two weeks later, she bawled me out and yelled something about Judas and told me to get out of the house. That was the end of Suzanna Lacey Delffs and scrappy little Teddy Bear Boone. We were together two weeks and two weeks only. Not so much as an over-the-jeans grope between us. I believe she married a nerd, Carr. A *nerd*: Just think of it. Women are fickle. And women you don't pay get *mouthy* when you break out of accordance with the gold standard . . . *Oh, not you, no, no, not you darling*," he tells the new girl on stage. She leans over the railing and turns Ted Boone's dirty red baseball cap to the side and then struts back to the pole and swings herself around it, her chestnut hair swaying in a fan behind her. "You know what thirty feels like, Carr? Of course you don't know what thirty feels like. Look at you staring back at me with your empty eyes and your poor empty head. You're as empty as a balloon. Go get a job in a balloon factory. You haven't lived and you don't know what it takes to be a man at odds with *man*, *nature*, and him*self*."

"How does thirty feel?"

"Thirty *felt*—it felt, past tense—like the world was ending. Like it *had* ended. I'd see these young girls . . . these beautiful young girls coming out of class in the evening from the window of my old apartment by Mesa College, and I'd think, Ted Boone, they see you as an *old man*. It doesn't matter that you still think of yourself as young and capable. It doesn't matter that if they read your in-progress writing, your candle-lit notes of *illumination*, they would soak their panties right then and there and bend over backwards to service you in all makes, variations, and modu . . . modu . . . modu*lations* of the word. What *they* see is an old man with loose flabby jowls, a face that has lost its elasticity. They see these *dull, beady* eyes and they hear that ragged, seasoned Boone voice, a *boozy* voice: Dulcet as it is (and it *is* dulcet), it is also boozy. This is the truth. Let's be honest here. And those girls, Carr, those perfect, little ripe young . . . these *junior college girls* . . . they would look at me and they would see their loser dirtbag of an uncle, their tall, shuffling, low-rent, potbellied, dark-eyed creepy uncle. (Like your uncle, Carr, who is a thousand years older than God himself and bald as a cock's head, but like your uncle I am *not*.) Or . . . or take high school girls."

"Come on, Ted Boone . . . ."

"They'd run past my work for track."

"Jeez."

"Those strong legs all tan in shorts, tight running tops, flat bellies, thick glossy hair in ponytails, everything bouncing but firm, 'way up firm and high.' My god. Sometimes in my darkest hour I would—*me*, Ted Boone, the dynamo, the unflagging *optimist*, the man of *measure*—I would see these amazing little high school track-stars running past the window in packs with those perfect teenage asses and I would do the math and there it would be plain as sunlight in clear sky . . . and it's hard to admit this . . . I was old enough to be their *dad*. And I would think, 'You're right, I am what you believe *because* you believe. The cover speaketh for the contents. You are right, right, *right*, I'm old enough to be your dad. I may have had you when I was twelve, but I'm your dad. You probably go home and say hi to your dad after school and he asks you 'Hey, how was school?' and you grunt your 'Same as always' and then his 'What did you learn?' and then your 'Nothing' and you go into your room to study or chat mindlessly on the computer or stare into the mirror at the wild hot deathless perfection that is you and your dad looks just like me, a young old man, deflated, fallen. I'm just as invisible—invisible in the sense of being *as* incompatible, *as* nonsexual of a creature, a total and confirmed *write-off* as a plausible, potential mate, impotent like Jake Barnes . . . me, here, strong, dashing, bold me . . . just as invisible as your dad is to you. I'm your dad. Your stale, boring, old-before-his-time, gray-around-the-edges *dad*.' You know what that does to a man?"

"But thirty isn't—"

"Thirty *is*. Whatever you were going to say, thirty *is*. You don't know yet, but you will. It will come sooner than you think and it will be a surprise attack in the dead of the night and it will knock you off your bearings and shake loose your ballast and it will *humble* you, it will humble you. You just wait, Carr. You have no idea how crushing it will be to turn thirty. Then . . . then thirty-one, the big three one. Even worse! At thirty-one, I was concerned with love in a spiritual sense. At thirty-one, I felt as if I had missed every opportunity I ever had of finding a woman who would marry me. I mean, not *any* woman, but the kind of woman I dreamed of, the kind every other guy would see and think, '*That* dude's got a prize.' I was washed up! The Ted Boone of thirty-one was a failure and he knew he was a failure and he'd see these famous actors on TV who were well-established, respected, *accomplished* at twenty-five and he'd read these books written by men ten years his junior and he'd *rage*, Carr. Fuck you Ellis! Fitzgerald! Rimbaud! He'd rage because, at thirty-one, he had nothing to *show for himself*. He had nothing to offer the kind of bride he so readily needed and *deserved*. He had done nothing with his life but work emasculating jobs, and no decent woman wants a man whose boss snips off his balls every morning as he walks through the door. 'Hello, Boone, you're early! Good man! *Team* player! Drop those drawers! This won't hurt a bit!' Snip! Oh, the indignity! Mr. Tambourine Man, where are you when I need you?! He would honestly and truly sit down on his couch in his apartment and he would cry over the loss of his youth! He felt so old that he started shaving every day and began to wear sneakers again and listen to youthful, spirited music—but to no avail. Carr, intelligent, cultured men my age stop listening to young music because it makes them feel old. They hear the voices of the singers and they see their faces in the magazines and on TV and it's not like they don't relate—*they relate*. The truth is that they feel threatened. They feel old listening to young music, so they start listening to old music because it makes them feel young in comparison. They want music so *gnarled* and *dusty* and *osssssified* that they feel like a blade of spring grass next to it. They get into jazz from the '40s and old Delta blues and they try to lose themselves in it and deny the cold, hard fact that rock 'n' roll is a young man's game. Carr, being the iconoclast that I am, I went the other way. Denial! *Maybe*. But I wanted so much to be young that I gave myself the trappings as best I could. After a few months of playacting, I knew it was no use. Your starry, godhead hero Bonnie "Prince" Boony would sit alone at the bar and the jukebox would play a song—anything—and he would try his best to drown it out. 'Turn that shit off, Timothy!' Timothy didn't care. 'Seal my ears with wax and strap me to the mast, Janica!' Janica just laughed. Argh! He . . . me

. . . he would shut his ears to the world because the world ceased to be his. He would cry because he would never be young again. Never, no matter *what* he did, or how well he lived. He'd cry for the death of the body, for material decay, and for the worst demon of all . . . time! The great and final hero killer!"

"Where do you come up with this stuff? Is your book like this?"

"You're teasing me again and I get that. I'm funny. I would tease you just as much if you had the guts to put yourself out there, but listen. Listen, Carr, the thirty-one-year-old Ted Boone would shake his meaty fist up to the stars (the stars being time) and he would dream the most beautiful dream of all in which he meets time incarnated in human form—Time as corporeal man, embodied as a robust young Mel Gibson—and he would challenge Time to fight! A fight to the death! And he'd win! He would destroy Time! He would punch Mel-Gibson-as-Flesh-Embodied-Time square in the chest and his fist would smash through the ribcage and burst through his organ meat and snap his spinal column and bust right out his back with a great spray of gore and Time would hang there dead on his outstretched arm like a sleeping scarecrow! He would kill Mel Gibson! Just think of it. He would stop Time, mid-march. He would stop the death procession! That was thirty-one. The next year, thirty-two, was back to petty sexual concerns. He . . . *I* would think of these college girls living in the apartments around me and how I *disgusted* them, Carr, and it killed what little confidence I had left. Me, here, thirty-two, working the register and bagging groceries at Ralph's, paying off a student loan for the degree I never finished, a shorn Sampson taking night school classes at City and getting *Cs,* me, the original and unbeatable Ted Boone, the one and only, the comet without a tail. I felt like a pariah—I *was* a pariah. (If your friend Chente's car was Mariah Carey, mine was Pariah Carry, because a pariah is what it carried.) I thought back on the, what are you, twenty-two, twenty-three, twenty-four? I thought back on the early-twenties Ted Boone as a god. Solar plexus of *steel*! I would shout, 'Hit me right here! See how it *feels*! Break your damn hand!' My body was that of a gladiator in his sun-kissed prime. Standing there in my sleeveless shirt drinking a forty and smoking a joint, *daring* the world to cross me. I could drink all night and I could fight six men at once and I could stay up for *days* on speed and nothing could touch me. I was a nonstick *pan*. And here . . . here we've got this *dried-up*, bloated, sour, farting, weak-eyed, heartburn-stricken thirty-two-year-old Ted Boone and sometimes he drinks a glass of wine and in the morning he has a hangover—a hangover! He's out of breath walking up the stairs to his depressing, nondescript apartment. His blind eyes bulge stupidly and his knees ache and he groans when he stands up from the couch and his shoulders make crackling sounds like a deer walking on dry leaves. His neck (once a thing of rope-corded muscle) is strained half the time and when it is it ruins his day at work but he can't complain because he's afraid he'll lose his job and never get another one and die on the street with a "work for food" sign and a dog that hates him for tying him to this dreary damn life! Mr. Tambourine Man, why hath thou forsaken me?! He sees homelessness as a distant but distinct possibility and he weighs his options for bailout and there are *none*. His family dead and scattered across the graveyards of El Centro and Needles and Calexico and Blythe, his brother doing tech support of all-things, his friends no longer friends, his bank account drained dry. He hooks up with a woman in his apartment building. A beautiful, complex, thick-legged, black-haired forty-year-old mother of three he's wanted to bleep all year and has thus been bleeping his bleep to for months in the dark of his apartment oh the shame! And when they sleep together, his manhood is so weak and floppy that he can't feel himself inside her; he can barely tell he's hard. He has to keep checking! He has to keep . . . keep (god) reaching down between their joined, thumping, sweating thighs to the place where two become one to see if it's hard enough to keep going! (It was like shooting pool with a rope, as they say.) And now, thirty-three, me at thirty-three, after the crap-storm of thirty-two, thirty-one, thirty. Me at thirty-three. You know who *else* was thirty-three?" Ted Boone is sweating. He fumbles for his cigarettes and lights one and offers the pack to Joey.

"Who?" Joey takes the pack and then decides against it and sets it on the counter.

"Jesus Christ. You may have heard of him. Middle name 'H.' Sometimes 'Fucking,' but only when you're mad, which is still a sin. Jesus Christ. In the Bible, the New Testament, Book . . . I don't know . . . Book something, Book Holy Moly Holly Jolly Jedediah Josiah Aunt Jemima humna humna googly moogly . . . that very book—the *best* book, the only book, the Great Human Comedy—tells us Jesus H. was thirty-three. He died when he was thirty-three. Dead, Carr. Suzy with a 'z's Jesus. My Jesus. Your Jesus. Everyone's Jesus. The most famous corpse in history. And you know what's coming December 25th?"

"Christmas."

"Yes, but my *birthday*. Carr, I'm going to be thirty-four on December 25th, and the fact that I'm going to make it past the age Jesus lived—on the *date* Jesus was born!—fills my heart with confidence and a fresh kind of strength and resolve I've not 'til this point *known*. I have dodged Pilot and Skull Hill and the Denials! I have been killed and killed again, then reborn by proxy! I have dodged the bullet by way of loophole and canceled check, and I have stepped back from the frame with the bullet between my fingers and I have looked at it close with my evil little pig-eyes and the bullet is *me*. 'Because I could not stop for death, He stopped for me!' Carr, the nearly thirty-four-year-old Ted Boone is a *deeply* powerful thing. The nearly thirty-four-year-old Ted Boone has survived by the sheer grit and bile in his oyster gut and he will live to see his enemies grow old and feeble and die, and *when* his enemies die he will sneak off to the graveyard in the blackest of night and he will . . . he will *stomp* and *dance* and beat a shovel upon on the pressed earth of their graves in a pure act of defiance! A *celebration* of defiance! Open resistance! Renunciation of what (and who) came before! He will use his shovel to dig up those bones and when he has their bones they will be his to use *however we wants*! He will buildeth a chair of their bones! A skeleton toilet to *expel* into! A boat to sail home in! A ladder up to heaven and once in heaven he will look God in the eye and he will say, '1, 2, 3, 4, I declare a thumb war! I'm kidding! Hug me! Now! I'm sad.' The Ted Boone of thirty-four will have lived thirty-four years because he is a thing carved of the *darkest* perversities! He is an animal unchecked! An evil Superman! A Tambourine Man ringing out infinite! Ready to go anywhere! Ready for to fade! An immoralist, a sensualist, a starman brought to Earth as a *babe* on the back of a dream! I can't expect you . . . I *don't* expect you to understand any of this, but, Carr, the Ted Boone of thirty-four will be a man who has known the depths, a man who has then *risen* to surreal heights thus uncharted by angel or demon!" He pulls his red baseball cap low over his eyes. "Carr, and this is why," he stops, slouching down in his seat, lighting another cigarette, his fingers shaking, "and this is why I *couldn't* be the mayor of San Diego. Great men are never seen as great men while they walk the proud land. Carr, I'm a monster. I'm Josef Stalin and malaria and the Creature from the Black Lagoon. I'm Pol Pott's malice and inhumanity distilled into humble Philip Seymour Hoffman Low-Paid Character Actor form. I'm a piece of dark matter spinning suspended over the ribbed and rocky tube down hell's fiery *maw*." He makes a claw with his hand. "I'm an ancient beast with claaaaws like taaaalons and a song on the lips, the golden translucent heart of a *lamb* beating in his chest, and those . . . those *Aryan puritans* who make the rules would have me run out of *town*. They'd cut me up in pieces and throw my evil chunks in the harbor. But I'd be back, Carr. I *always* come back."

HOME, NIGHT

By eight, Joey's apartment is packed and the stereo is playing a record that Rory brought over and people are getting stoned and shouting along with the song, screaming, "Ship to shore / Do you read? / SOS, JTB!" By nine, Curt comes over to sell ecstasy to Rory's boyfriend and half the party ponies up for a tab. By ten, Maggie and Joel are eating guacamole from a casserole dish with spoons and people who Joey doesn't know are doing cocaine in his bathroom. A few hours later, the party has cleared out and gone to a show at the Locust House and now it's:

Ted Boone: cleaned up for the night, wearing a nice new peacoat and dark pants, hair cut shorter and combed to the side like a Civil War soldier, mustache shaved off, face scrubbed pink; "FUN" written on the back of his hand in red Sharpie. In his peacoat pockets: one condom bought May 1999 and a pack of Tic Tac Freshmints that he offers to everyone, shaking it in the air ("Tic Tac? They're Freshmints"). Pants pockets: Sharpie marker, cigarette lighter, pack of Camel Lights, car keys, fourty-five dollars.

Maggie: tight gray jeans, no shoes, white belt, a black pearl snap cowboy shirt that her boyfriend bought her; hair in twin braids, thick and woven like coils of black rope, happy, talking a lot, comfortable, grabbing Joey's shirt and kissing him in the hallway. In her jean pockets: a white twist-tie from a loaf of Wonder Bread and her photo ID and ATM card.

Curt Santiago-Rieter: drug dealer, nineteen, big, hulking, quiet, mute stare, rap-star clothes, baggy pants, expensive sneakers, Kings Starter jacket, Dodgers hat cocked sideways. In his many pockets: canvas wallet, a small baggie of cocaine, a pill bottle with thirteen tabs of Mitsubishi ecstasy, a cigarette lighter, $980 in one-hundred dollar bills and twenties, a new canister of Binaca Blast, a cellphone, a tiny screwdriver, nail clippers, house keys, a quarter (1970), a green rubber band, a brand-new Kel-Tec P-32 pistol (unfired) with seven rounds (7.65×17 mm Browning SR, FMJ) in the clip, a light blue bead from a rosary.

Joey's sister, Macey: nineteen, tight jeans, blue oversized Kansas University sweater, long blonde hair, pale, loud Missourian accent, flirting with Curt and Ted Boone, mouthing off, chain-smoking, drunk since noon, five foot tall, in North Park to stay with Joey for the weekend. It's been years, and they're strangers now. Earlier in the night, she took ecstasy and, when it didn't work, she took another. Both kicked in an hour ago. In her pockets: a twenty dollar bill, a nickle (1986), a dime (2000), Cherry Chapstick with three applications left.

Joey: the host, happy, tired, half-drunk but too worried to go all the way. In his pockets: a lucky cat-eye marble with a green and yellow swirl, a pack of Wrigley's Spearmint gum, his switchblade, sixteen dollars in ones.

1:20 A.M.

A record that Ted Boone brought over of Southern chain gang music plays quietly on the turntable in the corner on the floor, the old, fuzzy chants and hammer clangs the only sound in the room. The five of them on Joey's L-shaped couch. Maggie and Joey and Ted Boone on the long side of the L. Macey and Curt on the short end. On the coffeetable, a bag of weed that Curt brought over ("Thunderboat Red Hair"), a yellow Bic lighter (Joey's), a Rosarita refried bean can for an ashtray, the remnants of the guacamole, a few scattered chips and pretzels, a tall red glass bong with a black and yellow 91-X sticker on it, and a dozen empty beer bottles. Under the table: more pretzels, beer caps, Joey's wallet (misplaced) under someone's baseball cap (Dodgers).

"What we need is a *beer run*," says Ted Boone breaking the silence. "A six-mile mud run to benefit beer cancer," he says, sitting on the edge of the couch holding an empty jug of wine in his lap, drumming his long nails on it. "A beer run run run," he sings quietly, "a beer run run." He rubs the place where his mustache was and his big hand drops back into his lap.

"That's what Ah'm talkin' about," says Macey, raising her coffee mug of wine over her head.

"The drunken, lazy Southern belle is right," says Ted Boone, standing up now and pacing in front of them, hands clasped behind his back. He brings his right hand forward and wags a finger at Joey. "And to get into the spirit, we're going to hop up off the sofa . . . right *now* . . . up, up, UP," he snaps his fingers at them, "and do shots from the bottle of evil brandy until the evil brandy is but a terrible memory rising . . . rising . . . rising . . . rising . . . rising like mist from the tops of the shaggy pine trees of the enchanted forest. Now . . . now, none of you know the evil brandy by name, but the evil brandy is in the trunk of my car (the Boonemobile) and when I get the evil brandy, your lives shall be transmogrified by the miracle of chemical science and scientific chemicals. The Evil Brand evil brandy is the reason for the season and you will be full of new wisdom and foresight . . . *extra*-extra sensory perception, which is double your pleasure and triple the fun." He turns to Macey. "You think *ecstasy* makes you love the world? You just *wait*." With that Ted Boone opens the door and steps outside.

"Whoa, man, that guy *rules*," drawls Macey. She shoves Curt's shoulder. "Wake up, Biggie Smalls! We got a friend who plays football for M.C. who looks just like you. We call him *Moose Ass*."

Curt looks at her with a sad, distant expression and says nothing. He pulls his ball cap down low over his eyes and turns it around sideways.

"Good answer," says Macey.

"You were right about him," Maggie says, cuddling up to Joey and rubbing his knee. "He's great but I think he's totally . . . he's *insane*. You know that, right? I mean, he's amazing but . . . whoa, dude, kookoo time." She makes three circles around her left ear with her pointer finger. "Kookoo *tiempo*."

Joey yawns. "He's . . . he's not insane. He's a talker. He likes to talk. He likes to say big, grandiose things even if it's complete nonsense. It's a performance. He's acting."

"Ah don't care if it's an act," says Macey, tucking a long strand of blonde hair behind her ear. "He's my type, big guys, tall guys, they can take care of you. Ah'd totally do him."

"Agh. Jesus, Macey. Gross," Joey says.

Maggie puts her head on Joey's shoulder. "Do you think he understands the stuff he says?"

"He can't. There's no way. It's a word game. He likes how it sounds."

"Still, whatever, he's great, Joey. I'm glad you invited him. This party . . . it was great. It was really fun."

"It's not over yet."

"I don't know, everybody's tired and— "

"Not me and B.I.G. here," drawls Macey. "We're *fun*."

Curt stares at her and looks away and sinks lower in the couch.

"Ted Boone'll bring it all back. He's a good guy for a party," Joey says, pushing a curl back from Maggie's forehead and kissing the top of her head.

"Get a *room*," says Macey. She puts her hand up for a high-five from Curt, who returns it without spirit.

Ted Boone comes back into the apartment with a small, crinkled-up brown paper bag in his arms. "The evil brandy!" he says happily. "Macetadon, get cups."

"The evil brandy!" shouts Macey. She pulls herself off the couch and pads barefoot into the kitchen.

"Ladies and gentlemen, up off the sofa! Up! Up! Up! Maggie! Carr! Kirk . . . *Curt*! Allow me to introduce . . . the *eeevilest* of evil, the darkest of dark, the dankest of dank, my brother and mentor and your new best friend with unseen agenda. Allow me to introduce," he lets the bag fall from the bottle dramatically and puts a finger along his lip to make a mustache, "*zee evul bran-day*!"

Macey lines up five Dixie cups on the island between the kitchen and living room. She knocks one over and then knocks the rest down and laughs. "Don't talk shit, y'all. Ah'm tryin'!"

"Darling," says Ted Boone, "you do the honor and pour. I think I'm falling in love with your clumsy little midget hands."

Macey stands the cups up again and pours five shots in a line, spilling brandy in the gap between the fourth and fifth cup. "Don't talk smack, y'all. Ah'm on drugs."

Joey and big, sullen Curt take their cups and hold them chest high. Curt nods at Joey and gives him a half smile and Joey nods back.

Maggie picks up hers. "I have to sip mine. I can't take it all in one swallow."

"Ah'll take *you* in one swallow," says Macey, slapping Maggie on the rear.

"Ow! Joey, tell your sister to be nice."

"Be nice, Mace Face."

"Ah don't care! Ah'm on *vacation*, y'all! We gettin' fucked up tahniiight! Ah'm on ecstasy, y'all! Woooo! Let's get wasted! K.U.! Woo!"

"To starting the heart again," says Ted Boone with a nod.

"To starting the heart."

"Starting the heart."

"Mumble" (Curt).

"To starting the heart."

They take their shots.

"Damn straight!" shouts Macey. "Woo, whoa."

"What's *in* this?" coughs Maggie, wincing and holding her throat. "This is *terrible*."

"It's a trade secret," says Ted Boone, winking at her. "Mace Face, pour another round. I think we got some nonbelievers in here."

"Ah'm on it, Cap."

"Maggie's right. It's awful," says Joey. "Is this really *brandy*? I thought brandy was supposed to be smooth. What is this?"

"It's the blood of a menstruating teen witch," Ted Boone says proudly, beaming at Joey. "It's curdled snake semen and essence of Nazi tears (which aren't tears at all, but rather an unconscious admission of guilt, as Nazis only cry in their sleep and when they're drunk). The origins of the evil brandy are humble but what I will tell you is I found it on the dusty back shelf of a Santería shop deep in the yeasty, crotchial, crotchtastic region of Mexico City and that I carried it over the border clutched close to my heart in the company of my faithful Aztec shaman, Toomectilan. He said, 'Hmm, Papa 'Merica, you no know what you getting you self into. Evil brandy plenty strong, plenty bad medicine.'"

"You really did all that?" says Macey.

"I did none of the above, you lovely hillbilly bride. Now, Maggie will appreciate this most out of anyone: This is *Mexican* brandy, which to the Jew is like honeycomb to the hungry bear. Alesanda . . . Carr, Alesanda, she's a Russian Jew. On our wedding day, this will be in the punchbowl. Maggie, *you*, you lovely Jewess, will be there as the maid of honor. Alesanda has no friends because all girls hate a truly beautiful woman, especially a Jew. The ceremony will be half-Santería, half-Jewish. You will serve as *aide de camp* for the celebratory Jewish American Princess part."

"Ah didn't know you were Jewish," says Macey.

Curt, sitting hunched over on the couch stares glumly at Macey's ass as she stands in front of him, kicking her legs side to side with nervous energy.

"I'm not Jewish," says Maggie, sitting down on the couch.

"No, you are and I *love it*," says Ted Boone.

"Ah love it, too," says Macey, her eyes glassy and drugged. "I know Ah'm on E, but Ah love alla you and Ah love the evil brandy and Ah love the Jews and ecstasy and Anne Frank's diary and San Diego."

"Jewish girls are the countesses of my countdom," says Ted Boone, "and the evil brandy is the official state-sanctioned drink. The Mexican death trip.

Adios, Motherfucker is what the Sonorans call it. The Mazatlan Handshake. And now our theme for the night—" He picks up his Casio keyboard off the floor, turns it on, and taps out the opening notes of "La Cucaracha." *Doot doot doot dooooo doo. Doot doot doot dooooo doo.* "And our motto: *Ahora es cuando, chili verde, le has de dar sabor al caldo.*"

"Up and at 'em, y'all!" shouts Macey. She spins around in a circle and falls down. "Ah feel amazin'!" she yells, rolling on the floor, rubbing her face on the carpet. "This carpet feels amazin'! Ecstasy is amazin'! Evil brandy is amazin'. Ah love alla you!"

"Oh, the *roads* you must be on," says Ted Boone, nodding down to Macey. "I love you more every day, more with every clumsy little stunt. Some are flustered by life (Carr, here) but some of us are desperate to live, and you and I, Mace Face, fall into the latter. We are wild to live and evil as the day is long, and that's why we're so *deeply* in love. Two good Southerners on a California romp. Two Colonels of the Commonwealth, leaders of the Honorable Order, happy and confident in high cotton."

"Up! Ah need up!" she shrieks, hands clawing up at him.

Ted Boone offers a hand and pulls Macey to her feet.

On the walk to 7-Eleven, Ted Boone leads the way, carrying the Casio and playing beer run theme music on the pre-programed setting. (Old tunes: "Guess I'll Go Eat Worms," "The Happy Wanderer," "Greensleeves," "Here We Go Loopty Loo.") Macey walks next to him, dwarfed by his towering bulk, as blonde and small as he is dark and large.

"Play somethin' faster!" shouts Macey, her little arm wrapped halfway around Ted Boone's waist. Curt shuffles along behind them, silent and impassive, Maggie and Joey a few yards behind Curt.

"You watching this?" says Maggie.

"It's amazing."

"Your sister's way too fucked up and Ted Boone's getting there. They're gonna do something stupid tonight. I can't believe she took that much ecstasy. Something bad's gonna happen. I can feel it."

"It's okay. Don't worry, baby."

"I guess I should relax and have fun, right?"

"It's fine. Me and you. We'll stay sober and watch out for everybody. Just say fuck it."

"Alright. Fuck it."

"Good work." Joey takes her hand and holds it and with her hand in his he feels strong.

"I'm a good guy for a party too, right?" she says.

"Of course, baby. You're a great guy for a party."

Outside 7-Eleven, they share a cigarette and discuss their new problem.

Joey has lost his ID and Ted Boone has forgotten his. The girls and Curt are too young to buy.

"I can go in and try," Joey offers, leaning against the phone booth. "I'll try and maybe they won't card me. I'm in here all the time. You guys hide in the phone booth."

"No, no, no. Lemons, lemonade," says Ted Boone. "I've hatched a plan. *Listen*. Maggie, you and MaceCapades go in and when you're in the back at the beer cooler, take off your shirts, pull your bras down—"

"That's what *you* think. Ah'm not *wearin'* one," drawls Macey, leering up at Ted Boone. She pulls her sweater over her head and begins to work the buttons of her plaid shirt. "You'll see." She starts to fall and Ted Boone grabs her by the arm.

"Whoops. Steady, Daisy Duke," he says, holding her up. "But, no, wait. Wait until you're inside. Element of surprise. Go up to the counter in full late-teenage bloom and that poor dumb boy won't know what hit him. He'll *give* you the booze. He'll *buy* it for you. He'll build a time machine out of Carr's phone booth here," he raps his knuckles on the glass, "and go back to the year negative-negative and invent booze just to come back and hand over the patent with a low swooping bow and a courtly, '*Anything* for you most excellent babes.' Okay? Quick now. This is a dire emergency and I've declared marshal law."

The boys wait outside while the girls go in.

"Look, there they go, sure as the river is wide," whispers Ted Boone in his affected drawl. "This is really happening. I'm a *wizard*." Ted Boone—stooped forward, looking at them through the big glass window. He taps on the window with his finger, his breath fogging the glass in a small round spot. "Look. Maggie's got her . . . she's unbuttoned her shirt," he wipes the glass with the cuff of his coat, "and so has your sister."

"Jesus. I can't look," Joey says.

Curt moves closer to the glass until his nose is touching.

Ted Boone claps his hands happily. "I see tits. Two, now four. God, it's a dream! Carr, it's better than a dream! Oh, okay, oh, now, look, okay, your sister and her lovely little sister tits have a case of Bud. Oh, no, wait, look, she must've read my mind. She's put it back and she's got Corona. Good girl. Southern intuition. Now . . . now Magic Maggie and her surprisingly . . . wow, surprising *large* ones are grabbing . . . oh, good . . . a couple bottles of red wine. Smart, smart. They're walking down the candy aisle . . . don't get sidetracked, girls . . . keep moving . . . keep—"

"Oh man," whispers Curt, nose to the glass, his breath fogging. "Y'all do shit like this all the time?"

"Always," says Ted Boone. "This is just the lemon next to the pie, my friend."

"Y'all's crazy. I'm hangin' out with you more often."

Through the window, they watch the girls carry their beer and wine to the counter and lay down a twenty. The clerk stands rail straight and listens, nodding while Maggie talks soundlessly. She shows him the twenty, holds it in both hands, snaps it tight in the air, and then stuffs it in Macey's back pocket and pats her butt.

"Glory, glory, hallelujah," whispers Ted Boone. "I can die now. 'Let us cross over the river, and rest under the shade of the trees.' I'm done. Bury me deep. 'Bury me at sea where no murdered ghost can haunt me.' Look at them. What are they saying? What could they be *saying*?"

They watch as Macey leans over the counter and cups her breasts in her hands and gives them a playful shake, then says something to the clerk with a mock-serious expression. The clerk nods his head yes and the girls turn to leave and Ted Boone whoops happily and claps his hands and hops around in a circle.

Maggie and Macey come out topless, carrying the booze.

"Mission accomplished!" shouts Maggie. "He *gave* it to us!"

"Ah'll give it to *you*," says Macey in a put-on trampy voice. "Naw, but you shoulda heard us in there. Me and Maggie gonna get ourselves a *racket* goin', huh girl."

"We're goin' into business." Maggie sets the wine bottles on the ground and unzips her jeans and begins to struggle out of them.

"Wait. What are you doing?" Joey says, horrified.

"Getting undressed," she says calmly. "We all are. C'mon everybody. Take it off."

"Hell yeah, *girl*," says Macey, undoing her jeans.

"Bingo!" shouts Ted Boone. "Biiiiiingo!" he sings. He drops his coat on the sidewalk and pulls off his t-shirt and throws it into the bushes. "Bingo! God is a flower! Every day above the ground is a beautiful pie baked in heaven! Bingo!" he shouts, his breath smoking in the air.

"C'mon everybody," says Maggie. "We're doin' this. We're walking back to our place like this."

Joey shivers and slowly, reluctantly, unbuttons his fly.

"Oh, lord. Oh, lord," shouts Ted Boone, dancing around in a circle. He undoes his belt and lets his pants fall and then pulls off his boxers and stands shivering and white and potbellied in front of the store windows, hands crossed in front of his crotch. The clerk stares out the window, wide-eyed. He picks up his cell phone and types in a number. "Everyone!" Ted Boone shouts. "Do like she says. Maggie's in charge here. I'll carry our clothes!"

While the clerk stares at them from inside, talking on the phone, they disrobe and pile their clothes on the sidewalk, Ted Boone and Maggie singing together, "He's related to you / He's related to you / He's dying to meet you! / He's related to you / He's related to you / He's related to you!"

"It's *cold*, yo," shivers Curt, walking in place and rubbing his fat arms.

"Macey, you naked little ape . . . you carry my instrument," Ted Boone says, handing the keyboard to her.

"*Ah'll* carry your instrument," she slurs happily.

"Haw haw, and I bet you will, darling." He bends down to pick up the pile of clothes.

Macey plays a stream of nonsense noise on the keyboard and then hits an automatic drum setting, which beats out a loud, tinny snare beat. She begins to march in place, small and naked and white under the yellow lights of the 7-Eleven.

"You young, dumb, ripe thing," says Ted Boone, shaking his head happily.

"I'm not drunk enough for this," says Joey.

"Hold on." Ted Boone drops the armload of clothes on the ground, squats down, and digs through them until he finds his coat. He takes the red Sharpie marker out of his pocket. "Macey, come here, you beautiful little racist dickhead." She marches up to him, and he takes her little chin in his hand and draws three red lines along each cheek while she stares up at him. "Now you're ready. Let's go!" He throws the Sharpie out into the parking lot and they start the long walk home.

On the way there, Maggie and Joey walk in the back, holding hands.

"I can't believe you left your coat on, nerd."

"It's cold."

"It's not that bad. Look at me. Look at them."

"That's all I've got on."

"Doesn't count."

"Alright." He pulls his coat off and wraps it over his shoulders like a towel.

"*There* we go."

"I can't believe this is happening."

"I can. Look at this, Joey. *Look* what I did. You see this?"

In front of them, Macey and Curt and Ted Boone walk, pale white and stark nude, the boys large and out of shape, Macey small and slim with a high-school swimmer's build, Ted Boone singing at the top of his lungs, "He's related to you! / He's related to you!" Curt energized now, trying to sing along without knowing the song, Macey jogging circles around them as they walk, shadow-boxing at them, shouting, "Look at me: Ah'm nekid! Look at me! Look at me!"

HOME, 2:30 A.M.

Back at the apartment, Joey turns up the heater and then opens beers and they drink, everyone shivering and rosy-faced and rubbing their arms to warm up.

"Let's make some soup! Joey, where y'keep the *soup*?" shouts Macey, going through Joey's cupboards, then singing. "'Ooh that dress so *scandalous* / And you know another woo-hoo can't *handle* this.'"

In the kitchen, Maggie pours one of the bottles of wine into five mason jars and everyone takes a jar.

When the wine is gone, the evil brandy is brought back and they pass it around until the bottle's empty and then they're glowing drunk. (Joey, in an attempt to numb himself to the sight of his naked sister and the way the boys are looking at her, has drunk more than anyone: three of the new 7/11 beers, his mason jar of wine and half of Maggie's, four shots of evil brandy, and the last trickle of Malibu Caribbean [modified by Macey with a black marker to read CARRibean.])

"Okay, listen up." Maggie looks around the room. "Time for naked party tricks. Everybody come up with something you can do and let's see what you got!"

"Me first!" says Curt, excited, drunk. "The Running Man, yo. I'm gonna do the naked *Running Man*." And he does it and Macey shrieks in horror.

"Good work. Good work. Joey?" says Maggie.

Joey sitting on the couch, half-conscious now, smoking a cigarette. "Uh . . . I don't know. That's not really my—"

"C'mon, baby," says Maggie, "for me. Do it for rock 'n' roll."

"Okay. The . . . uh . . . the drunk naked somersault . . . without dropping my cigarette."

"Ah'd like to see you do it," Macey says. "You'd break your neck," and with that Joey sticks the cigarette in his mouth and lets himself tumble forward off the couch and somersault into a sitting position, the cigarette hanging from his lips.

"Like that. Like I said." He pulls the cigarette back and blows out a cloud of smoke.

Maggie claps. "Good work, baby."

Ted Boone looks around worried. "I don't know! I don't know. What . . . what . . . uh . . . the naked hug of Carr's sister" and before she can stop him, Ted Boone lurches forward and bear hugs Macey.

"Whoa man, whoa, no, ew, you're all sweaty," says Macey, pushing him away.

"Macey . . . what's yours?" says Curt with a happy gleam in his eye, staring at her tits.

"This." Macey takes Maggie's hand and leads her to an empty spot on the carpet by the wall. They sit, cross-legged in front of each other, knee to knee, and Macey leans in and they kiss.

Ted Boone's legs give out and he kneels down next to the girls. "Oh lord, oh lord," he drawls reverently, ringing his hands. "You two could make me richer than God. You two could make me the next Boone President."

Maggie pulls back. "You kiss like your brother," she whispers. "Whoa, sorry, that was weird."

"Shh, girl."

Maggie touches Macey's hair. "Sorry. That was a dumb thing to say." She leans in and kisses her chin.

Macey puts her hands on Maggie's shoulders and pulls her closer. "It's all good." Kiss. "It's okay." Another kiss.

"Okay, cool."

"Yeah."

Maggie kisses her neck and puts her hands on Macey's chest.

"Whoa, no, slow down, girl." Macey pulls away and shakes her head. She laughs. "Whoa, man. This's some crazy spring break shit."

Maggie stands up and laughs. "Whoa, right?

"Ah ain't never done shit like this," says Macey.

"Here," Maggie reaches down and Macey takes her hand and she pulls her up.

The room is quiet. Joey on the couch watching, smoke rising up from his cigarette. Curt and Ted Boone sitting on the floor.

"That was it," Macey says with a smile. "My trick. Most places you'd pay cash *money* to see that kinda stuff. What about you, Mags?"

"My trick was getting you all naked," she says.

Macey says, "Fair enough. Maggie wins."

Joey opens another beer. Curt and Ted Boone get up.

"What now, y'all?" says Curt, and Macey reaches up and grabs his face, pulling him down to her, and then they're kissing. The rest happens fast. Curt and Macey move to the floor. Maggie pulls Joey off the couch and they lie down on the carpet next to Macey and Curt—Macey, tiny and crushed beneath Curt, his hands all over her chest, pulling her knees up to him.

Maggie watches them, big-eyed, disconnected, drunk, while Joey sucks on her neck.

"Don't give me a hicky."

"Sorry."

"No, it's okay. You can. You . . . you can fuck me, if you want."

"Not now. We're . . . we're too drunk."

"Come on, Joey."

"Not in front of everybody. It's too weird."

"Alright."

"Later. I promise."

"Okay."

Macey and Curt get up and she leads him by the hand into the bedroom.

"Maggie, we should stop."

"No, why?"

"We should. It's too weird."

"Yeah. We should. Look." She nods at Ted Boone in the hallway looking through the linen closet. "It's gonna get awkward."

"Sure, of course."

Ted Boone comes back from the hall closet wrapped in a white sheet. "Beers?" he says quietly. He has three of them held by the neck.

Maggie goes to the closet and gets a wool blanket and she and Joey sit with it wrapped around them and open their beers. She flicks the cap at the wall and it curves through the air and hits the window blinds and falls behind the stereo. Ted Boone sits on the floor next to the couch and sips his beer and stares down at the turntable on the carpet and spins the record with his finger. "What a night." There's no drawl anymore. His voice is quiet and sad and clear.

"I think that was too much for me," Joey says. "I mean, to be honest. That got heavy, quick." He hears the sound of Macey giggling in his bedroom. "Wow, no, no, no."

"I'll drink to that," says Maggie. She holds her beer by the neck but she doesn't drink it.

"I guess the only thing to do is to get . . . totally fall-down *wasted*," says Ted Boone. He doesn't drink, either.

"Yeah." Maggie cuddles up to Joey and puts her head on his lap and then she's asleep.

Macey is loud now, shouting something, laughing.

Joey drinks his beer, and then Maggie's, and tries to blot it out.

"Oh, god!" he hears Macey say. "Oh, fuck! Oh, god! No, stop!"

Joey lurching forward to get up but then Macey's laughing again, "You freak! Dude, you so *crazy*." He settles back into the couch.

Ted Boone lies on his back on the carpet and stares up at the ceiling and his eyes close and he's out.

Joey sets Maggie's bottle down on the carpet and reaches for Ted Boone's and then turns the record player on.

4:12 A.M.

When Joey wakes up, he's blurry drunk and Ted Boone is passed out next to the record player. He can hear Macey laughing from his bedroom again.

Maggie's awake.

"Okay. Now," she says, taking his hand. "Now. In the bathroom."

"Maggie, you sure?"

"Yeah, I'm sure."

She leads Joey down the hall and shuts the bathroom door.

"Maggie, I don't know." Joey tries to compose himself but the room is spinning. "I'm really, really drunk. I don't know if I can."

"It's okay. It's fine. Get a condom."

He digs through one of the drawers until he finds a box of Trojans.

Maggie spreads an orange beach towel on the floor and lies on her back and stares up at him.

The towel has a faded picture of Garfield on it: Garfield with a bubble caption next to him, 'Lasagna on Monday? It's a miracle, John!'

"Now, quick," she whispers.

Joey lies down next to her and then he wakes up again lying on the linoleum and she's sitting in the bathtub with her arms wrapped around her knees, crying.

"You *passed out* on me," she says.

Joey tries to tell her to come back. He says No, no, no over and over again.

She gets up and steps out of the tub and she's all raven-black hair and bright white skin and he fights to keep his eyes open, but then she's there below him and he's there too and all is okay and all is good.

6 A.M.

Joey wakes up again to a knock at the bathroom door. Maggie—curled up asleep, wrapped in the Garfield towel.

Daylight is coming through the space between the linoleum and the door.

"Knock, knock, knock. It's me, Ted Boone. I'm going home. I'm going . . . I'm driving home."

Maggie is awake now and she sits up and tucks the Garfield towel around her and rolls it tight at the chest. She stands up and leans over the counter to look at her face in the mirror.

Joey gets up, pulls the condom off, and drops it in the bathroom trash. "I'm opening the door, Ted Boone. We're coming out."

Joey opens the door and Ted Boone comes in and closes the door behind him and sits on the toilet. He has the Casio keyboard in his lap and he's dressed again—coat on, scarf wrapped neatly around his neck. He looks down at the condom in the trash. "Maggie, Carr. I mean, you guys in here, them in there. I'm kind of the odd man out. I'm just here, by my lonesome. Stranger in a strange land. I'm driving home, alright? Thanks for inviting me, but I should—"

"No, no, no," says Joey. "Ted Boone, no, it's cool. Let's go back in the living room and have a cigarette. Let's get dressed. Maggie, get dressed. We'll make coffee. Coffee? Tea?"

"Tea," he says happily. "With milk."

Back in the living room Ted Boone takes a 7" record out of his shoulder bag and sets it on the turntable and Joey gets dressed. Ted Boone sings along with the record, quietly, his voice rich and husky and low, "And now his ghost is a rising host above the briny blur / I would that soon some maid would swoon and his soul would capture her / He's still a fine kid what with all he did / He's a fan of mine." And then the slow, aching solo, and Ted Boone shuts his eyes and plays a tiny air guitar in the middle of his chest.

Maggie makes tea and then puts on one of Joey's big t-shirts and tosses the Garfield towel back in the bathroom.

"Ted Boone." Maggie hands Ted Boone a cup of tea and he takes it with a smile.

He sips it and his eyes close happily. "Ahhh, 'Power and the passion / Temper of the time.'"

And then Joey's bedroom door is creaking open and Macey shuffles out wrapped in a dark green flannel bed-sheet, her hair a mess. "Whas goin' on?" she says, squinting, puffy-eyed.

"We decided to get dressed," Joey says, lighting a cigarette. The cigarette tastes dirty. He snubs it out in a coffee mug. "Sit down, relax. I think the party's over."

"Thas cool," she says, and then smiles wickedly, cupping her mouth and whispering, "He wants to *fuck* me," she nods back toward the bedroom, "But Ah *can't*. Ah have a *boyfriend*. This ain't cool. He went down on me and then he tried to lick my ass and Ah was like, 'Nooo, dude, no way.' Dude's a *freak*. Ah just wanted to have a good—"

"Okaaay," Joey says, "I don't think we need to hear any more of that. Here, smoke a cigarette and talk about something else. Kittens. Talk about kittens."

"Mewl, mewl, muhfucker." Macey sits down on the couch next to Ted Boone, pulls the green sheet up around her, and lights a cigarette. "Ah was a cat in another life." She puts her head in his lap, trailing her arm and the cigarette hand off the couch. "This cool, Daniel Boone?" she whispers.

"Course darling," he says, petting her head, the smoke twisting up around them.

Curt comes out of the bedroom, naked and big and disoriented, shielding his eyes from the sunlight. "What's up, y'all? Y'all are dressed. We drinkin'?"

"Sure," Joey says. "Have a beer."

"Awright." He sits cross-legged on the floor, then curls up on his side and he's asleep.

Maggie goes into the bedroom and comes back with a blue comforter and covers him up. "I think we blew his mind tonight."

Joey opens the blinds and the sun comes in the window, cold and bright and hard. He looks out into the parking lot and he hears the sound of birds in the trees. "I'm still drunk. We're gonna feel like crap." He pulls the blinds shut.

"*Thank* you," says Macey.

"What Macey said," says Ted Boone. "Well . . . well, I think it's time to sleep. Come on, Mace Face, let's take the bed since your brother was so kind to offer. Meet me there. Get it toasty for me."

"I didn't offer anyth—" Joey starts to say. "That's fine. Take it."

"'Kay," she mumbles, sitting up, pulling the sheet around her. Macey gets up and walks, unsteady down the hall. She staggers to the side and drops her sheet and continues, naked, into the bedroom. "We can mess around but you aren't allowed to fuck me," she calls back to Ted Boone, who's still on the couch. "Those are the rules. Love it or leave it, Daniel Boone."

Ted Boone laughs and shakes his head. "Carr, I've said it before and I'll say it again, women are strange machines. Carrtoosh Carr, Magic Bullet Maggie, it's been good, wonderful, amazing, life-affirming." He stands up and shakes Joey's hand and then Maggie's and then Joey's again. "Carr, in the name of full disclosure, I plan to talk your sweet little sister into letting me rub one out onto her sweet little sister tits and slash or face before I sleep, which—"

"Oh, god. Ted Boone, come on. Don't tell me shit like that."

"—which . . . which in this time zone is *not* considered cheating on your boyfriend but rather a nice, healthy, new-age sleep aid and skin-toner . . . and I have the *public records* to prove it." He stands before them, shaking his head, smiling. "You teenage girls and your inconsistent, fluctuating morals," he wags his finger at Maggie. "Though a man of the cloth, an evil Boone like myself cares not for Judeo-Christian standards of morality. Grey areas and black holes." He gives them a low bow. "Yes, fuck the world, fuck the Austrians, fuck the whales, fuck everyone except the gang of us here. Goodbye, goodnight, I have been . . . *Ted Boone*."

APARTMENT, 5:30 P.M.

It's getting dark early now and by the time Joey wakes up, it's night outside. After Ted Boone and Curt left at half past three, Macey took the couch and gave Joey and Maggie the bed. Joey walks past her now, a brown and white Mexican blanket pulled up to her chin, eyes closed and her mouth open. In her hair, a tiny white clot of dried come and Joey knows it's come and he tries to ignore it but it makes him sad and angry and lonely all at the same time. He goes into the bathroom and gets a wash cloth and runs it under the hot tap and comes back out into the living room and (gently, so as not to wake her) he picks up the strand of hair and loosens the stain with the washcloth and then drops the washcloth in the kitchen trash. Macey stirs in her sleep and says, "Ohhf," and rolls onto her back and now she's still again.

Joey leaves the apartment and goes to the store for Gatorade and tangerines and returns and the place smells like cigarette smoke and stale beer.

He opens the window in his bedroom (Maggie cocooned into the blankets, just her face showing, like a painting of Mary) and lights a stick of Nag Champa. The tangerines go in a wooden bowl that his aunt gave him as a moving-out gift. He sets the mail on the counter and goes through it. Phone bill for the previous tenant (Janey King-Newsom), Trader Joe's flyer ('Trader José's Jalapeño Cheese Tamales, $3.99!'), a notice from AmVets, a Pizza Hut coupon pack, an Oriental Trading catalog, and two postcards: 1) Chicago skyline, industry, steel, tall buildings, and 2) A desert scene—cactus, empty blue sky, orange rockland. 'Visit Us In Arizona!' in looping white lettering.

Joey picks up the first postcard and flips it over. It's from Ben Frank. He looks at the second one. The same.

In tiny handwriting across both sides, hard to read:

Card 1)

Dear Fruit Picker Upper G.I. Joesph McCarr(thy) File Clerk,
Hello from freezing Chicago. [illegible] noon here and I'm sitting in the big room with the TV on writing this. [illegible] says something along the lines of us, "Look at her, Frahhnk," and points at a TV commercial, "her face looks like a *man's* face." Nate's next to me on the sofa, reading one of the books I stole from Crown. He reads aloud, "'How often have I lain beneath rain on a strange roof, thinking of home.'" Nate's on heroin, he thinks no one knows, and I must admit he's pulling it off. [illegible] Peter's been sleeping with a kid called Leo Hauser who works as a runner for a big insurance firm. Leo stays at our place and shoots speed all night [illegible] never sits down and looks like a ghoul, saying, "All you guys do is sit around and watch TV like a bunch of damn zombies." Snow, snow, cascades of white dandruff falling. (They all say it's beautiful but to me it's dead skin.) I can hear a churchbell tolling somewhere out in the streets. Doom! Doom! Doom! That's more like it. (Cont.)

Card 2)

Doom! Yesterday I woke up with one of Byron's songs in my head and walked down the hallway in my boxers and the window was open and there was a dead bird lying on the bathroom floor. I dropped my drawers (you sleep fully clothed here) and sat on the toilet, shivering in the blue light from the window and rapidly shat out a gallon of booze and dumpstered chicken and stared at the bird. My feathers, his feathers, me alive, him gone. Heartbreak and no greater delight. The old awe at being organic and still moving [illegible] despite everything. I promptly [illegible] into Jana's room and fell into her bed like a man into a pool and [illegible] and then I watched while she fixed and tied off with her sparkly silver belt and nodded out, icy and flatchested and purple red green blue haired, her head like a snow cone. Joey, the big news on TV today is I'm coming back to San Diego for the holidays. I'll call when I'm at the Greyhound station Downtown and you will pick me up with a bottle of wine and a pack of cigarettes and a pepperoni pizza the size of the Mayan Calendar (I have no money; I'll starve the whole way over. Fix it). Following that, the two-week party shall begin at my La Jolla office squat and your pertinacity shall be rewarded. Until then, war-mad, wild-hearted, stomping on the rutted corpse of mankind, BenGazi Frank aka [illegible] Mr. Dalloway aka your friend

1980

OCTOBER 3RD

Rose Morning Manor has been hit by wedding madness, so Channy and I are staying away as much as possible. On days when I'm not helping with the farm, we borrow Bettie, Issy's beautiful blue and white '64 Mercury Comet, and take the kids down to P.B. to see Jacob and Sorel. Jake and I are getting along fine these days. Sorel and I don't talk much, but it's not awkward and she's taken well to Channy.

Last week, we bundled up the kids and walked down to the beach and sat on lawn chairs by the lifeguard tower while the kids played in the sand.

Jacob has quit drinking and smoking pot, but he's looking older. He has gained weight since our trip and now his hair is speckled with gray. (He's also starting to lose it. His hair, I mean. It's thinning in the front and for some reason that scares the hell out of me. My brother can't be getting old. I hate that.) Sorel looks the same and now I see what I missed back then. Sorel was (she is) *beautiful.* Still, whatever I once felt for her is gone. Was it love? Now I'm sure it was. I loved Sorel, but the only thing left from our time together is guilt.

OCTOBER 7TH

[Note: Bottom half of page burnt and unreadable.]

OCTOBER 10TH

Tonight we left the kids with Morgan and took the Comet down to P.B. to eat at Roman Oh's. The owners of Bozic's Ocean Floor (RIP) now run an abalone processing plant in the backroom so once a week you can get these great abalone *rellenos* as a two buck special. Abalone Tuesdays. When it's on, the place is packed.

Channy and I have become regulars and we've gotten to know the owner, Roman Angelo, and his whole staff and family. It's nice to have a hangout, a place you can go and get the same thing every time, a place that's a steady thing in your life.

Tonight, after Benny the waiter took our order and Veta the hostess (Roman's wife) brought our bread, Bozic's little boy James ran out of the back and stopped at our table. He stared at us, three feet tall, toe-headed and serious, frowning, then grabbed the breadbasket off our table and ran right out the front door.

Benny and Veta went after him like some kind of slapstick silent movie and Channy and I laughed and I missed the kids and wanted nothing but to leave and go back to the farm and confess everything to Channy and stay there forever, just the four of us, sheltered, sequestered like monks in the dark wood halls. Agh.

After dinner, we went to Jacob's and walked into the middle of a raging party. People on couches smoking pot. The stereo blasting awful rock 'n' roll songs from the '60s, and the living room full of drunk people dancing close and all over each other. I was instantly off-guard.

Channy broke away from me when she saw Sorel and they went out back to talk.

"Hey! Hey, baby brother," said Jacob, emerging from the crowd. He had a joint in his hand and he offered it to me.

"Jacob, you know I don't."

"I know, I know. I just figured—"

"I thought you *quit*."

"It's a party, Mercander. I'm allowed to go off the res *sometimes*. Merc, 'It's impossible to describe what is necessary to those who do not know what horror means.' Tonight's my blow-off night. I'm blowin' it off. Blowin' it away."

"But I thought—"

"Yeaaah, yeah, baby bro, hey listen," talking low, "you and Channy swing?"

"No, god, no. Of *course* not. How could you even *ask*?"

"That's what I figured but . . . this party . . . it's one those kinds of . . . *you know*."

"Oh, wow. Okay. We just came to say hi."

"Just wanted you to know what you were getting yourself into—oh, hey Gracie, hey babe." A young black girl in a white mini dress kissed Jake on the cheek then walked past us into the kitchen. "See that ass? Gracie and me tonight. Sorel and Gracie's guy Kev. You know, Kev K. Smith, the R&B singer. 'You Got The Glory / You Got The Love'? 'Partners in Crime'?"

"No."

"Friend of Herm's. Anyway, you figure it out ahead of time. It's easier that way. Less hurt feelings when people start going off alone together."

I looked around the room, the red lights and bottles, the fog of pot smoke. "Hey Jake, it was good to see you, but I think I'm . . . I'm gonna go find Channy and we're going to—"

"Sure, no problem. I understand. Hey, Merc . . . thanks for stopping by." He hugged me hard and held on for a long time and then broke away and danced into the crowd with the joint held over his head.

Out in the backyard, Channy and Sorel were sitting on the top step of the deck laughing at something, Sorel's head on Channy's shoulder.

I started toward them, then turned and took the brick path out into the dark part of the yard.

From the house, I could hear music and laughter and a swirl of voices.

I knelt down in the wet grass and looked up at the stars, sprawling out immense and countless above me. *Tomorrow.*

OCTOBER

[Note: The date and top half of entry are fire damaged, following three intact, but unreadable, pages]

"Channy, I need to tell you something and I'm really sorry you have to hear this and I'm sorry I couldn't tell you earlier."

"You and Sorel?"

"How'd you know?"

"I've always known, I guess. I mean I could just *tell*."

"Really? How?"

"How you guys acted around each other. (Or didn't act.) How she talked about you when she . . . when she very, *very* rarely did."

"It never happened when we were together."

"I know."

"It only happened—"

"Merc, I know. I know you wouldn't do that to me."

"I'm sorry, Channy. I've wanted to tell you . . . for a long time."

"Why'd you wait?"

"I didn't want you to—"

"What? Leave you?"

"I guess. Yeah."

"Merc, don't forget that the reason you went away the first time was because I told you to go."

"It's not your fault."

"Merc, it is. It was."

"But I—"

"The second time . . . Merc, we know whose fault that was."

"No, it was mine. I should've been there. I shouldn't have worked so much. You wouldn't have been so alone all the time and you wouldn't have had to—"

"Merc, you were twenty. You were a kid."

"People used to be grownups at fifteen."

"They aren't anymore. People take longer to grow up now. You were twenty. We were kids."

"Channy . . . there's something else. When I was down in Mexico—"

"Baby, you don't have to tell me. We're here now."

"When I was down in Mexico I was with a couple of different—"

"A couple?"

"Prostitutes."

"Prostitutes, Merc?"

"Yeah."

"Really? Merc, prostitutes? Like *hookers?*"

"You're laughing."

"Yeah, I'm sorry, I can't believe . . . I mean, I can. Wow, that's funny."

"Stop laughing."

"You're laughing, too."

"I know."

"Merc, you should know me well enough to know that I don't *care* about any of this stuff. We'll never be who we were again."

"Channy, I'm so sorry. About all of this."

"The only thing I'm sorry about is all the time we spent apart. Whenever we're apart, I'm just waiting until we're together again. It's wasted time."

"I feel the same way. God, I love you so much, Channy Morning Greene."

"Channy Carr."

"I don't care. That's how I see you still. I love the sound of your name. I love saying it."

"Well, I'm proud to have your name, so you better get used to it, buddy. I'm in this for the long haul."

"Channy Carr . . . I'm proud of it too."

"I'm sorry you kept it in so long. I mean, telling me about Sorel and all that."

"It feels great to have off my chest. No more secrets. I feel amazing right now."

"I bet. Merc, I'm just happy being here. Me and you. It's all I want."

"I'm so glad to hear you say that."

"Merc . . . do you . . . do you want to know who the baby's father is?"

"As far as I'm concerned, it's me, and that's all anyone'll ever know."

"You sure?"

"It's buried. Family secret. As long as it wasn't Jake or any of his friends."

(Silence) "Merc . . . it was Jake."

"Channy . . . do we—"

"I'm kidding! No, no, no. It wasn't Jake or anyone he hangs out with. Jeez. Don't worry."

"You had me going for a sec."

"I'm sorry."

"I'll get you back for that. If not today, if not tomorrow—"

"Merc, I love you so much that it's just ridiculous."

"Channy, come here."

OCTOBER 16TH

The bricks were still warm from the sun. It was dusk and the work was done and the farm was quiet. Everything was in its place. I finished my Coke and went back into the barn. It was dark under the hayloft, but sunlight filtered in through the cracks while slated pencils of yellow light came through the nailholes in the walls. I set the hay fork in its 'u' on the wall and took off my gloves and stood in the doorway and looked out across the fields—a mist creeping over the lake, the big wall of trees so featureless they were almost black. Back at the farmhouse, someone was turning on the lights on the lower floor. They blinked on one by one. The windows in the parlor were pure yellow now and you could see figures moving inside. And there was Channy. I could see her slim shape, and in her arms the boy and girl. She stood at the window and then she was gone. I tucked my gloves in my belt and began the long walk back to the house.

[Note: another page, dated OCTOBER 18TH, lost to fire damage]

OCTOBER 31ST

Tonight will be the boy's first real Halloween. His sister's too young to know what's going on, but we're dressing her up, too, and she looks great in her fat little pumpkin outfit. The boy is Greedo from *Star Wars*. His favorite character. We got a plastic mask at Sav-On and Channy made him a little green space suit complete with green gloves and boots, and Gus built him a laser gun out of PVC piping. The boy calls his costume "Giddo." "Giddo, daddy, Giddo. Hoween."

Dear Joey and Macey,

Happy Halloween, kids. (I'm going to get a photo of you in your costumes to include with this one.) The plan is to take you guys and Morgan down to P.B. early in the Comet, pick up my brother and his wife, get dinner at Pernicano's (Son, you're into the pizza, but you like sitting in the gondola table more than anything), then trick-or-treating in Jake's neighborhood.

Jake asked me a few days ago if I wouldn't rather leave you two with he and Sorel so that your mom and I could go off and do something on our own. Kids, when you become a parent, you take a backseat to your children. Or at least you should, and if you're any kind of person, you enjoy it. If you bring a child into the world, you have a duty to be the most giving version of yourself, and that means you need to be a little selfless.

Take Jake's friend, Herman King, for instance. Herman and his wife Jennifer live in a beautiful mansion on the seaside of Mount Soledad. Herman sells rare palm trees for a living and his business affords him certain luxuries, the best amongst those is the free time to stay home with his kids and Jenn [Note: Small burnt area obscuring approximately three lines.] Jennifer does a lot of cocaine (which is a horrible thing that you should never, *ever* try) and spends most of her time making these immense wall-sized self-portraits in her backroom studio.

Herman lives on the phone in his kitchen. He wears brown-tinted sunglasses in the house and he has a long dropping mustache like Jake used to have and he isn't comfortable unless he's stoned out of his mind with the radio blaring, the plastic kind of music that people are into these days. Kids, maybe Herman will be a better person by the time you two are old enough to know him, but I have my doubts and I'm hoping that by then he's not in our lives anymore. Jenn's a good person. The problem is she's married to Herman and he treats her like a Labrador and because of that she hates her life. Hence, the drugs. Show me someone who does drugs who isn't dissatisfied with his or her lot in life and I'll be surprised. Kids, drugs are for people of weak character. Some people use them to enjoy things more—music, films, food—but once you start doing that, the things you love will never be the same once you're sober. A good, strong, intelligent person has no need for vice. Life should be good enough and if it isn't you fight until it is. You push and you keep your hands on that plow and you sweat and bleed until you have what you want. The two best things you can be in life are honest and a fighter. I've not always been both but I'm trying to walk the line. I *want* to be better and I think that's an important step.

Herman and Jenny have two girls who you play with sometimes. Dinah and Janey. The girls are three and five and they sit in the house unattended, morning to night. After breakfast—Jane makes hers and Dinah's—they turn on the giant TV and sit there until it's time for bed. If there's nothing on TV, they go outside and roam around the neighborhood without anyone knowing where they are. Officially, they're "homeschooled," but no one teaches them anything and the man in charge of checking up on them is the man who sells Jenn her cocaine. And there's Herman in the kitchen yelling into the phone and Jenn coked out of her mind in the back room painting her own portrait over and over and over again because Herman stopped seeing her for what she is and she needs to build herself everyday to remember she's there. The girls are like scenery, but they're scenery that their parents don't notice anymore. In that house, no one sees anyone. They're all together as some kind of copy or reproduction of a "family," but they're all like ghosts on different planes, moving through the place without touching.

[Note: Fire damage in middle of page, cutting off short paragraph.]

Tonight, I'm going to give you guys the best Halloween that I can. Anything you want, it'll be yours. I want to give the two of you and your mother the best possible life I can. I want you to feel respected and nourished. To hell with Herman and Jenn and the whole aging, rotting "Love Generation" and their faulty ideals. Freedom means being in charge of yourself and acting selflessly and finding the most fulfilling life you can for the people you love; it's not sitting around doing whatever the hell you want. I feel sorry for my brother and his friends. The '60s ruined them. We can be better than that.

Your daddy,
Merc

NOVEMBER 1ST

Halloween was perfect. The streets were dark and full of parents walking kids from house to house, and all the kids in the cutest costumes. For Halloween I was always a cowboy or a soldier but last night I saw neither. Most kids were either witches or ghosts but I saw two Cylons from *Battlestar Galactica*, a couple hobos, a '50s greaser, one clown with big shoes and sad makeup, and a lot of *Star Wars* stuff.

It was a warm night and the air was rich with jasmine and honeysuckle and we took it slow and let Morgan (Strawberry Shortcake) and our little Giddo lead us wherever they wanted.

At home, we went through their candy bags and picked out a few that the boy could eat and finished the rest ourselves. We don't give the kids much sugar, but, like Jake said, you gotta go off the reservation sometimes.

After we put the kids to bed, Issy and Morgan made caramel apples and hot apple cider and Gus and I sat out on the back deck and drank coffee.

Gus let me in on his plans for the wedding, and Channy was right after all, he is the secret Victorian. The funny thing is that it's respectable. This serious man in his denim and wool rancher's coat and Stetson hat talking about wait staff and meal courses and suit cuts—it works. There's nothing absurd, unbecoming or at all unmanly about it.

The thing about Gus is that around him I want to be a better man, and that's one of the best things you can ask for in a friend. Still, talking to him I know that I've got a lot of work left. Someone like Gus will show you your weak and hypocritical sides, and what you see will hurt. Talking to Gus, I realize that I'm judgmental in the areas of my life where I feel most lacking. The reason I'm uncomfortable around people like Herman and Jenn is that I see their flawed parts in me. When someone holds a mirror up, you can either look away or break the glass, pick up the pieces, and build the life you've always wanted. The question is: Do you have the courage to do the latter?

NOVEMBER 15TH

It's November and the whole valley is orange and red and brown. Fall is here in full force, but it's a different kind of fall than the one I knew back east. It's not as sudden, and it doesn't precede a hard winter, but it's beautiful nonetheless, my favorite season of the year, the great slowdown and mellowing.

Today, Channy and Issy went down to Chula Vista to look at bridesmaid dresses and Issy dropped some news on her. Issy's great-aunt Sara left Issy property in Georgia and a good bit of money when she passed eleven years ago, but she made one important stipulation: Issy wouldn't see a penny until she married. If that wasn't big enough news, Issy told Channy that she and Gus have decided to move to Georgia and run Issy's family estate, a former cotton farm outside Atlanta, the second largest in the area. Twenty-four bedroom plantation house, servants' dorm, a fifteen-horse stable with a polo green, hunting land, three lakes, more acreage than anyone in their right mind would know what to do with. The plan is to put Rose Morning up on the market and move out to Georgia by the end of the year. Gus is already hiring staff. Farm hands and a groundskeeper, a butler and two men under him, maids, a cook and a six-piece kitchen staff.

Rose Morning Manor is the first real home I've had. Channy and I talked about getting a bank loan to buy the place, but neither of us have credit (or any money in our own immediate families) and even this far inland the property will come with a considerable asking price. Beyond that, it would be calling in family favors, and we don't want to do that. Issy has been good enough to us already. We want to live beholden to no one. Even someone we love.

As of now, we have a month and a half left on the farm and then our plan is to find a place in the city. I'll miss Rose Morning, and the knowledge that we'll be leaving soon hangs heavy. The fields, the horses, the farmhouse and all its dark wood and hidden rooms and big windows . . . the whole thing is just heartbreaking.

Moving to the city will be a big life-change. I'll need to get a job, and without Issy's large extended family around us, we'll need to look into things like daycare and babysitters for the children. Life out here in the country was a steady, grounded, dependable thing. As long as I have Channy and the kids with me, it'll be a good life, but still, the idea of going back to the city scares the hell out of me.

Oh, I almost forgot! Last night, Jake's friend Herman told Jake that he was the palm tree arsonist from two years ago. Said he used to get coked out of his mind and drive all around town scouting out trees to burn then come back at night to finish them off. (It was something about breaking outside the role he was given.) I asked Jake if he mentioned my *Midtown* stories, but he didn't.

[Note: Burned section. Three pages unreadable. Two more possibly torn out.]

DECEMBER 3RD

This past week was all big family meals and rushing around in a million different directions at once. A few days before Thanksgiving, the people began to arrive. Family from both sides of the wedding flew in from all over the country. They arrived in wild mobs with armloads of food and luggage and gifts. Extended family from Texas and New Mexico and Louisiana and Michigan, Issy's aunt the paleontologist and her three redheaded daughters whose names all rhyme, the usual girl cousins, an uncle I later heard was a "fallen senator from the wrong part of Arkansas."

By Thanksgiving, Rose Morning Manor was packed and the kitchen was full of chattering girl cousins chopping vegetables and making broth and rolling dough. Dinner that night stretched from the dining room into the living room and on into the parlor, with cardtables set up next to the main table, a picnic table carried in from the fields, a dozen people eating at chairs against the wall with their plates on their laps and their drinks on the floor between their feet.

The meal was four dressed turkeys, three honey-baked hams, a roast, Yorkshire pudding, three yam casseroles, a dish of green beans and fried onions, nine breaded trout from the lake, four pots of mashed potatoes, nine bowls of gravy, a vat of cranberry sauce, a platter of corn on the cob, three plates of summer squash baked with marshmallows and kale, a desert called "the pink stuff," Idiots' Delight, assorted pies (pumpkin, apple, rhubarb, blackberry, cherry, banana cream, sweet potato, pecan), cookies (chocolate chip and walnut, sugar cookies, peanut butter, Mexican wedding cookies, ginger cookies, oatmeal raisin), baskets of sourdough rolls and buttermilk biscuits and black bread, popovers, fresh butter brought by Johnston's son Frank, a platter of green Julian apples sliced and drizzled in caramel and butterscotch, and a dozen glass bowls full of filberts, walnuts, pecans, hazelnuts, peanut butter chocolate drops, and candied pears.

Issy and Gus sat at the head of the main table and Gus held up the conversation, running from cattle stock to rare gem collecting to the tragedy of Clipperton Island. (The men of the island killed off and the corrupt lighthouse keeper declaring himself "king" and enslaving all the women as his harem. Killed later by the widow of the island's governor *just as* the Naval rescue ship arrived. High drama.)

The meal went long into the night and, one by one, the friends and family members excused themselves or drifted off into other rooms or went out onto the porch to smoke the Cuban cigars that Gus' father brought up from Havana in 1950.

At the end of the night, it was just Channy and me and Gus and Issy, both of them quite drunk.

I raised my glass for a toast. "To the end of an era."

We drank the toast and Gus pushed himself from the table and rocked back in his chair, satisfied and full. "So, the city."

"That's the plan," said Channy, the sleeping baby in her arms.

"You don't sound as excited as you did."

"We are," she said. "I mean," she looked at me, "It's different. It's something new. And it's not like we haven't lived in the city before."

"You know the offer stands," said Issy, elbows on the table, face in her hands, her eyes glittering and her cheeks flushed with drink.

"We've talked it over," I said, nodding at Channy. "It sounds nice and in a perfect world . . . but these past couple years have been *busy*. We'd like to stay put for a while. Let the kids meet friends. Find a neighborhood that we like. Speaking for myself, I mean, I'm *tired*. I don't know why I am, but I am. I feel *old*. The idea of pulling up stakes again is—"

"Daunting," said Channy, nodding.

"Daunting."

"You two are *young*," said Gus. "What are big life-changes for but the young?"

"I know but . . . I mean, aren't you guys kinda heartbroken to leave the place?"

"Yeah," Issy nods. "I've . . . I'm mean I've worked hard and I had a *plan* for Rose Morning. But . . . sometimes you have to make sacrifices to take things to the next stage. It's gonna hurt. I won't lie."

"Anyway, Merc, look," says Gus. "Regardless, you're the perfect age to set off and try things out for a while. You need to come along with us and see how it goes. Let's all be proper *Southerners* together. We have a chance to build something that could last for *generations*."

We agreed that it sounded good, but our plans were set.

Channy got up to check on the boy and Issy went into the kitchen to help clean up and it was just Gus and me.

"I'm telling you, Merc, this is an opportunity, and one day you'll regret all the chances you didn't take."

"I appreciate the offer, Gus. Don't get me wrong. You and Issy . . . it's *exciting*. You're starting a new life and that has to feel . . . I mean, I can *tell* by looking at you it feels great. We just need some time to settle down and do things on our own and not depend on anyone. You guys have money. That's you. We need to find our own way."

"I respect that. I do. I just . . . I just hope you're not acting out of fear."

"Maybe I am. Maybe we are, but everything seems to be pointing to . . . like, *all signs point to stop* or whatever the saying is. Channy and I need to set a base of operations for a while. She's nearly done with the book and I think she's going to try to get it published."

"She should."

"She needs a few months still. Plan right now is to take a week off in December and go to Keith Martin's cabin in Alpine where she can finish it."

"He Roger Martin's boy?"

"Yeah. He and Channy went to school together at Clairemont and we caught up with Keith and Lupe at the bowling alley a while back. He bought the cabin with his artichoke money."

"He and his brother have some acres up in Watsonville, don't they?"

"He's farming there and in Castroville, Salinas, and La Selva Beach. He's done well and he told us, y'know, any time we want we can stay at the place. He and Lupe and their kids never use it and K.M. says it's beautiful this time of year with all the snow on the trees and the fireplace going. Channy wants to head out there and finish typing the manuscript and then start editing when we get home. After that, who knows."

"You know, my brother Billy owns a big press in New York City. Calibre Dale Press. They started small in the '50s and now they're doing well—what with Ed Distler's books selling so fast these days."

"I *love* Distler."

"They did *A Book of Lists,* two novellas, and his first novel, *Ghosts and The Amazon*. Distler's my first cousin. His parents were killed in a streetcar accident when he was twelve, and after that we grew up together. My parents raised him after he lost his."

"Really? I mean . . . Jesus, I had no idea. *Ghosts and The Amazon* is fantastic. I read *Ghosts* in school. Ed *Distler*. I'm impressed. Were you . . . I mean, were you there when he—"

"No, no, no. He went off and did that himself when most of us were out at the Denver stockshow. Just Eddie . . . alone out in the fields with his favorite shotgun. We all took it pretty hard, as you might imagine."

"God, I'm sorry. This is all news to me."

"Well, anyway, right . . . the past. Sometimes it's hard to believe it's real when you don't see it every day. My brother Bill . . . Bill's a good man and his printing house is solid and he loved that story of Channy's that Miracle Press put in their anthology.

"'The Girl on the Bed and The Man by The Mirror.' One of her best."

"He asks about her a lot. If I'd known she was so close to finishing, I would've put in a word earlier. I bet he'd love to take a look at her manuscript. Last time I talked to him, he told me he thought Channy had a lot of McCullers in her, and that's high acclaim coming from Bill."

"Well, she'll be excited about that. To say the *least*. She and I were just talking about *Ghosts*. There's a scene during the Battle of Berlin—"

"I know the one."

"—where the Greek boy is digging through the rubble and in the rubble he comes across a stone in a red glass bottle."

"A glowing red stone."

"A glowing red stone, dark red like a ruby with a light shining from it and he breaks the bottle it's in and he kneels there in the ruins of Berlin with the shells dropping all around and he reads the inscription on the stone . . . what does it say . . . I always meant to look it up . . . it says *thana*—"

"'*Thanatos ouden diapherei tou zen*.'"

"What does it mean?"

"It means, 'Death is no different than life.' It's from Thales of Miletus.'"

"The Father of Science."

"Right." Gus held his amber wine glass to the light and shut one eye and stared into it. "He was the first mathematician. He was a Hylozoist, if you know what that is."

"I don't."

"Deals with abiogensis, biological life rising from inorganic material. He believed that all matter was alive. He also theorized that earthquakes were a result of the land itself floating on water, that the earth shook because it was rocked by waves, like pieces of an ice flow, or a lake dock moved by boat wake."

"'Death is no different than life.'"

"It makes sense when you look at the boy's experiments later in the book."

"It does. Channy and I were just talking about that . . . about the quote."

"Alright, listen, buddy, I'm *bushed*. I'm off to bed. Promise me . . . promise me you'll at least . . . *think* about it. Keep the thought of moving out there with us in mind. If not now, later, in the future. There's no expiration date on this."

"I will."

"You and Channy are too smart to live in the city. You know what I mean? Paying city rents for a room the size of a shoebox just so you can be near things to *buy*. You want that?"

"I guess not."

"Breathing all that *bad air*. Everyone working all day like slaves to afford a house they're never at because they're *working* all day. Listen, Merc, you don't have to promise anything. Just think about it."

The wedding was a few days after Thanksgiving: a Roman Catholic ceremony at St. Martin's. Issy, dark and gorgeous in a train of lilac and pale blue. Gus, looking proud and serene and satisfied in his Italian suit.

The reception was held at Karn Marshall Galloway's famous dining hall, a room he had built after the armistice, in the English medieval style.

The party went long into the night and by the time the desserts were served, Channy and I had a new plan. We'd regroup for a month or two in town and then as soon as Channy's book was finished editing, we'd pack up the kids and follow Issy and Gus out east and start our new life.

Dear kids,

I'm writing this as your mother drives. The weekend in the cabin was just what we needed. I drew up plans for our move back east and your mother finished typing her book.

It's dark outside the car and the snow is eerie blue on either side of the road and your mother's playing her tape of Elton John's *A Single Man*.

It's the near-instrumental track, the piano piece, "A Song for Guy." An achingly beautiful song, sad and longing and hurt, but almost spiritual in its optimism.

Your mother's handwritten manuscript is in the trunk and the typewritten book sits on the seat between us, six-hundred pages, bound with a thick red rubber band across the middle.

As of now we're an hour out, but it's nice driving with Channy and listening to her favorite music and taking it slow.

"Merc, when we move out to Gus and Issy's, I want to take up archery."

"I'll buy you the stuff for it."

"And chopping wood. For exercise."

"You're not out of shape."

"But you know, two kids."

"You'd be cute chopping wood. *The little lumberjack*."

"Merc, you rat, are you *writing down everything I'm saying*?"

"Yeah."

She laughs. "*Turkey*."

"I think it was a left back there."

"Oh. I didn't see the sign."

"It was there."

"Really?"

"It was a way's back."

"Hey baby, Issy's friend Dawny told me this one—"

"Okay."

"When is a women and her child the warmth of the sun?"

She holds the wheel at ten and two and looks at me, smiling in the dark—radiant, beautiful.

2000

DON DIEGO EXPO HALL, DEL MAR FAIRGROUNDS, 4 P.M.

Joey looks up at the airplane hanger ceiling of the expo hall with its metal rafters and beams, the aisles of vendors' booths, the rows of cliplights above product displays, the horse trailers and decorative blocks of straw. He looks up because he's guilty. He wants to forget about Tyler walking next to him and all the things he's going to tell him on the drive back to Clairemont.

'Three Weeks of Equestrian Pageantry!' says the banner across a feed display. Joey and Tyler are here for Tyler's Intro to Marketing class (Professor Ned Gallagher, prostate cancer survivor, divorced, secret writer of haiku in the Gary Snyder style). Tyler tells Joey all about the assignment on the drive up the coast. "Create a viable hypothetical strategy involving a vendor at the Del Mar Fairgrounds' annual horse show. Delineate (and elaborate upon) five points of potential success. Propose path and estimate trajectory of financial arc. Anticipate areas of failure and offer plan for pragmatic preemptive strike. BRAINS: Believe, Research, Act, Impress, Navigate (to) Success."

On the way up to Del Mar, they hot-boxed the car with the weed that Curt left at Joey's apartment and they stepped out into the blinding sun of the parking lot crushingly stoned.

It was cold and breezy but Joey broke out in a sweat as he made note of: 1) The curve of the big valley, 2) The flat expanse of sea below the fairgrounds to the west, 3) The flags snapping in the breeze (and how the sound made him think of a] flags on castle turrets, b] a Naval yard, and c] something vaguely reminiscent of Crown Point Elementary School.) Finally, and as a side-glance, 4) The brown hills and old wetlands to the east. In summary: Too much before them and too much behind and all the parked cars with sun on their windshields and all the people walking toward the hall and everyone in English riding wear or Western gear, checked shirts, hats, boots, and/or jockey caps.

Joey lit a cigarette as they walked to the ticket box.

"Tyler, I think I'm too stoned for this."

"Put your sunglasses on."

"I forgot them."

"In the car?"

"At home."

"Want mine?"

"No, no, it's okay."

To fit in, Joey bought a cowboy hat at the first booth inside the hall. A nice, hard yellow-straw Stetson with a handsome black band. Not comfortable, but something big and sturdy to hide beneath. (Some people are happier as someone else.)

They walk past a booth offering samples of colorful rope. The man sitting behind the table is slouched back in his chair, arms folded over his chest, Tractor Supply ballcap pushed low over his eyes, asleep. Tyler takes a business card and a sample of pink and purple rope and twists it in his hands as they walk.

"This rope is campy," he says.

"Huh?"

"Nothing."

"Oh, campy, right."

"Joey, where've you been all week? I called your apartment like six hundred million times."

"I don't know, busy I guess."

"It's alright. I just—"

"I know."

Tyler and Joey haven't spoken in weeks. Today is no different. When Tyler asks where Joey's been, why he hasn't called back, the guilt hits and Joey tries to change the subject and makes jokes and offers plans as distractions.

"Hey Tyler . . . we should . . . let's get a drink. On me. I think I saw the Horsemen's Club had mint juleps."

"Mint what?"

"Julep. A mint julep. It's a Southern drink. It's bourbon . . . or whiskey . . . what's the difference between whiskey and bourbon? Anyway, one of those and I think sugar and mint leaves mashed up together."

"Yum."

"Yeah, they're great. Makes you feel like that cartoon Southern rooster, you know, 'Ah say, Ah say, Ah say, Ah do say, bring me my duuueling pistol, son. You, *suh*, have offended my awe-nah.'"

Tyler laughs and does his own Southern rooster impression. "I say! I do say! Bring me my dueling pistol, my good sir!"

"That sounds British."

"It does. It does. Hey, look more twelve-year-old girls!" Tyler says, pointing to a mass of tiny bodies in English riding suits coming toward them. "Daddy," he says in a high and girlish voice as the girls divide and pass into two packs and move around them, "Daddy dear, buy me some Mexicans and some black slaves to comb my stallion. Daddy I want amigos *and* negroes for Christmas! Comb my stallion, daddy!"

"Tyler, Jesus, don't, please."

"Comb my *thoroughbred*!" He laughs. "Thoroughbred's a funny word, isn't it? I'd like to be a horse person just so I could say 'thoroughbred' all the time. 'Oh *Bunny*, have you seen my thhhhoroughbred anywhere? I think I've misplaced my thoroughbred. *How sahhhd*.' I bet I'd make a good horse person. What do you think?"

"Tyler, you can't just—"

"I *can*."

"You don't even know what I'm going to say. What I was going to *say* is you can't just keep pointing out *twelve-year-old girls* wherever we go."

"One over there. One over there."

"Tyler . . . Tyler, people are going to think you're," whispering, "Tyler, they're going to think you're a *pedophile*."

"Pedophiles are funny."

"Oh yeah? How so?"

"They are."

"Wow, they're *really* not. You can't just . . . *ironically like pedophiles*. That's too much."

"Whatever. I think they are, so they are. Scary stuff is funny. It's fun to laugh about scary stuff. Look at all . . . like, all the funny Hitler movies . . . *The Producers*? Totally funny," singing, "Springtiiiiime for Hitler in—"

"Please, Tyler. You're freaking me out. I'm gonna have a panic attack."

"Lighten up. Fun is fun. Do you like fun? I like fun. Fun is fun. Fun's pretty okay. Look!" laughing, "That's . . . that one's like the White Aryan Resistance twelve-year-old g—"

"Jesus, Tyler. At least call them . . . use a *code*."

"A code?" Tyler turns to Joey and stops walking. "I love codes. I'm the best at codes. What kind of code?" His eyes bright and happy. "Give me a code they won't crack."

"Call them . . . call them . . . uh, okay . . . T.Y.O.Gs."

"What's T—oh, right, yeah, hahaha. Hellooo T.Y.O.Gs and thoroughbreds!" Tyler shouts happily, arms raised above his head, turning a half circle. "I am Tyler Monahan! 'Do you see that I am your friend? Can you see that you will always be *my* friend?'"

"*Jesus,* Tyler, you're killing me."

"*Dances with Wolves* reference, mothafuckaaaah." Tyler shakes his head and laughs, happy and satisfied that he's done something bad.

They walk past an indoor corral where a young girl in a silver rhinestone cowboy outfit rides a tall black horse along the circumference of the fence.

Tyler pulls a yellow Kodak disposable out of his messenger bag and snaps a photo of her without looking into the viewfinder. Click. "One for the files!" he announces to the people around the three-bar fence. "One more for the files." He leans in and whispers to Joey, "the *pedo*philes."

"Tyler, please. I'm too stoned for this. You're *seriously* freakin' me out. Please don't—"

"What, I've got nothing to hide," shouting, "Attention citizens of the Del Mar Fairgrounds! We are here on a mission from the Church of Jesus Christ of Latter Day Saints! We seek T.Y.O.G. wives and thoroughbreds to put them on!"

"No, Tyler, pleeeeease."

"People of the Farigrounds!"

"No. No, no, no."

"Give us what we want! Cough it up!"

A thin, gray-faced man standing at the gate in a black Stetson and a dark tight suit turns to glare at them. His eyes narrow at Tyler, and he shakes his head. Tyler smiles, waving. "Jus' doin' the waaark of Jaaaysus Chriiist!"

"Please, Tyler. I'm starting to—"

Joey feels the room tightening in around him. He walks faster to get away from Tyler but Tyler jogs back up to him, laughing. "They love me in this place. That guy back there fell in love with me." Tyler looks back at the man and gives him a floppy wave. The man looks down at his left boot and knocks the toe of it against the fence. "Joey? You there?" Tyler waves his hand in front of Joey's face as they walk and makes a radio static sound and pretends to talk into his fist. "Tsssht. Tsssht. Earth to Joey Carr. Come in, Joey Carr. You there? Ground Control to Maaaajor Carr. Ground Control to Ma—"

"Yeah, whoa, I'm just . . . whoa . . . I'm just really, really . . . how did I get so stoned?"

"You sure you're okay?"

"Yeah, I'm fine. I'm okay. Ohhh man. Hold on. I need to—"

"You've been quiet and kind of, I don't know, different or weird or something. Look at those T.Y.O.Gs!" He snaps a picture of them and they look in the direction of the flash. "They're like a school of rich retarded fish. Private school fish. Get it?"

Joey goes pale and stops walking.

"Joey, what?" he says, laughing. "That was *funny.*"

The lights around Joey go dark and then bright again. "Yeah, I need to . . . whoa—"

"You okay?"

"I need to stop for a second and catch my br—"

Joey, bent over now. Hands on his knees. Breathing hard. Sweat dripping on the floor. Drops of sweat from his face dotting the concrete. His hat falls off. He tries to pick it up, swaying to the side.

"Joey? You okay? Joey do I need to do something? Joey!"

"Tyler . . . Tyler, where was the . . . ohh, I can't breathe . . . the . . . the restroom?"

Beads of sweat on his forehead.

Wipes them off with his sleeve.

"Joey what's going *on*?!"

"Oh man. Oh god. Restroom . . . where is it?!"

"Oh! Wait! Back at the hotdogs! Right by the hotdogs!"

Tyler points to the left of them and Joey staggers off.

At the bathroom sink he takes off his cowboy hat and drops it in the trash next to him and grips the edge of the sink and holds on.

"Y'awright, son?" says the man next to him washing his hands. The man turns off the tap, shakes his hands at his sides and then pulls a paper towel from the dispenser and rubs them dry. He wads up the towel and drops it in the trash next to Joey's hat. "Son? You need me to—"

You're having a panic attack. That's all. Look at the man next to you. Forget about yourself and concentrate on him and it'll pass. Don't think about yourself. The man: string tie with a silvery abalone shell center, long-sleeve denim shirt with embroidered horse heads on the shoulders, cowboy hat, tan or yellow or something, not important, no, this is important, tan, yes, tan cowboy hat, pink skin, white hair, shirt buttoned at the wrists with black stone snaps, slacks, boots, blue eyes, worried, why is he worried, what's he worried, about? No, no, sticker label on his shirt, "Hello, My Name Is Frank Johnston J-E Tack and Feed, Lakeside, CA," his company's name, okay, turn on the cold water, yes, do it, no, turn it on, reach for it, turn it, okay, good, yes, splash your face.

"Son?"

Joey runs his hands through his hair and slicks it back and looks in the mirror.

Who is that in the mirror? It's not him. It's you. You've had a stroke, no, a panic attack, don't forget, you're having a pani—no, you're not here, the bay, okay, sitting on the catamarans, October, the dusk over the water, slow down, breathe, slow, slow, the ghost shrimping women, they're walking along the shore in white pants and tops and straw hats like umbrella tops, it's choreographed, good, okay, good, breathe, good, big elegant steps like a tai chi class at Balboa Park, no it's not, it is, they're dancing on the shore to put on a show for you, how nice, the music is a . . . swelling . . . throb of . . . strings and trilling pan flute, a zither plunked once, the rowboat pulled up onto the sand and you're walking back to the house to get lunch for you and Nicole to go rowing and no, no rowboat, there was never a rowboat to begin with because this is earlier and the rowboat was never built, the rowboat is a tree somewhere, tall and strong with its leaves up in the wind, branches were baby birds are born, shade for flowers, in ten years it will be lumber, no, no tree, no boat, just you and your friends you miss so much now and your toes in the sand, your feet are small and dark brown and your toes are tiny and your toenails bright white, you're just a kid, you play with toys and battery operated squirt guns that look like Uzis and M-16s and you make your action figures talk and they all have their own voices and favorite meals and catchphrases. Shipwreck is the sailor's name and he has a little plastic parrot you lost as soon as he was out of the box from Susan's Toys, though you looked for it for weeks in the garden (he loved to eat fish and chips and drink beer), and there's Duke the leader you always liked him (dependable, honest) and Bazooka what did he do, he had a bazooka, boring, you traded him for the Marine, the Marine what was the Marine's name? Leatherhead, Face, Man? Neck! Leatherneck! He was boring, but you could rely on him to whup some Cobra ass. Shipwreck was the best. Wisecracking, funny, had a pirate's soul, settled things with his fists, "full of juice" like your second cousin used to say about your mom. No, your cousin said nothing. No cousin. There was a girl Joe—Scarlett. Red hair. Oh, two of them. Scarlett and Lady Jaye. Right. You used to make them kiss and you'd get erections in your shorts and you didn't know why and you felt horrible about it. No, you were okay. That was fine. The girls, they were in love. You had a wedding for them and you told "Tall" Tim about it and he called you"stupid and crazy" and you went home and threw both of them out into the yard and didn't go looking for them for a week. You were so embarrassed. No, it was okay, you were fine. You were unsure but you were safe and you were happy and no one was angry with you about anything. Scarlett and Lady Jaye. They were in love and they would hump. Hump you called it because that's all you knew. Your uncle saying, "Boys have poles and girls have holes. Poles go into holes once they're married and that's humping and when they hump there's a baby in nine months end of story done ask your aunt about the rest leave me alone." Lady Jaye was your favorite of the two. If you thought about it too much Scarlett would remind you of the fever and the fever meant you burned the Velveteen Rabbit and that was horrible because it might happen to your stuffed lamb you named Pindo Lapillo. But that never happened. Pindo's still in a shoebox under your bed (minus one eye and most of his wool) and the Velveteen Rabbit went to a farm in either England or New England and lived with a farmer who loved him. You didn't have scarlet fever but you had the flu and you know how the flu was, a week in bed that felt like a year, fantasy books all around you, the boy in the forest with his wisecracking assistant beast, the mice that lived in a church abbey and had wars and ate feasts of cheese and elderberry wine and harvest soups and kept piles of nuts and made bread and you had a cup of soup you were so hungry thinking about it. Chicken and Stars! You loved the kid's books that made you want to eat and you loved soup and you loved Chicken and Stars more than anything besides tomato but that came later, after Harriet the Spy when all-things tomato were wonderful. The flu was alright. Stare straight ahead and breathe in and watch the bay-water, a sheet of silver, the ripples of boat wake splash up on the shore but just barely, a tremor in the mercury you can feel in your blood. A pelican skimming the surface, slow and weightless with hollow bones like soda straws, and sitting on the catamaran you stand up balancing on the light hull and close your eyes and stretch your arms out like the pelican's wings and "Tall" Tim says, "Koo Koo," like a clock, "Koo Koo! Koo Koo!" But it's you in the bathroom mirror staring back. And it isn't the nice one. It's the monster-you, the one who lies and can't own up and doesn't care about anything but doing whatever he wants, that's who you are, you're in the bathroom at the fairgrounds, standing in front of the sink, the bay sand washed off your feet, December, late fall, the fluorescent lights are terrible and you can hear the lapping of the bayshore deep in your ears, the man standing next to you, he's looking at you, he's concerned, he hates you because you're not a man to him, you're not that nice wholesome kid anymore and he knows it, you do drugs and have gross thoughts and weird fantasies about sex and you lie and hurt the people you love and maybe you don't them love after all, maybe you hate everyone in the world, maybe you're using everyone, using them and throwing them away, looking out for what's best for you, you're a snake, a robot without feelings, a spray of acid in the pretty girl's face, a crooked lawsuit, a vengeful ex, a con-man scheming, a knife in the dark, a shot in the back, a corporate raider destroying families, you're the Nazis, the Plague, AIDS, a wriggle of maggots beneath the dead deer's skin, no, it's you in the mirror, the nice you and the monster, Joey Carr, son of Cowboy Merc the Julian Jerk. Mercander Carr, who died driving home and took your mother too. Hit by a drunk driver in Alpine and off the road into ditch. Just like that and then two sides of the family fighting, and you off to live with your aunt Sorel and uncle Jacob and your sister to the Midwest to live on your great-aunt Clara's farm. A trucker found both cars in the morning but it was too late. The drunk driver's Buick in the middle of the road, his body shot out the window, thirty feet away, face down, still hanging on, then a coma, dead a week later. Your parents . . . burned up in their car, their car burnt down to the tires. You were two and Macey was a baby, staying with your mother's cousin Morgan. Your mom and dad, you have no memories of them, they were no one to you. You never knew them. But you're not a Lost Boy on the Lost Boy island. That's too easy. You're starting over. You're something new. Become an island. No. Let it sink. The island is a hill and the hill is underwater.

Swim.

EPILOGUE

The words on the wall are written in blood. Dried brown letters, drawn on with a fingertip. "College Night Flexitime!" Maggie asks Joey what it means and he shrugs. She says she likes it anyway and Joey kisses her forehead and she tells him that she's cold. Joey hugs her for a long time and then he gives her his jean jacket and she gives it back but he insists and she takes it and puts it on and Joey buttons it up high and says Better and she says Better too. Above the doorway to the stairwell another one: "You win, pal, I'll cut you up with my sword and put you on a pizza." They laugh. A lot of blood, she says, and he nods and says that it must've taken days. She tells him it's her favorite because it sounds like something he would say, the pizza stuff, the sword stuff, the violence but friendship at the core, and Joey says her name to himself, her whole name. He says it because he knows he's hers even if she's not his, and he says it because he's coming down and *god* he's tired. He's so tired that he could lie down in the corner and turn to stone and then dust . . . the dust collapsing.

The office lobby is dark except for a dozen saint candles arranged to light the entrance. At the entrance to the hall, a moldy slice of pizza with a pentagram of red tea lights around it. They look closer. Pennies arranged on the pizza like pepperoni. Joey holds his cigarette lighter up as they walk, the flickering light on the wall like the tomb of a pharaoh: "I'll make a suitcase out of your dad's ties." "I shit gold into your ears, conquistador." She whispers that one, tracing the letters just short of touching them. Maggie asks Joey if Ben Frank did all these himself and Joey says he did. He tells Maggie that this is Ben Frank's secret hideout and that he lives here when he's in town. He tells her that Ben Frank has no parents and she says that she knows and tells him to remember that he was her friend first and that he's always telling her things she knew first. Joey laughs and says maybe he does and then he says Ben Frank's a Lost Boy and she says that maybe he's not a Lost Boy, maybe he's Peter Pan and of course that's obvious and true, and he smiles at the thought of it.

She takes Joey's hand and holds it tight and says, Take me to the party, and he's brave now and he leads the way and now he's not tired. He could've slept forever but now he's awake. Hers, but not his. This is okay.

Joey's lighter cuts out and he tries to flick it on again, but it's dead and he sticks it in his back pocket.

They feel their way down a dark section of hall and into a large room lit with candles. The lair. Ben Frank's friends sitting on tossed-out Lay-Z-Boys and lawn chairs and standing in groups drinking forties. Ratty Indian carpets and milk-crate bookcases. In one corner, a pile of blankets and a blonde girl wearing a fast food uniform asleep with her arms wrapped around a backpack. Bottles everywhere. A smashed-up model ship on the floor with plastic rigging. More writing in blood. Just words now. 'Banned.' 'Soda.' 'Mutant.' They stand inside the doorway and no one sees them. Another set of words in blood: 'Steel.' 'Trees.'

'Doorway' (above the door). Across the room, a mirror propped up on the floor and Maggie and Joey standing in it looking back at themselves. Maggie's head on Joey's shoulder. Her arms around his chest. Joey whispers that they're Scrooge McDuck and the ghost of Christmas Whatever and they're watching their lives without them. She tells him that this isn't their life and he yanks one of her braids and she kisses his neck.

Kids milling about. Candles the size of Pringles cans. Platters of dumpstered food. Red grapes. Baguettes. Leroy Harris sitting on the floor (calm, patient) taking the strings off a red sunburst Les Paul. May in a ripped-up felt coat and a short dress collecting money in a Maxwell House can. Nate, standing in the middle of the room wearing boxers, a sleeveless black t-shirt, pink-framed sunglasses, and a big pair of neon green ski gloves.

"Okay! Listen up!" he says loud enough for everyone to hear. "The game is called High Stakes Pants Traders. What happens is that everyone takes off their pants and trades with someone else. Now, when I say go, drop your pants and find somebody to trade with. Alright? Okay, go!" Nate picks up a toy megaphone from a cardboard box on the floor. He turns it on and hits the siren. "High! Stakes! Pants! Traders!" he yells through the megaphone and does the siren again.

A small, redheaded girl standing next to Nate unbuttons her fly and struggles out of her pink jeans and throws them aside. She picks up Nate's big black pants and steps into them and pulls them high around her chest and yanks the belt snug and says, "I'm you," and walks off. Nate takes her tiny jeans and tries to push a leg into them but they're too small. He kicks his leg into the pants and hops on one foot and falls backward onto the sleeping girl and the pile of blankets. "High Stakes Pants Traders!" he shouts, lying on his back, the pink jeans hanging off his foot, the sleeping girl startled awake, flailing at him, beating her fists on his head, laughing and screeching. She pushes him off and he flops over onto his belly and she gets up and stands on him like a surfboard, then steps off him and walks away.

In one corner, Ben Frank and two boys wearing Halloween masks are smashing a line of beer bottles with a golf club. The wolfman and a vampire. All three in their boxers and nothing else.

"Forrrrrre!" screams one of the boys. He swoops just over the top and tries again and this time the bottle sprays into shards against the wall. He pulls the mask up on the top of his head like a hat. "Fore," he says proudly. "Fore, fore, fore, fore." He hands the golf club to Ben Frank and takes a pair of bright blue tights from the floor and holds them up to his belt-line.

Ben Frank brings the club over his shoulder and with a signature shout of "Ben Frank!" he slices it through a line of bottles.

Maggie grabs Joey's hand and whispers that they should go explore and he says, definitely, and they run back down the hall.

The building is a maze of corridors. Some of the smaller rooms are too dark to see into, but most are lit by the moon and the streetlights outside. They take the stairs up to the third floor, their shoes echoing in claps behind them as they run, Maggie a few steps ahead of Joey, her braids bouncing on her shoulders and back, and then into the third floor hall.

As they run past each room, Maggie shouts what they'll be once she owns the company. One will be the music room. A mattress on the floor. Speakers below it like box springs and you lie down and turn on the volume and it thunders below you. The stab room. A file cabinet full of steak knives. Stab holes in the walls to blow off steam. She tells Joey that this is what his job would be like if she had her way, ghost-town office, ghost job, and we'll run away together and go somewhere we've never been. Sit on couches in the desert. Live in a tree house and shoot arrows and run across the forest floor.

And now the hallway dead ends into a large open room full of empty desks, white metal glowing in the moonlight, each identical to the next.

Joey—bent over, hands on his thighs, catching his breath. His heart pounds. It opens and shuts like a hand and he feels old.

"Joey, this one's horrible. Let's go back."

"Hold on." He walks alone into the middle of the room. "No, no, *look at this. This* is where I work. The exact same . . . the same exact layout without the cubicals. Weird. Right here. This is my desk. Look, Maggie. There's Marcus before he left and that's the door to Rob's office and that's Yesenia at hers, filing her nails a million miles an hour and looking bitchy. Across there is where the Jeffs would be."

"Joey, let's go. This room's bad."

Joey climbs up onto one of the desks. "Bad?"

"Yeah, bad." Maggie stands below him, looking up, the moon on her face.

Joey helps her onto the desk and she's next to him and now her arms are wrapped around his chest and he's warm and he feels her heart beating next to his.

"I hate this place, Joey. Let's go, okay?"

"I'm going to tell him."

"I know you will."

"Maggie, I mean soon. Tomorrow."

"Can we go home, Joey?"

"Yeah. Of course."

But they stay where they are.

The metal legs of the desk creak below their feet and the air is damp and the ceiling crumbling and the lights of La Jolla sprawl out through the big wall of windows, the darkness of the coastline and the sea beyond, a sliver of dark purple on the horizon, wavering, a dim light against the black.

"Joey . . . you know I love you, right?"

The moonlight on her face, pale and silver. Her eyes shine up at him in the darkness. She looks at him, nervous, expectant. *My Maggie, Tyler's Maggie, her boyfriend's, her own, no one's.*

"Yeah."

"Say that you know it."

"I do."

"No, *say* that you know it."

"I know it."

"And you believe me, right?"

They stand in the middle of the room, the world turning around them, and Maggie and Joey steady, a pinnacle, a place where the orbit has no pull. Outside, the earth dips into the sea, the end of the coast and continent, the end of the world.

"I believe you."

"Good, because I want you to believe me."

"I do."

They climb down from the desk and leave the party and drive back home.

Supporters

This first printing of *Caveworld* was crowd-funded by a number of good eggs, including:

Jacqlynn Asherman
The Book Shop
Chris Cooke
Jay Duquette
John N. Duquette
Al English
Linda Farmer
Amanda de Frias
Anthony Gallo
Arlene Gnade
Rikka De Herrera
Katarina Marelja
Benno Martens
Russ Maxwell
Drew Packham
Joseph Phelps
The PNW Contingent
Mary Roche
Michael Schuster
Jeremy Staples
Dayna Sterlachini
Michael Woods

And many more generous contributors.

ABOUT THE AUTHOR

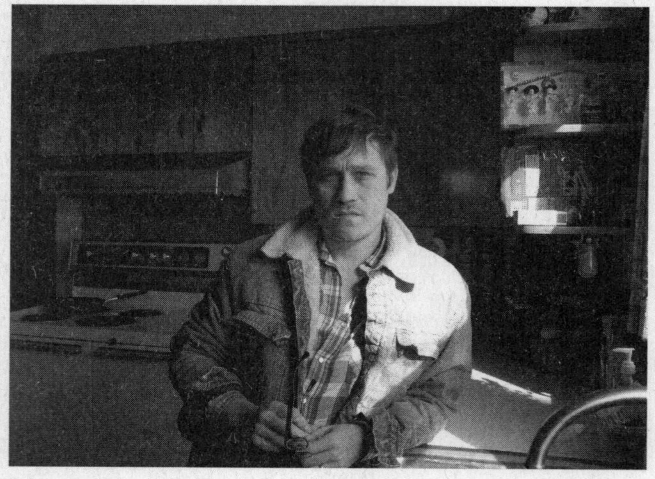

Adam Gnade's (*guh•nah•dee*) work is released as a series of books and records that share characters and themes; the fiction writing continuing plot-lines left open by the self-described "talking songs" in an attempt to compile a vast, detailed, interconnected, personal history of contemporary American life. This is his second novel.